Animal Health and Welfare: A Medical Guide

Animal Health and Welfare:
A Medical Guide

Editor: Herbert Dunda

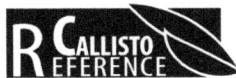

R CALLISTO REFERENCE

www.callistoreference.com

Callisto Reference,
118-35 Queens Blvd., Suite 400,
Forest Hills, NY 11375, USA

Visit us on the World Wide Web at:
www.callistoreference.com

ISBN: 978-1-64116-150-3 (Hardback)

Cataloging-in-Publication Data

Animal health and welfare : a medical guide / edited by Herbert Dunda.
     p. cm.
Includes bibliographical references and index.
ISBN 978-1-64116-150-3
1. Animal health. 2. Animal welfare. 3. Veterinary medicine. I. Dunda, Herbert.
SF740 .A55 2019
636.089--dc23

Table of Contents

Permissions

List of Contributors

Index

Preface

The state of health and welfare of an animal is understood from the different parameters of longevity, immunosuppression, disease, behavior, physiology and reproduction. There are various threats to animal welfare such as animal testing, blood sport, abandonment, cruelty, overpopulation, etc. Animals suffer from a wide variety of diseases, such as bacterial diseases, fungal diseases, viral diseases and genetic diseases. The field of medicine that studies all aspects of animal health and welfare is known as veterinary science. It is concerned with the diagnosis, treatment and prevention of animal diseases. Different specializations exist in veterinary science such as animal physiotherapy, animal dentistry, etc. Health monitoring in livestock, maintenance of good physical and mental health of pets, control of zoonotic diseases, etc. are all within the domain of veterinary science. This book unravels the recent studies in the field of animal health and welfare. Also included is a detailed explanation of the various concepts and advancements in veterinary science. This book will serve as a reference to a broad spectrum of readers.

After months of intensive research and writing, this book is the end result of all who devoted their time and efforts in the initiation and progress of this book. It will surely be a source of reference in enhancing the required knowledge of the new developments in the area. During the course of developing this book, certain measures such as accuracy, authenticity and research focused analytical studies were given preference in order to produce a comprehensive book in the area of study.

This book would not have been possible without the efforts of the authors and the publisher. I extend my sincere thanks to them. Secondly, I express my gratitude to my family and well-wishers. And most importantly, I thank my students for constantly expressing their willingness and curiosity in enhancing their knowledge in the field, which encourages me to take up further research projects for the advancement of the area.

Editor

Occurrence of Newcastle Disease and Infectious Bursal Disease Virus Antibodies in Double-Spurred Francolins in Nigeria

Daniel Oladimeji Oluwayelu,[1] **Adebowale Idris Adebiyi,**[1] **Ibukunoluwa Olaniyan,**[1] **Phyllis Ezewele,**[1] **and Oluwasanmi Aina**[2]

[1] *Department of Veterinary Microbiology and Parasitology, University of Ibadan, Ibadan 20005, Nigeria*
[2] *Department of Veterinary Anatomy, University of Ibadan, Ibadan 20005, Nigeria*

Correspondence should be addressed to Daniel Oladimeji Oluwayelu; ogloryus@yahoo.com

Academic Editor: Carlos González-Rey

The double-spurred francolin *Francolinus bicalcaratus* has been identified as a good candidate for future domestication due to the universal acceptability of its meat and its adaptability to anthropogenically altered environments. Therefore, in investigating the diseases to which they are susceptible, serum samples from 56 francolins in a major live-bird market (LBM) in Ibadan, southwestern Nigeria, were screened for antibodies against Newcastle disease (ND) and infectious bursal disease (IBD) viruses. Haemagglutination inhibition (HI) test and enzyme-linked immunosorbent assay (ELISA) revealed 25.0% and 35.7% prevalence of ND virus (NDV) antibodies, respectively, while 5.4% and 57.1% prevalence of IBD virus (IBDV) antibodies was detected by agar gel precipitation test (AGPT) and ELISA, respectively. This first report on the occurrence of NDV and IBDV antibodies in apparently healthy, unvaccinated double-spurred francolins from a LBM suggests that they were subclinically infected with either field or vaccine viruses and could thus serve as possible reservoirs of these viruses to domestic poultry. Furthermore, if they are to be domesticated for intensive rearing, a vaccination plan including ND and IBD should be developed and implemented.

1. Introduction

Newcastle disease (ND) and infectious bursal disease (IBD) are the two most dreaded viral diseases of poultry in Nigeria as they cause severe economic losses in domestic and wild bird populations resulting from illness, reduced egg production, immunosuppression, and death following infection with pathogenic strains of their respective causative viruses. Despite efforts to prevent and control them over the years, circulation of the causative virus among free-roaming and wild birds has been reported as one of the factors responsible for the sporadic outbreaks of ND and IBD among free-roaming village chickens as well as commercial poultry flocks [1, 2].

Newcastle disease (ND) is an acute, highly contagious, rapidly spreading viral disease affecting birds of all ages [3] and is characterized in chickens by respiratory, circulatory, gastrointestinal, and nervous signs [4]. The clinical signs seen in infected birds vary widely and are dependent on viral factors like pathogenicity (which depends on virulence and tropism of the virus), host factors (species, age, and immune status), concurrent infections, route of exposure, duration and magnitude of the infection dose, and external factors such as social and environmental stress [5]. According to Docherty and Friend [6], it is capable of infecting over 230 species from more than one-half of the 50 orders of birds. These include domestic poultry [7, 8] and wild birds such as house sparrows, hawks, crows, double-breasted cormorants, and waterfowls [9–13]. Wild birds constitute a natural reservoir of low-virulence viruses, while poultry are the main reservoir of virulent strains. Exchange of virus between these reservoirs represents a risk for both bird populations [13]. The most virulent form of ND virus (NDV) causes up to 100 percent mortality in affected flocks [6].

On the other hand, infectious bursal disease (IBD) is a highly contagious immunosuppressive viral infection of chicks (3–6 weeks old) causing severe economic and production losses worldwide [14]. Although turkeys, ducks, guinea fowls, and ostriches may be infected, clinical disease occurs solely in chickens [15]. However, serological evidence of the infection has been reported in free-living wild birds such as cordon bleu and village weaver [16], wild water birds [17], Antarctic penguins [18], cattle egrets [19], and wild turkeys and cranes [20]. Moreover, IBDV antibodies were detectable in the sera of sedentary and migratory wild bird species in Japan, suggesting that they play a key role in the natural history of IBD [21] while the virus was isolated from wild birds in Korea [22].

Although several studies have been conducted on francolins in South Africa [23–25], sparse information exists on the West African-based double-spurred francolin, *Francolinus bicalcaratus* (synonym: *Pternistis bicalcaratus*), which is a gamebird in the pheasant family Phasianidae of the order Galliformes. It is a resident breeder in tropical West Africa and feeds on insects, vegetable matter, and seeds [26]. According to Keith et al. [27], seven Afrotropical francolin species including the double-spurred francolin have been found in Nigeria where they are widely consumed as bush meat. In a comparative biochemical study of meat quality and digestive enzymes, their meat was reported to be tastier, juicier, more palatable, and richer in protein than domestic chicken meat [28]. Based on these desirable qualities of francolin meat, it is needful to consider them as an alternative source of affordable animal protein to the ever-increasing Nigerian human population. Moreover, although they are found mostly in the wild, Mbinkar et al. [29] noted that the species is considered a good candidate for future domestication due to the universal acceptability of its meat and its adaptability to anthropogenically altered environments, which may be occasioned by extensive bush burning and intensive grazing of grasslands. Therefore, since studies on their biology and ecology, which can provide a basis for their eventual domestication, have been conducted [28–31], there is a need to also investigate the infections to which they are susceptible. Apart from few studies which showed that francolins are affected by diseases such as Marek's disease [32], coccidiosis [33], toxoplasmosis [34], and bacterial sinusitis [35], there is sparse information on viral diseases such as ND and IBD in francolins. This study was therefore designed to investigate the presence of NDV and IBDV antibodies in free-living double-spurred francolins caught in the wild and sold at a popular live-bird market (LBM) located in Shasha, Ibadan, southwest Nigeria.

2. Materials and Methods

The study was conducted in Ibadan (latitude $7° 23'$ N and longitude $3° 56'$ E), the capital city of Oyo State, southwest Nigeria. This region is the core of the Nigerian poultry industry with Ibadan being a major city from where poultry (day-old chicks, broilers, and point-of-lay pullets) and poultry inputs (drugs, vaccines, and feed ingredients) are distributed to other parts of the country. The city also has some LBMs, of which the one located at Shasha is popular as it is a sales point

for diverse bird species brought by peasant farmers from adjoining rural communities and traders from the northern part of the country that transport cattle, sheep, and goats to southwest Nigeria.

Blood samples collected via the jugular vein between April and August 2012 from 56 double-spurred francolins at Shasha live-bird market were poured into sterile sample bottles without anticoagulant and allowed to clot at room temperature. Separated sera were harvested and stored at $-20°$C. Although larger sample population of spurred francolins existed in the market and prior consultations were made with the traders on the importance of the project, the number of birds available for bleeding was restricted to 56 in view of the refusal of traders to have their birds bled. The ages of the birds could not be determined.

The 56 sera were screened for antibodies to NDV and IBDV using the haemagglutination inhibition (HI) test and agar gel precipitation test (AGPT) as described by Durojaiye and Adene [36] and Hirai et al. [37], respectively. Positive control ND and IBD sera were obtained from the National Veterinary Research Institute, Vom, Nigeria. Antibodies to NDV and IBDV were also detected and quantified in 42 francolin sera (the remaining 14 sera had been exhausted) using commercial ND and IBD enzyme-linked immunosorbent assay (ELISA) kits (ProFLOK Plus, Synbiotics Corporation, Kansas City, USA), respectively, according to the manufacturer's instructions. Positive and normal control ND and IBD sera were used to validate the tests. As specified by the kit manufacturer, a serum dilution of $1:50$ was used and optical density (OD) values were read at 405 nm with an ELx800 universal microplate reader (Bio-Tek, Vermont, USA). Valid NDV or IBDV ELISA results were obtained when the average OD value of the normal control serum was less than 0.250 and the corrected positive control value range was between 0.250 and 0.900.

Data obtained were analysed with column statistics using GraphPad prism version 5.0 (GraphPad software, San Diego, CA, USA) and P values < 0.05 were considered significant.

3. Results and Discussion

Prevalence of NDV antibodies in the tested francolin sera was 25.0% (14/56) and 35.7% (15/42) using the HI and ELISA tests, respectively (Table 1). The HI antibody titers ranged from $1:2$ to $1:32$ while mean NDV antibody titer obtained with the ELISA was 3206 (95% CI: 1261–5152). There was a 59.5% agreement between the HI test and the ELISA. Only 3 (5.4%) of the tested sera were positive for IBDV antibodies with the AGPT while 24 (57.1%) were positive using ELISA (Table 2). Mean IBDV antibody titer obtained with the ELISA was 5735 (95% CI: 2919–8550) and there was a 50% agreement between the AGPT and ELISA. Using the ELISA, 28.6% (12/42) of the tested sera had antibodies to both NDV and IBDV.

This study investigated the presence of NDV and IBDV antibodies in free-living double-spurred francolins caught in the wild and sold at Shasha LBM, which is a trading centre where different avian species including indigenous chickens, pigeons, guinea fowls, turkeys, and francolins are sold in

TABLE 1: Correlation of HI and ELISA for NDV antibodies.

Test	Positive	Negative	Total
HI	10	32	42
ELISA	15	27	42

TABLE 2: Correlation of AGPT and ELISA for IBDV antibodies.

Test	Positive	Negative	Total
AGPT	3	39	42
ELISA	24	18	42

Ibadan, Oyo State, southwest Nigeria. To our knowledge, there is no information available on viral diseases of double-spurred francolins which have been suggested as a good candidate for domestication in order to meet the animal protein needs of the Nigerian populace [29]. Therefore, this first report on the detection of NDV- and IBDV-specific IgY antibodies in the sera of free-living francolins in Nigeria is an indication of previous exposure of these birds to the two viruses. Since they were not routinely vaccinated, it is possible that the birds acquired their ND and/or IBD seropositive status through exposure to other infected wild or domestic birds that were shedding the viruses. The seropositivity detected could be due to circulating ND and IBD vaccine viruses which the birds might have contracted through interaction with vaccinated free-range birds or even through operating occasionally around commercial poultry farms. Karesh et al. [38] noted that wild birds in the pet or exotic bird trade have the potential to transmit parasites, bacteria, and viruses which may or may not be pathogenic in their normal host but pose threats when introduced to new geographic locations and new host species. In this study, we observed that wild and domestic bird species were kept by the traders in the same cages and this is consistent with a previous report that ND, for example, is spread by contact between birds and exacerbated by birds being mixed together in rural markets [13]. As the francolins were usually kept at the LBMs for about 3-4 weeks before being sold, it is likely that they acquired the viruses from infected domestic or wild bird species with which they were kept in the same cages.

Moreover, the francolins tested in this study were all apparently healthy except for one that showed signs of torticollis at the time of sample collection (Figure 1). Therefore, the detection of NDV and IBDV antibodies in their sera suggests that they were subclinically infected and could serve as reservoirs shedding the viruses into the environment. Previous studies have implicated wild birds as possible reservoirs/vectors of these viruses for domestic poultry [16, 21, 39]. It is also possible that the birds possess some host factors responsible for resistance. Moreover, Kim et al. [40] suggested wild-type virus transmission between wild and domestic birds as the origin of the similarity of NDV strains found in wild birds and domestic birds in LBMs.

It is noteworthy that 28.6% (12/42) of the sera tested by the ELISA technique had high titres of both NDV and IBDV antibodies, which is an indication that the birds were coinfected with the two viruses. Additionally, the detection

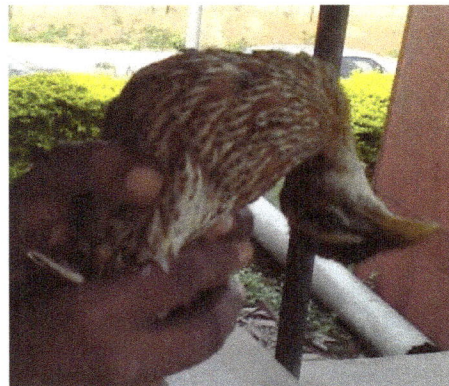

FIGURE 1: Francolin showing sign of torticollis at the time of blood collection.

of a higher proportion of positive samples by the ELISA technique compared to the HI test and AGPT shows that it is more sensitive than the latter two tests for detecting NDV- and IBDV-specific antibodies, respectively, in francolin sera. This is consistent with the reports of Bell et al. [41] and Marquardt et al. [42] who also found that the ELISA was more sensitive than the HI test and AGPT for detection of antibodies to NDV and IBDV, respectively.

4. Conclusions

This study has shown that free-living double-spurred francolins are susceptible to infection with NDV and IBDV and can serve as reservoirs of these viruses, thus acting as a means of transmission to domestic poultry. Therefore, if they are to be domesticated for intensive rearing as an alternative source of animal protein, a vaccination programme which includes ND and IBD vaccinations should be developed and implemented to protect them from clinical disease. In addition, the detection of NDV and IBDV antibodies in francolins sold at LBMs where they have close interaction with commercial and village chickens and other wild birds warrants continuous surveillance for these diseases because of increased concerns that low-virulence wild bird viruses could become more virulent in domestic bird populations. Further studies to isolate the two viruses from francolins and determine their level of pathogenicity should be conducted.

Conflict of Interests

The authors declare that there is no conflict of interests regarding the publication of this paper.

References

[1] E. N. Okeke and A. G. Lamorde, "Newcastle disease and its control in Nigeria," in *Viral Disease of Animals in Africa*, A. O. Williams and W. N. Masiga, Eds., CTA/OAU/STRC/Publication, Lagos, Nigeria, 1988.

[2] O. J. Ibu, A. Aba-Adulugba, M. A. Adeleke, and A. Y. Tijjani, "Activity of Newcastle disease and infectious bursal disease

viruses in ducks and guinea fowls in Jos area, Nigeria," *Sokoto Journal of Veterinary Sciences*, vol. 2, pp. 45–46, 2000.

[3] P. A. Abdu, "Evolution and the pathogenicity of Newcastle disease virus and its implications for diagnosis and control," in *Proceedings of the Workshop on Improved Disease Diagnosis, Health, Nutrition and Risk Management Practice in Poultry*, Ahmadu Bello University, Zaria, Nigeria, November-December 2005.

[4] N. J. MacLachlan and E. J. Dubovi, "Paramyxoviridae," in *Fenner's Veterinary Virology*, N. J. MacLachlan and E. J. Dubovi, Eds., pp. 299–325, Academic Press, London, UK, 4th edition, 2011.

[5] J. B. McFerran and R. M. McCracken, "Newcastle disease," in *Newcastle Disease*, D. J. Alexander, Ed., pp. 161–183, Kluwer Academic, Boston, Mass, USA, 1988.

[6] D. E. Docherty and M. Friend, "Newcastle disease," in *Field Manual of Wildlife Diseases: General Field Procedures and Diseases of Birds*, M. Friend and J. C. Franson, Eds., pp. 175–180, USGS-National Wildlife Health Center, Madison, Wis, USA, 1999.

[7] P. H. Jørgensen, K. J. Handberg, P. Ahrens, O. R. Therkildsen, R. J. Manvell, and D. J. Alexander, "Strains of avian paramyxovirus type 1 of low pathogenicity for chickens isolated from poultry and wild birds in Denmark," *Veterinary Record*, vol. 154, no. 16, pp. 497–500, 2004.

[8] B. S. Seal, M. G. Wise, J. C. Pedersen et al., "Genomic sequences of low-virulence avian paramyxovirus-1 (Newcastle disease virus) isolates obtained from live-bird markets in North America not related to commonly utilized commercial vaccine strains," *Veterinary Microbiology*, vol. 106, no. 1-2, pp. 7–16, 2005.

[9] H. Takakuwa, T. Ito, A. Takada, K. Okazaki, and H. Kida, "Potentially virulent Newcastle disease viruses are maintained in migratory waterfowl populations," *Japanese Journal of Veterinary Research*, vol. 45, no. 4, pp. 207–215, 1998.

[10] O. J. Ibu, J. O. A. Okoye, E. P. Adulugba et al., "Prevalence of newcastle disease viruses in wild and captive birds in central Nigeria," *International Journal of Poultry Science*, vol. 8, no. 6, pp. 574–578, 2009.

[11] W. Zhu, J. Dong, Z. Xie, Q. Liu, and M. I. Khan, "Phylogenetic and pathogenic analysis of Newcastle disease virus isolated from house sparrow (*Passer domesticus*) living around poultry farm in southern China," *Virus Genes*, vol. 40, no. 2, pp. 231–235, 2010.

[12] D. G. Diel, P. J. Miller, P. C. Wolf et al., "Characterization of newcastle disease viruses isolated from cormorant and gull species in the United States in 2010," *Avian Diseases*, vol. 56, no. 1, pp. 128–133, 2012.

[13] C. J. Snoeck, M. Marinelli, E. Charpentier et al., "Characterization of newcastle disease viruses in wild and domestic birds in Luxembourg from 2006 to 2008," *Applied and Environmental Microbiology*, vol. 79, no. 2, pp. 639–645, 2013.

[14] H. Müller, M. R. Islam, and R. Raue, "Research on infectious bursal disease—the past, the present and the future," *Veterinary Microbiology*, vol. 97, no. 1-2, pp. 153–165, 2003.

[15] Office Internationale des Epizooties, "Newcastle disease," in *OIE Manual of Standards for Diagnostic Tests and Vaccines*, pp. 221–232, OIE, Paris, France, 2008.

[16] D. R. Nawathe, O. Onunkwo, and I. M. Smith, "Serological evidence of infection with the virus of infectious bursal disease in wild and domestic birds in Nigeria," *Veterinary Record*, vol. 102, no. 20, article 444, 1978.

[17] G. E. Wilcox, R. L. P. Flower, W. Baxendale, and J. S. Mackenzie, "Serological survey of wild birds in Australia for the prevalence of antibodies to egg drop syndrome 1976 (EDS-76) and infectious bursal disease viruses," *Avian Pathology*, vol. 12, pp. 135–139, 1983.

[18] H. Gardner, K. Kerry, M. Riddle, S. Brouwer, and L. Gleeson, "Poultry virus infection in Antarctic penguins," *Nature*, vol. 387, no. 6630, p. 245, 1997.

[19] O. A. Fagbohun, D. O. Oluwayelu, A. A. Owoade, and F. O. Olayemi, "Survey for antibodies to Newcastle disease virus in cattle egrets, pigeons and Nigerian laughing doves," *African Journal of Biomedical Research*, vol. 3, no. 3, pp. 193–194, 2000.

[20] K. L. Candelora, M. G. Spalding, and H. S. Sellers, "Survey for antibodies to infectious bursal disease virus serotype 2 in wild Turkeys and Sandhill Cranes of Florida, USA," *Journal of Wildlife Diseases*, vol. 46, no. 3, pp. 742–752, 2010.

[21] M. Ogawa, T. Wakuda, T. Yamaguchi et al., "Seroprevalence of infectious bursal disease virus in free-living wild birds in Japan," *Journal of Veterinary Medical Science*, vol. 60, no. 11, pp. 1277–1279, 1998.

[22] W.-J. Jeon, E.-K. Lee, S.-J. Joh et al., "Very virulent infectious bursal disease virus isolated from wild birds in Korea: epidemiological implications," *Virus Research*, vol. 137, no. 1, pp. 153–156, 2008.

[23] J. H. van Niekerk, "Social and breeding behaviour of the crested francolin in the Rustenburg district, South Africa," *South African Journal of Wildlife Research*, vol. 31, no. 1-2, pp. 35–42, 2001.

[24] J. H. van Niekerk and D. J. Verwoerd, "Avian pox in Swainson's francolin in South Africa," *South African Journal of Wildlife Research*, vol. 32, no. 1, pp. 43–48, 2002.

[25] A. C. Uys and I. G. Horak, "Ticks on crested francolins, *Francolinus sephaena*, and on the vegetation on a farm in Limpopo Province, South Africa," *Onderstepoort Journal of Veterinary Research*, vol. 72, no. 4, pp. 339–343, 2005.

[26] Birdlife International, "Francolinus bicalcaratus," IUCN 2013, IUCN Red List of Threatened Species, Version 2013.2, 2012, http://www.iucnredlist.org/.

[27] S. Keith, C. H. Fry, and E. K. Urban, *The Birds of Africa*, vol. 2, Academic Press, London, UK, 1993.

[28] P. C. Onyenekwe, *Biochemical studies on the meat quality and digestive enzymes of double-spurred francolin Francolinus bicalcaratus [M.Sc thesis]*, Ahmadu Bello University, Zaria, Nigeria, 1988.

[29] D. L. Mbinkar, A. U. Ezealor, and S. J. Oniye, ""Food habits of the double-spurred francolin Francolinus bicalcaratus (Linnaeus) in Zaria, Nigeria," *Journal of Biological Sciences*, vol. 5, no. 4, pp. 458–462, 2005.

[30] A. U. Ezealor, *Ecological profile of a Nigerian Sahelian wetland: toward integrated vertebrate pest damage management [Ph.D. thesis]*, Virginia Polytechnic Institute and State University, Blacksburg, Va, USA, 1995.

[31] J. T. C. Codjia, M. R. M. Ékué, and G. A. Mensah, "Ecology of the double-spurred francolin Francolinus bicalcaratus in the southeast of Benin," *Malimbus*, vol. 25, pp. 77–84, 2003.

[32] J. R. Pettit, P. A. Taylor, and A. W. Gough, "Microscopic lesions suggestive of Marek's disease in a Black Francolin (*Francolinus f. francolinus*)," *Avian Diseases*, vol. 20, no. 2, pp. 410–415, 1976.

[33] D. F. Adene and M. Akande, "A diagnosis of coccidiosis in captive bushfowl (*Francolinus bicalcaratus*) and identification of the causative coccidian," *African Journal of Ecology*, vol. 16, no. 4, pp. 227–230, 1978.

[34] T. M. Work, J. G. Massey, D. S. Lindsay, and J. P. Dubey, "Toxoplasmosis in three species of native and introduced Hawaiian birds," *Journal of Parasitology*, vol. 88, no. 5, pp. 1040–1042, 2002.

[35] W. Yanhong, Y. Yuehui, Z. Shouchang, and L. Wenbo, "A report on sinuitis of francolin," *Journal of Animal and Veterinary Advances*, vol. 10, no. 19, pp. 2499–2500, 2011.

[36] O. A. Durojaiye and D. F. Adene, "Newcastle disease and egg drop syndrome '76 in guinea fowls (*Numida meleagris galeata* Pallas)," *Journal of Veterinary Medicine: Series B*, vol. 35, no. 2, pp. 152–154, 1988.

[37] K. Hirai, S. Shimakura, and M. Hirose, "Immunodiffusion reaction to avian infectious bursal virus," *Avian Diseases*, vol. 16, no. 4, pp. 961–964, 1972.

[38] W. B. Karesh, R. A. Cook, M. Gilbert, and J. Newcomb, "Implications of wildlife trade on the movement of avian influenza and other infectious diseases," *Journal of Wildlife Diseases*, vol. 43, no. 3, pp. S55–S59, 2007.

[39] E. Schelling, B. Thür, C. Griot, and L. Audigé, "Epidemiological study of Newcastle disease in backyard poultry and wild bird populations in Switzerland," *Avian Pathology*, vol. 28, no. 3, pp. 263–272, 1999.

[40] B.-Y. Kim, D.-H. Lee, M.-S. Kim et al., "Exchange of Newcastle disease viruses in Korea: the relatedness of isolates between wild birds, live bird markets, poultry farms and neighboring countries," *Infection, Genetics and Evolution*, vol. 12, no. 2, pp. 478–482, 2012.

[41] J. G. Bell, D. Ait Belarbi, and A. Amara, "A controlled vaccination trial for Newcastle disease under village conditions," *Preventive Veterinary Medicine*, vol. 9, no. 4, pp. 295–300, 1990.

[42] W. W. Marquardt, R. B. Johnson, W. F. Odenwald, and B. A. Schlotthober, "An indirect enzyme-linked immunosorbent assay (ELISA) for measuring antibodies in chickens infected with infectious bursal disease virus," *Avian Diseases*, vol. 24, no. 2, pp. 375–385, 1980.

An Antioxidant Dietary Supplement Improves Brain-Derived Neurotrophic Factor Levels in Serum of Aged Dogs: Preliminary Results

Sara Sechi,[1] Francesca Chiavolelli,[2] Nicoletta Spissu,[1] Alessandro Di Cerbo,[3] Sergio Canello,[2] Gianandrea Guidetti,[2] Filippo Fiore,[1] and Raffaella Cocco[1]

[1]Department of Veterinary Medicine, Pathology and Veterinary Clinic Section, Via Vienna 2, 07100 Sassari, Italy
[2]SANYpet S.p.a., Research and Development Department, Via Austria 3, Bagnoli di Sopra, 35023 Padua, Italy
[3]School of Specialization in Clinical Biochemistry, "G. d'Annunzio" University, Via dei Vestini 31, 66100 Chieti, Italy

Correspondence should be addressed to Raffaella Cocco; rafco@uniss.it

Academic Editor: Antonio Ortega-Pacheco

Biological aging is characterized by a progressive accumulation of oxidative damage and decreased endogenous antioxidant defense mechanisms. The production of oxidants by normal metabolism damages proteins, lipids, and nucleotides, which may contribute to cognitive impairment. In this study 36 dogs were randomly divided into four groups and fed croquettes of different compositions for 6 months. We monitored derivatives of reactive oxygen metabolites (dROMs) and biological antioxidant potential (BAP) levels in dogs' plasma samples as well as brain-derived neurotrophic factor (BDNF) serum levels at the beginning and at the end of the dietary regime. Our results showed that a dietary regime, enriched with antioxidants, induced a significant decrease of plasma levels of dROMs ($p < 0.005$) and a significant increase in BDNF serum levels ($p < 0.005$) after six months. Thus, we hypothesized a possible role of the diet in modulating pro- and antioxidant species as well as BDNF levels in plasma and serum, respectively. In conclusion the proposed diet enriched with antioxidants might be considered a valid alternative and a valuable strategy to counteract aging-related cognitive decline in elderly dogs.

1. Introduction

Biological aging is characterized by a progressive accumulation of oxidative damage and decreased endogenous antioxidant defense mechanisms [1]. The production of oxidants by normal metabolism damages proteins, lipids, and nucleotides which may contribute to neurodegeneration and, subsequently, cognitive impairment such as Alzheimer's (AD) and Parkinson's diseases (PD) [2, 3]. Although the body normally has sufficient protection producing endogenous antioxidants enzymes, such as catalase, glutathione and superoxide dismutase, an imbalance in the pro-oxidant/antioxidant species could increase the risk for lipid peroxidation DNA and protein damage. Oxidative damage also affects neuron function and may contribute to a cognition decline with age. The excess of reactive oxygen species in neuronal level can lead to irreversible damage of cytoskeleton and the microtubular network [4]. Microtubules, important dynamics polar formations of the cytoskeleton, are abundant in neurons, where they provide a scaffold also for their dendrites. Because of oxidative stress conditions the peroxynitrite may react with tyrosine to form 3-nitro-L-tyrosine (3NT). This final product may be selectively incorporated into the α-tubulin, resulting in an irreversible blocking of the characteristic dynamics of microtubules causing morphological changes, neuronal death and consequent onset of neurodegenerative diseases. Several experimental evidences have shown the importance of polyunsaturated fatty acids (PUFAs) in human and animal nutrition and development [5]. Further, an omega-3 and omega-6 deficiency likely correlates with the development of behavioral disorder [6].

Thus we hypothesized that a valid alternative and valuable strategy to counteract aging-related cognitive decline and neurodegeneration in aged dogs might be a dietary supplementation with antioxidants. Recent studies of animal models of neurodegenerative diseases suggest that dietary restriction can increase neurons endurance to age-related and disease-specific stresses [7]. Neurotrophic factors, including nerve growth factor (NGF) and brain-derived neurotrophic factor (BDNF), can protect neurons against death, as observed for *in vivo* and *in vitro* models of acute (stroke, trauma, and seizures) and chronic (Alzheimer's and Parkinson's diseases) neurodegenerative diseases [8].

Our interest in the neurological effects of age stems from a more general concern with the development of a canine model of human cognitive aging. Dogs show age-related pathology similar to that observed in elderly humans, like learning and development impairments [9]. Although the exact mechanisms have not been established so far, recent evidences indicate that a combination of an antioxidant-enriched diet with essential fatty acids, like omega-3 and omega-6, can be used to reduce age-dependent impairments and cognitive decline in aged dogs [10]. We focused on BDNF due to its role in supporting the survival and growth of many neuronal subtypes and in mediating the synaptic efficacy, neuronal connectivity and plasticity [11].

We hypothesized that BDNF serum levels might be modulated by an antioxidant-enriched diet.

In humans, BDNF mRNA and protein are decreased in the cortex and hippocampus in mild cognitive impairment (MCI) and AD [12] and are also decreased in cognitive decline [13]. In animals, decreased BDNF serum levels result in a LTP and memory deficit, thus increasing BDNF availability in the brain may be a viable strategy to counteract cognitive decline with aging.

The canine model provides us with an opportunity to test the relationship between cognitive impairment in aging, related to a decrease in BDNF serum levels, and the effects of non-pharmacological interventions.

The aim of this study was to evaluate the effects of a novel dietary supplement endowed with antioxidant properties as an adjuvant in the prevention of oxidative stress conditions and neurodegenerative disorders in aged dogs. The supplement consisted in a mixed formula of fished or chicken proteins, rice carbohydrates, *Grifola frondosa*, *Curcuma longa*, *Carica papaya*, *Punica granatum*, *Aloe vera*, *Polygonum cuspidatum*, *Solanum lycopersicum*, *Vitis vinifera*, *Rosmarinus officinalis* and an Omega 3/6 ratio of 1 : 0.8.

Grifola Frondosa is a culinary-medicinal mushroom that may play an important role in the prevention of many age-associated neurological dysfunctions, including Alzheimer's and Parkinson's diseases. The mushroom shows neuroprotective, antioxidant and anti-(neuro)inflammatory effects; in fact it reduces beta amyloid-induced neurotoxicity, neurite outgrowth stimulation, and nerve growth factor (NGF) synthesis [14]. It can be considered a useful therapeutic agent in the management and/or treatment of neurodegenerative diseases [15]. It was suggested that there could be an overall improvement in cognitive abilities of subjects when incorporated in their daily diet [16].

Curcuma Longa is a naturally occurring phytochemical compound endowed with powerful free radical scavenging activity [17]. Farinacci et al. observed that curcumin, polyphenol derived from *Curcuma longa*, reduced neutrophils adhesion and superoxide production *in vitro* [18]. Moreover, it resulted beneficially in improving spatial attention and motivation deficits associated with impaired cognition in aging and AD, in both humans and dogs [19]. Head et al. observed that 9 aged beagles provided with a medical food cocktail containing 95% of curcuminoids for 3 months had significantly lower error scores and were more accurate across all distances, suggesting an overall improvement in spatial attention [20]. da Rocha et al. demonstrated that *C. longa* had neuroprotective effects *in vitro* and *in vivo* by targeting biochemical pathways associated with neurodegenerative disorders that include cognitive impairments, energy/fatigue, mood and anxiety [21, 22].

Carica papaya is a natural compound with a high phenolic and flavonoid content which explains its free radical scavenging and antioxidant potential [22–24]. Mehdipour et al. demonstrated its antioxidant effect *in vitro* and reported a significant decrease in blood lipid peroxidation, while the blood total antioxidant power resulted significantly increased ($p < 0.001$) [24].

Punica granatum is a plant containing some species of flavonoids and anthocyanins, for example, delphinidin, cyaniding and pelargonidin, which have been shown to have an antioxidant activity *in vitro* [25] and *in vivo* [26]. The antioxidant action of *P. granatum* is related to its free radical scavenging activity against superoxide ions, mainly due to the presence of anthocyanins and to the ability to form metal chelates [25]. Rehydration effects have been also reported [27].

Aloe vera and its extracts have medicinal properties attributed to the active components such as anthrone, chromone, aloe verasin and hydroxylation [28, 29]. Sahu et al. demonstrated that *Aloe vera* had different degrees of antioxidant activity [30]. The antioxidant properties of this plant may depend on the radical scavenging activity. Moreover, life-long dietary supplementation of *A. vera* was shown to suppress many age-related consequences *in vivo*. Due to the presence of phenolic acids, polyphenols, sterols, fatty acids and indoles, *A. vera* may result to be effective in relieving symptoms associated with or preventing neurodegeneration [31].

Polygonum cuspidatum is an important natural source of resveratrol [32]. Due to its numerous pharmacological activities it has been used as an antioxidant [33]. Antioxidant activities of *P. cuspidatum* have been reported both *in vivo* and *in vitro* study [34]. Moreover, three of its dimers, parthenocissin A, quadrangularing A and pallidol, have shown strong free radical quenching and selective singlet oxygen scavenging activity [35]. Trans-resveratrol has been used as antidepressant in chronically stressed rats, probably by acting on the monoaminergic systems, such as the serotonergic and noradrenergic [33]. In fact, chronic treatment with trans-resveratrol was found to inhibit monoamine oxidase-A (MAO-A) activity in all the four brain regions, particularly in the frontal cortex and hippocampus [36].

Solanum lycopersicum is rich of vitamins C and E, lycopene, beta-carotene, lutein and flavonoids such as quercetin, phenols, ascorbic acid (AsA) and dehydroascorbic acid (DHA). It is considered an important plant able to prevent chronic diseases and improve energy balance and antioxidant activity [37]. Both direct and indirect antioxidant activity, as indicated by reduced malondialdehyde (MDA) and nitric oxide (NO) production and increased glutathione peroxidase (GPx) and superoxide dismutase (SOD) activity, support the conclusion that tomatoes containing anthocyanins can potentially provide better protection against oxidative stress related chronic diseases [38].

Vitis vinifera can be considered as a potential source of natural antioxidants, due to the presence of carotenoids such as lutein, beta-carotene and polyphenols [39]. The antioxidant activity of grape extracts is due to their reducing power [40]. The grape seed flavanol/procyanidin compounds may act as similar as reductones by donating electrons and reaching with free radicals to convert them to more stable products and terminating the free radical chain reaction [40]. Antioxidant activities of *V. vinifera* were also assessed by their capacity to prevent Fe^{2+}-induced lipid peroxidation in microsomes and their action on Cu^{2+}-induced lipid peroxidation in low-density lipoproteins [41]. Astringin, a stilbenoid present in *V. vinifera*, is endowed with an important antioxidant effect and a higher radical scavenger activity [41].

Rosmarinus officinalis is known to exert an antiproliferative, antioxidant and antibacterial activity [42]. The crude extract also has shown antioxidant and anti-inflammatory activities inhibiting NO production and reducing proinflammatory cytokines (IL-1β) and enzymes (COX-2) mRNA expression in LPS-activated cells thus highlighting its chemopreventive potential [43]. Afonso et al. showed that phenolic compounds from *R. officinalis* protected against hypercholesterolemia-induced oxidative stress, increasing the activities of antioxidant enzymes [44]. Several literature reports have demonstrated that *R. officinalis* exerted multiple benefits for neuronal system and alleviated mood disorders [45]. In particular its active compounds, luteolin, carnosic acid and rosmarinic acid, exhibited neurotrophic effects by improving cholinergic functions [46] and showed neuroprotective properties by inhibiting amyloid precursor protein synthesis and higher brain-derived neurotrophic factor production in hypothalamus cells [45]. Antidepressant-like effect of *R. officinalis* may be mediated by an interaction with the dopaminergic system, through the activation of dopamine D1 and D2 receptors [47].

Omega 3/6 fatty acids: a good balance of the Omega 3/6 fatty acids ratio in the food is a basic requirement to improve the inflammatory and neurological background [48]. More in detail, n-3 polyunsaturated fatty acids, usually found in fish oil, such as eicosapentaenoic acid (EPA) and docosahexaenoic acid (DHA), are known to both decrease the production of proinflammatory mediators and inhibit natural killer cell activity [49]. Moreover preclinical studies suggested that low plasma omega-6 and omega-3 fatty acids levels were associated with accelerated decline of peripheral nerve function with aging [50]. Intake of PUFAs, mainly omega-3 and omega-6, was shown to increase BDNF production in brain [50, 51]. Docking studies on PUFAs and their

TABLE 1: Dogs' diet groups and their features.

Group	Pet food	Sex	Mean age ± SEM
1	Organic chicken	2M, 6F	9 ± 0.08
2	Chicken + antioxidants	5M, 3F	7 ± 0.25
3	Fish	6M, 2F	9 ± 0.63
4	Fish + antioxidants	3M, 5F	9 ± 0.94

Antioxidants added in groups 2 and 4 are *Grifola frondosa*, *Curcuma longa*, *Carica papaya*, *Punica granatum*, *Aloe vera*, *Polygonum cuspidatum*, *Solanum lycopersicum*, *Vitis vinifera*, and *Rosmarinus officinalis* an Omega 3/6 ratio of 1 : 0.8.

metabolites with BDNF revealed that PUFAs metabolites, mainly LXA_4, NPD1 and HDHA, had more binding affinity towards BDNF [51]. These metabolites of PUFAs are also responsible for modulation of BDNF activity [51].

2. Methods

2.1. Subjects. Thirty-six dogs of different breeds were randomly and equally divided into four groups based on age and diet (Table 1). First group, made up of 8 dogs (three males and five females, age 9 ± 0.08, mean ± standard error of the mean), was fed a control diet with organic chicken. Second group, made up of 8 dogs (three males and five females, age 7 ± 0.25, mean ± standard error of the mean), was fed a chicken-based food enriched with natural antioxidants. The third group, made up of 8 dogs (four males and four females, age 9 ± 0.63, mean ± standard error of the mean), was fed a fish-based meal and the fourth one was made up of 8 dogs (three males and five females, age 9 ± 0.94, mean ± standard error of the mean) and was fed a fished-based meal enriched with natural antioxidants.

d-ROMs and BAP tests (Free Radical Analytical System FRAS 4, H&D s.r.l., Langhirano PR, Italy) were performed before (T0) and at the end (T1) of the treatment in all animals in order to determine the oxidative stress status. The four diets were administered for a six-month period.

2.2. Sample Collection and Analysis. Blood samples were collected from each dog before the new dietary regime (T0) and at the end of the treatment (T1) after six months from cephalic vein and stored in two tubes, one with heparin and the other without anticoagulant. Heparinized plasma samples and serum samples were obtained by blood centrifugation at 4000 g× 1,5 min at 37°C.

The derivatives of reactive oxygen metabolites (dROMs) and the biological antioxidant potential (BAP), as indicators of oxidative stress, were measured by portable spectrophotometer (Free Radical Analytical System FRAS 4, H&D s.r.l., Langhirano PR, Italy) on plasma samples. In the dROMs test, reactive oxygen metabolites (primarily hydroperoxides) of the sample, in presence of iron released from plasma proteins by an acidic buffer, generate alkoxyl and peroxyl radicals, according to the Fenton reaction. Such radicals then oxidize an alkyl-substituted aromatic amine (N,N-dietylparaphenylendiamine), thus producing a pink-colored derivative which is photometrically quantified at 505 nm [52]. The dROMs concentration is directly proportional to the colour intensity and is expressed as U.CARR (Carratelli Units). One U.CARR corresponds to 0.8 mg/L hydrogen peroxide. The reference values of dROMS are summarized below:

(i) reference value 50–90 U.CARR;

(ii) threshold borderline: 92–95 U.CARR;

(iii) condition of mild oxidative stress: 100–120 U.CARR;

(iv) condition of oxidative stress: 140–200 U.CARR;

(v) condition of strong oxidative stress: 220–300 U.CARR;

(vi) strong oxidative stress: over 300 U.CARR.

In the BAP test plasma samples were added with a colored solution, obtained by mixing a ferric chloride solution with a thiocyanate derivative solution, which causes a discoloration, whose intensity is measured photometrically at 505 nm and it is proportional to the ability of the plasma to reduce ferric ions. The results are expressed as μMol/L of reduced ferric ions. Both tests were validated for canine species [53]. Range values of BAP are listed below:

(i) reference value 2000–4000 μMol/L;

(ii) optimal values: >2200 μMol/L;

(iii) threshold borderline: 2200–2000 μMol/L;

(iv) discrete deficiency state: 2000–1800 μMol/L;

(v) deficiency state: 1800–1600 μMol/L;

(vi) strong deficiency state: 1600–1400 μMol/L;

(vii) very strong deficiency state: <1400 μMol/L.

2.3. BDNF Analysis. BDNF analysis was performed with BG BDNF ELISA kit (Blue Gene Biotech CO., LTD, Shanghai, China) designed for the quantitative determination of canine BDNF. The ELISA test reaction was performed using Crocodile mini Workstation (Totertek Berthold, Pforzheim, Germany). The kit utilizes a monoclonal anti-BDNF antibody and BDNF-HRP conjugate. The assay sample and buffer are incubated together with BDNF-HRP conjugate in precoated plate for one hour. After the incubation period, the wells are washed five times. The wells are then incubated with a substrate for HRP enzyme. The product of the enzyme-substrate reaction forms a blue colored complex. Finally, a stop solution is added to stop the reaction, which will then turn the solution yellow. The intensity of color is measured spectrophotometrically at 450 nm with a microplate reader. The intensity of the color is inversely proportional to the BDNF concentration since BDNF from samples and BDNF-HRP conjugate compete for the anti-BDNF antibody binding site. Since the number of sites is limited, as more sites are occupied by BDNF from the sample, fewer sites are led to bind BDNF-HRP conjugate. A standard curve is then plotted relating the intensity of the color (O.D) to the concentration of standards. The BDNF concentration of each sample is interpolated from this standard curve.

2.4. Statistical Analysis. All data are presented as the mean $\pm$ SEM. An unpaired 2-sample Student's t-test was used to compare the differences in plasma dROMs, BAP, and BDNF levels between the four groups. All statistical analyses were performed with GraphPad Prism 6 (GraphPad Software Inc., San Diego, CA, USA). $p < 0.05$ was considered significant.

3. Results

3.1. Oxidative Stress Status Evaluation. We firstly analyzed dROMs and BAP levels as a measure of the oxidative stress status of dogs. Analysis was made on dogs plasma in all of the four groups before starting the new dietary regime (T0) and at the end, after six months (T1).

As shown in Figure 1, a significant decrease in plasma levels of dROMs, after six months of feeding regime, in groups 2 and 4 (food supplemented with antioxidant) was observed ($p < 0.005$). dROMs levels remained unaltered in the first (control group) and third groups (fish-based meal, without antioxidant addition).

These data indicate that a diet enriched with natural antioxidant might be able to promote a decrease of reactive species in plasma of aged dogs.

Antioxidant influence, evaluated with BAP analysis, remained unchanged in all groups of dogs after the diet (Figure 2).

Natural antioxidants seemed to modulate the balance between pro- and antioxidant species through the decrease of dROMs without increasing natural antioxidant defense.

3.2. BDNF Evaluation. Literature reports have shown a decrease in BDNF serum levels to negatively correlate with cognitive decline and deficits in LTP and memory in dogs [13]. BDNF is a neurotrophic factor that can protect neurons against death supporting the survival and growth of many neuronal subtypes [8]. An increase in BDNF serum levels is one of the factors underlying improvements in learning and memory [8, 54]. Increasing BDNF availability in the brain, by diet, may be a viable strategy to counteract cognitive decline with aging [7, 55, 56].

We reported a significant BDNF serum levels increase in groups of dogs that received a diet enriched with antioxidant, $p < 0.005$ (Figure 3), while in the other groups BDNF serum levels remain unchanged.

4. Discussion

The purpose of this study was to evaluate the possible potential ability of a long-term dietary antioxidant supplementation in controlling the oxidative stress and the general health status of aged dogs. Moreover we demonstrated a possible modulation of BDNF serum levels by a diet with antioxidant supplementation.

Environmental stress and aging may induce psychological stress that possibly influences also the nutrition of pets. An unbalanced diet deficient in essential nutrients may represent a risk factor of degenerative diseases. Among the several

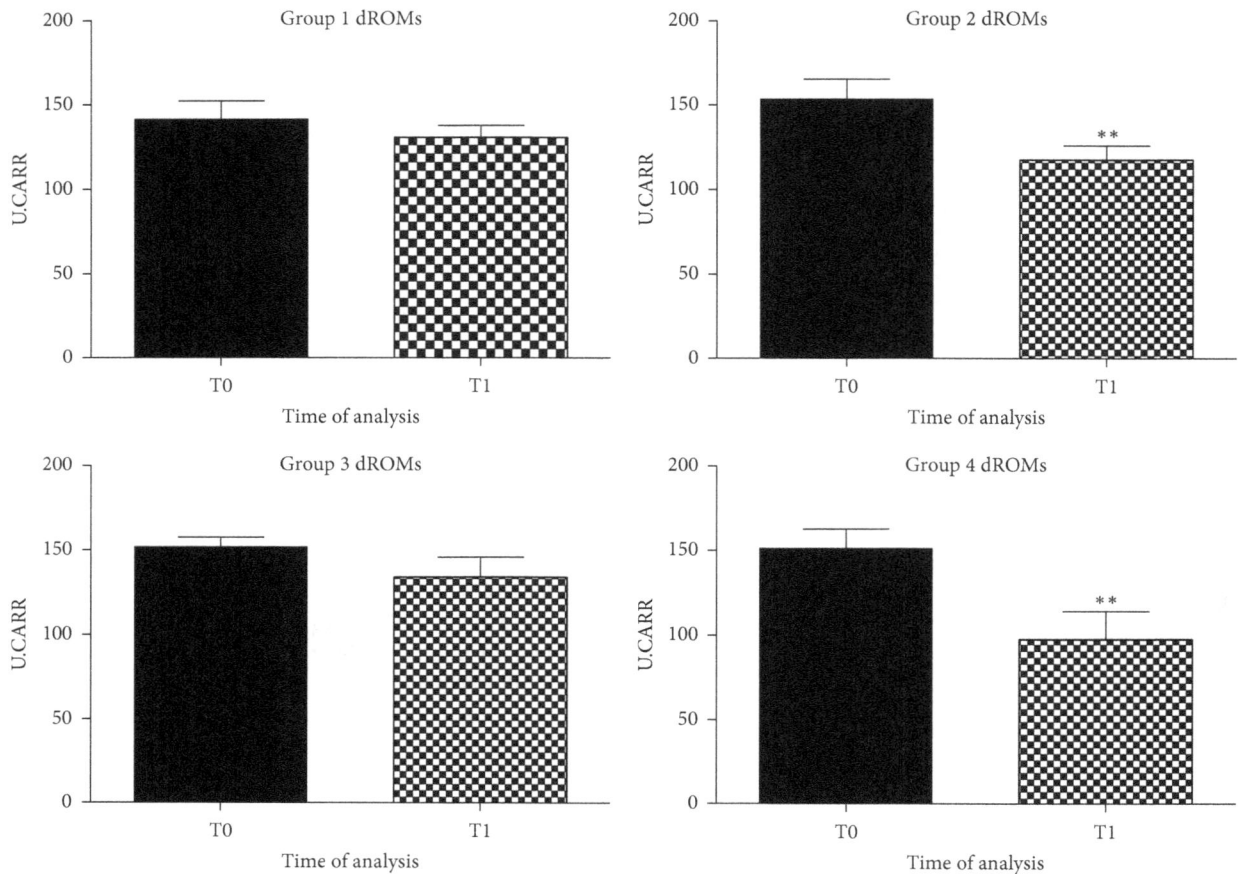

FIGURE 1: Graphical representation of dROMs in plasma of aged dogs before and after the 6 months of the dietary regime. A significant decrease of dROMs levels was observed in dogs fed with antioxidant supplementation, in the second group ($^{**}p < 0.005$) and in the fourth group ($^{**}p < 0.005$), respectively.

mechanisms by which nutrients influence the health status, the balance of oxidative stress has a relevant role. Constantly, in the animal species, metabolic oxidative reactions take place. The goal of these reactions is to balance free radicals production with antioxidants molecules.

The inhibitory activity of antioxidant molecules was observed in *in vitro* studies using plants derivative compounds such as flavonoids, anthocyanins and other poliphenols evaluating their effects on the converting activities of α-amylase, α-glucosidase and angiotensin-converting enzyme (ACE). They all have shown an inhibitory activity on α-amylase, α-glucosidase and ACE [57].

Furthermore, a significant reduction in dROMs values in the experimental diet enriched with natural antioxidants was observed. In apparently healthy dogs, serum levels of the dROMs ranged between 50 and 90 U.CARR. These values were in agreement with those reported by Pasquini et al. [53]. The antioxidant supplementation significantly decreased dROMs levels from 155 U.CARR (T0) to 120 U.CARR (T1) in the second group and from 150 U.CARR (T0) to 95 U.CARR (T1) in the forth group. Differently, dogs fed

the control diet, deficient in antioxidant nutrients, did not modulate the oxidative stress status. The antioxidant status revealed by BAP test was not affected by nutrition and values were at optimal levels throughout the observational period. Probably antioxidant supplements only affected dROMs species but not the endogenous antioxidant components of dogs, which remained in the initial optimal condition. This might be related to the really efficacy of the experimental diet in modulating the oxidative stress.

The antioxidant formulation employed in this experiment was based on *Grifola frondosa, Curcuma longa, Carica papaya, Punica granatum, Aloe vera, Polygonum cuspidatum, Solanum lycopersicum, Vitis vinifera* and *Rosmarinus officinalis* extracts.

All these compounds contain anthocyanins and polyphenols with antioxidant effects [7].

With this study we showed a decrease in dROMs species following the administration of the analyzed antioxidant formulation.

Our study reporting the scavenger activity of an antioxidant supplementation in dogs diet is in agreement with

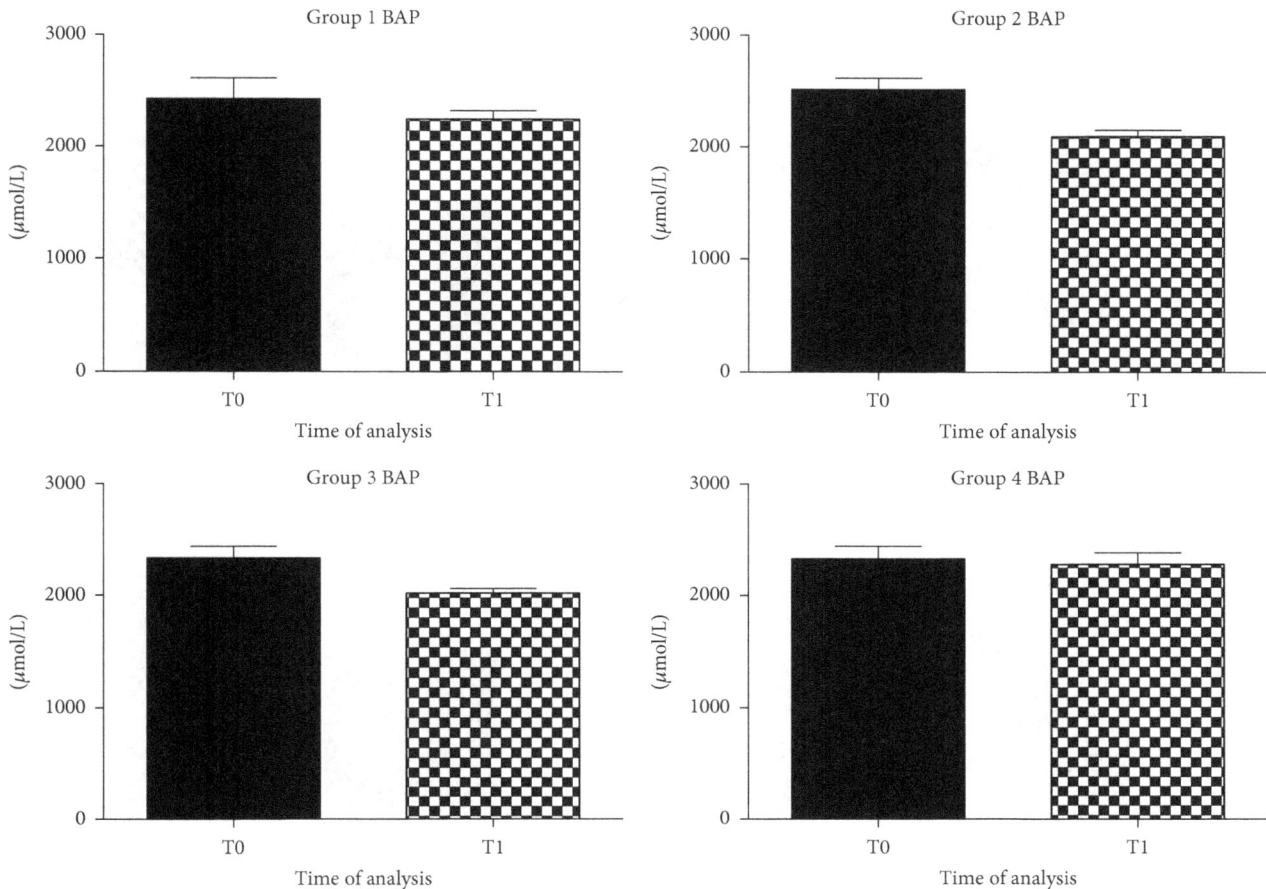

FIGURE 2: Graphical representation of BAP in plasma of aged dogs before and after 6 months of the dietary regime. BAP levels did not show significant modifications in all groups of dogs after the diet.

other studies about antioxidant effects of singular active principles included into an antioxidant supplementation [58]. The anthocyanins and polyphenols have antioxidant effects in some pathological conditions, such as metabolic disorders, aging-related diseases, cardiovascular diseases cancer, and inflammatory-related disturbs, as well as carotenoids and flavonoids [39, 59]. These compounds are inhibitors of lipid peroxidation probably by interfering with the glutathione activity [60].

Resveratrol (3,5,4′-trihydroxystilbene) is a polyphenol naturally present in grapes, berries, peanuts, and other vegetables [61], with therapeutic and neuroprotective functions [7]. Moreover trans-resveratrol, which is highly presented in *Polygonum cuspidatum*, could modulate BDNF levels through the monoaminergic system activation [36]. In our study we observed that a diet enriched with natural antioxidants was able to increase BDNF serum levels from $100 \pm 0.5 \, \text{pg/mL}$ to $180 \pm 0.8 \, \text{pg/mL}$, while in the other groups remained unchanged. As to *Grifola frondosa*, an improvement in cognitive abilities in aged dogs was observed

when adding *Curcuma longa* and *Aloe vera* to a daily diet through a stimulation of the BDNF synthesis [16]. According to what was observed by Sasaki et al., luteolin, carnosic acid, and rosmarinic acid, from *Rosmarinus officinalis*, exerted a neuroprotective activity probably modulating the neurotrophic metabolic pathway in the neuronal system [46]. Finally, Kumar et al. observed that PUFAs, like omega-3 and omega-6, along with their metabolites, had more binding affinity towards BDNF [51]. Further, the serum level increase of both fatty acids might be modulated by these metabolites which in turn could regulate the BDNF production in the brain. Neurotrophic factors, such as BDNF, can protect neurons against death and be a preventive approach in neurodegenerative conditions [7, 8].

By means of this new canine model of aging, we showed that providing antioxidants within a specific dietary supplement it was possible to restore the balance between pro- and antioxidants species, possibly modulating also BDNF serum levels. Future studies in both aged humans and dogs will be more effective if antioxidants combinations will be

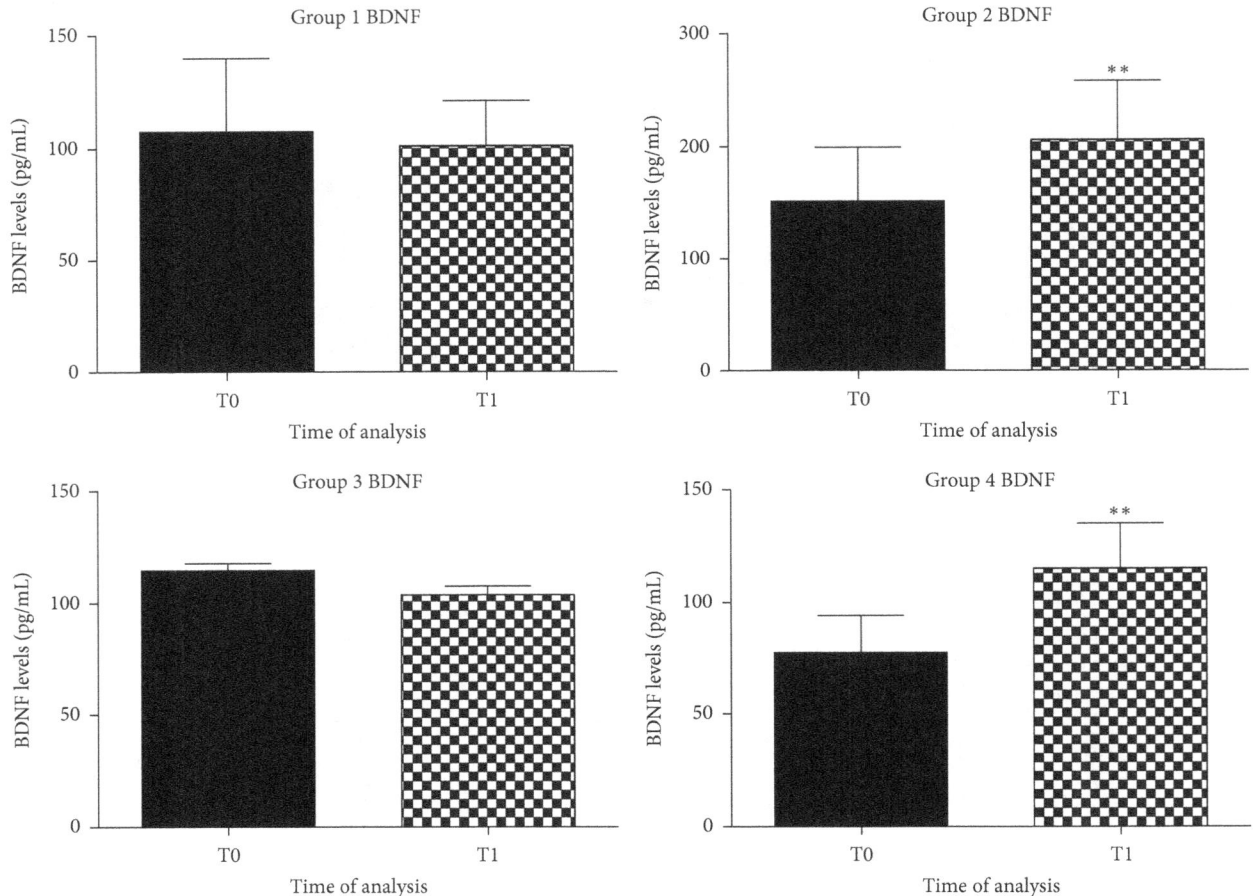

FIGURE 3: Graphical representation of BDNF in plasma of aged dogs before and after the 6 months of the dietary regime. A significant increase of BDNF levels was observed in dogs fed with antioxidant supplementation, in the second group ($^{**}p < 0.005$) and in the fourth group ($^{**}p < 0.005$), respectively.

evaluated along with additional lifestyle improvements such as cognitive training and physical exercise.

Conflict of Interests

None of the authors has any financial or personal relationship that could inappropriately influence or bias the content of the paper.

Acknowledgment

This paper was supported in part by grants from Regional Law 7 August 2007 n°7, "Promozione della Ricerca scientifica e dell'innovazione tecnologica in Sardegna".

References

[1] T. M. Hagen, D. L. Yowe, J. C. Bartholomew et al., "Mitochondrial decay in hepatocytes from old rats: membrane potential declines, heterogeneity and oxidants increase," *Proceedings of the National Academy of Sciences of the United States of America*, vol. 94, no. 7, pp. 3064–3069, 1997.

[2] M. Tavakkoli, R. Miri, A. R. Jassbi et al., "*Carthamus, Salvia* and *Stachys* species protect neuronal cells against oxidative stress-induced apoptosis," *Pharmaceutical Biology*, vol. 52, no. 12, pp. 1550–1557, 2014.

[3] X. L. Wang, G. H. Xing, B. Hong et al., "Gastrodin prevents motor deficits and oxidative stress in the MPTP mouse model of Parkinson's disease: involvement of ERK1/2-Nrf2 signaling pathway," *Life Sciences*, vol. 114, no. 2, pp. 77–85, 2014.

[4] K. Fukui, A. Masuda, A. Hosono et al., "Changes in microtubule-related proteins and autophagy in long-term vitamin E-deficient mice," *Free Radical Research*, vol. 48, no. 6, pp. 649–658, 2014.

[5] R. Molteni, R. J. Barnard, Z. Ying, C. K. Roberts, and F. Gómez-Pinilla, "A high-fat, refined sugar diet reduces hippocampal brain-derived neurotrophic factor, neuronal plasticity, and learning," *Neuroscience*, vol. 112, no. 4, pp. 803–814, 2002.

[6] T. Murphy, G. P. Dias, and S. Thuret, "Effects of diet on brain plasticity in animal and human studies: mind the gap," *Neural Plasticity*, vol. 2014, Article ID 563160, 32 pages, 2014.

[7] W. Duan, J. Lee, Z. Guo, and M. P. Mattson, "Dietary restriction stimulates BDNF production in the brain and thereby protects neurons against excitotoxic injury," *Journal of Molecular Neuroscience*, vol. 16, no. 1, pp. 1–12, 2001.

[8] M. P. Mattson, S. Maudsley, and B. Martin, "BDNF and 5-HT: a dynamic duo in age-related neuronal plasticity and neurodegenerative disorders," *Trends in Neurosciences*, vol. 27, no. 10, pp. 589–594, 2004.

[9] A. L. S. Dowling and E. Head, "Antioxidants in the canine model of human aging," *Biochimica et Biophysica Acta*, vol. 1822, no. 5, pp. 685–689, 2012.

[10] R. J. Kearns, M. G. Hayek, J. J. Turek et al., "Effect of age, breed and dietary omega-6 (n-6): omega-3 (n-3) fatty acid ratio on immune function, eicosanoid production, and lipid peroxidation in young and aged dogs," *Veterinary Immunology and Immunopathology*, vol. 69, no. 2–4, pp. 165–183, 1999.

[11] D. K. Binder and H. E. Scharfman, "Brain-derived neurotrophic factor," *Growth Factors*, vol. 22, no. 3, pp. 123–131, 2004.

[12] B. Michalski and M. Fahnestock, "Pro-brain-derived neurotrophic factor is decreased in parietal cortex in Alzheimer's disease," *Molecular Brain Research*, vol. 111, no. 1-2, pp. 148–154, 2003.

[13] S. Peng, J. Wuu, E. J. Mufson, and M. Fahnestock, "Precursor form of brain-derived neurotrophic factor and mature brain-derived neurotrophic factor are decreased in the pre-clinical stages of Alzheimer's disease," *Journal of Neurochemistry*, vol. 93, no. 6, pp. 1412–1421, 2005.

[14] S. Ling-Sing Seow, M. Naidu, P. David, K.-H. Wong, and V. Sabaratnam, "Potentiation of neuritogenic activity of medicinal mushrooms in rat pheochromocytoma cells," *BMC Complementary and Alternative Medicine*, vol. 13, article 157, 2013.

[15] C.-W. Phan, P. David, M. Naidu, K.-H. Wong, and V. Sabaratnam, "Therapeutic potential of culinary-medicinal mushrooms for the management of neurodegenerative diseases: diversity, metabolite, and mechanism," *Critical Reviews in Biotechnology*, 2014.

[16] V. Sabaratnam, W. Kah-Hui, M. Naidu, and P. David, "Neuronal health—can culinary and medicinal mushrooms help?" *Journal of Traditional and Complementary Medicine*, vol. 3, no. 1, pp. 62–68, 2013.

[17] S. Prasad, S. C. Gupta, A. K. Tyagi, and B. B. Aggarwal, "Curcumin, a component of golden spice: from bedside to bench and back," *Biotechnology Advances*, vol. 32, no. 6, pp. 1053–1064, 2014.

[18] M. Farinacci, M. Colitti, and B. Stefanon, "Modulation of ovine neutrophil function and apoptosis by standardized extracts of *Echinacea angustifolia, Butea frondosa* and *Curcuma longa*," *Veterinary Immunology and Immunopathology*, vol. 128, no. 4, pp. 366–373, 2009.

[19] D. Chin, P. Huebbe, K. Pallauf, and G. Rimbach, "Neuroprotective properties of curcumin in Alzheimer's Disease—merits and limitations," *Current Medicinal Chemistry*, vol. 20, no. 32, pp. 3955–3985, 2013.

[20] E. Head, H. L. Murphey, A. L. S. Dowling et al., "A combination cocktail improves spatial attention in a canine model of human aging and Alzheimer's disease," *Journal of Alzheimer's Disease*, vol. 32, no. 4, pp. 1029–1042, 2012.

[21] M. D. da Rocha, F. P. dias Viegas, H. C. Campos et al., "The role of natural products in the discovery of new drug candidates for the treatment of neurodegenerative disorders II. Alzheimer's disease," *CNS and Neurological Disorders—Drug Targets*, vol. 10, no. 2, pp. 251–270, 2011.

[22] G. Srikanth, S. Manohar Babu, C. H. N. Kavitha, M. E. Bhanoji Rao, N. Vyaykumar, and C. H. Pradeep, "Studies on in-vitro antioxidant activities of Carica papaya aqueous leaf extract," *Research Journal of Pharmaceutical, Biological and Chemical Sciences*, vol. 1, no. 2, pp. 59–65, 2010.

[23] K. Imao, H. Wang, M. Komatsu, and M. Hiramatsu, "Free radical scavenging activity of fermented papaya preparation and its effect on lipid peroxide level and superoxide dismutase activity in iron-induced epileptic foci of rats," *Biochemistry and Molecular Biology International*, vol. 45, no. 1, pp. 11–23, 1998.

[24] S. Mehdipour, N. Yasa, G. Dehghan et al., "Antioxidant potentials of Iranian *Carica papaya* juice in vitro and in vivo are comparable to α-tocopherol," *Phytotherapy Research*, vol. 20, no. 7, pp. 591–594, 2006.

[25] N. P. Seeram, R. N. Schulman, and D. Heber, *Pomegranates: Ancient Roots to Modern Medicine*, Taylor & Francis, Boca Raton, Fla, USA, 2006.

[26] K. N. Chidambara Murthy, G. K. Jayaprakasha, and R. P. Singh, "Studies on antioxidant activity of pomegranate (*Punica granatum*) peel extract using in vivo models," *Journal of Agricultural and Food Chemistry*, vol. 50, no. 17, pp. 4791–4795, 2002.

[27] P. C. Pande, L. Tiwari, and H. C. Pande, "Ethnoveterinary plants of Uttaranchal—a review," *Indian Journal of Traditional Knowledge*, vol. 6, no. 3, pp. 444–458, 2007.

[28] M. D. Boudreau and F. A. Beland, "An evaluation of the biological and toxicological properties of *Aloe barbadensis* (Miller), Aloe vera," *Journal of Environmental Science and Health—Part C Environmental Carcinogenesis and Ecotoxicology Reviews*, vol. 24, no. 1, pp. 103–154, 2006.

[29] K. Eshun and Q. He, "*Aloe vera*: a valuable ingredient for the food, pharmaceutical and cosmetic industries—a review," *Critical Reviews in Food Science and Nutrition*, vol. 44, no. 2, pp. 91–96, 2004.

[30] P. K. Sahu, D. D. Giri, R. Singh et al., "Therapeutic and medicinal uses of *Aloe vera*: a review," *Pharmacology & Pharmacy*, vol. 4, no. 8, pp. 599–610, 2013.

[31] F. Nejatzadeh-Barandozi, "Antibacterial activities and antioxidant capacity of *Aloe vera*," *Organic and Medicinal Chemistry Letters*, vol. 3, article 5, 2013.

[32] L. Chen, Y. Han, F. Yang, and T. Zhang, "High-speed counter-current chromatography separation and purification of resveratrol and piceid from *Polygonum cuspidatum*," *Journal of Chromatography A*, vol. 907, no. 1-2, pp. 343–346, 2001.

[33] Y. Xu, Z. Wang, W. You et al., "Antidepressant-like effect of trans-resveratrol: involvement of serotonin and noradrenaline system," *European Neuropsychopharmacology*, vol. 20, no. 6, pp. 405–413, 2010.

[34] X. Q. R. Sheela and V. A. Raman, "*In-vitro* antioxidant activity of *Polygonium barbatum* Leaf extract," *Asian Journal of Pharmaceutical and Clinical Research*, vol. 4, supplement 1, 2011.

[35] I. Gülçin, "Antioxidant properties of resveratrol: a structure-activity insight," *Innovative Food Science and Emerging Technologies*, vol. 11, no. 1, pp. 210–218, 2010.

[36] Y. Yu, R. Wang, C. Chen et al., "Antidepressant-like effect of trans-resveratrol in chronic stress model: behavioral and neurochemical evidences," *Journal of Psychiatric Research*, vol. 47, no. 3, pp. 315–322, 2013.

[37] M. Dorais, D. L. Ehret, and A. P. Papadopoulos, "Tomato (*Solanum lycopersicum*) health components: from the seed to the consumer," *Phytochemistry Reviews*, vol. 7, no. 2, pp. 231–250, 2008.

[38] H. Li, Z. Deng, R. Liu, S. Loewen, and R. Tsao, "Bioaccessibility, *in vitro* antioxidant activities and in vivo anti-inflammatory activities of a purple tomato (*Solanum lycopersicum* L.)," *Food Chemistry*, vol. 159, pp. 353–360, 2014.

[39] C.-I. Bunea, N. Pop, A. C. Babeş, C. Matea, F. V. Dulf, and A. Bunea, "Carotenoids, total polyphenols and antioxidant activity of grapes (*Vitis vinifera*) cultivated in organic and conventional systems," *Chemistry Central Journal*, vol. 6, article 66, 2012.

[40] G. K. Jayaprakasha, R. P. Singh, and K. K. Sakariah, "Antioxidant activity of grape seed (*Vitis vinifera*) extracts on peroxidation models in vitro," *Food Chemistry*, vol. 73, no. 3, pp. 285–290, 2001.

[41] B. Fauconneau, P. Waffo-Teguo, F. Huguet, L. Barrier, A. Decendit, and J.-M. Merillon, "Comparative study of radical scavenger and antioxidant properties of phenolic compounds from *Vitis vinifera* cell cultures using *in vitro* tests," *Life Sciences*, vol. 61, no. 21, pp. 2103–2110, 1997.

[42] A. I. Hussain, F. Anwar, S. A. Shahid Chatha, A. Jabbar, S. Mahboob, and P. Singh Nigam, "*Rosmarinus officinalis* essential oil: antiproliferative, antioxidant and antibacterial activities," *Brazilian Journal of Microbiology*, vol. 41, no. 4, pp. 1070–1078, 2010.

[43] S. Cheung and J. Tai, "Anti-proliferative and antioxidant properties of rosemary *Rosmarinus officinalis*," *Oncology Reports*, vol. 17, no. 6, pp. 1525–1531, 2007.

[44] M. S. Afonso, A. M. de O Silva, E. B. Carvalho et al., "Phenolic compounds from Rosemary (*Rosmarinus officinalis* L.) attenuate oxidative stress and reduce blood cholesterol concentrations in diet-induced hypercholesterolemic rats," *Nutrition and Metabolism*, vol. 10, article 19, 2013.

[45] C. Ramachandran, K.-W. Quirin, E. Escalon, and S. J. Melnick, "Improved neuroprotective effects by combining *Bacopa monnieri* and *Rosmarinus officinalis* supercritical CO_2 extracts," *Journal of Evidence-Based Complementary and Alternative Medicine*, vol. 19, no. 2, pp. 119–127, 2014.

[46] K. Sasaki, A. El Omri, S. Kondo, J. Han, and H. Isoda, "*Rosmarinus officinalis* polyphenols produce anti-depressant like effect through monoaminergic and cholinergic functions modulation," *Behavioural Brain Research*, vol. 238, no. 1, pp. 86–94, 2013.

[47] D. G. MacHado, V. B. Neis, G. O. Balen et al., "Antidepressant-like effect of ursolic acid isolated from Rosmarinus officinalis L. in mice: evidence for the involvement of the dopaminergic system," *Pharmacology Biochemistry and Behavior*, vol. 103, no. 2, pp. 204–211, 2012.

[48] A. P. Simopoulos, "The importance of the ratio of omega-6/omega-3 essential fatty acids," *Biomedicine and Pharmacotherapy*, vol. 56, no. 8, pp. 365–379, 2002.

[49] R. Verlengia, R. Gorjão, C. C. Kanunfre et al., "Effects of EPA and DHA on proliferation, cytokine production, and gene expression in Raji cells," *Lipids*, vol. 39, no. 9, pp. 857–864, 2004.

[50] F. Lauretani, S. Bandinelli, B. Bartali et al., "Omega-6 and omega-3 fatty acids predict accelerated decline of peripheral nerve function in older persons," *European Journal of Neurology*, vol. 14, no. 7, pp. 801–808, 2007.

[51] Y. P. Kumar, G. S. Srinivas, Y. Mitravinda E, L. Malla, and A. A. Rao, "Agonistic approach of omega-3, omega-6 and its metabolites with BDNF: an In-silico study," *Bioinformation*, vol. 9, no. 18, pp. 908–911, 2013.

[52] A. Pasquini, E. Luchetti, V. Marchetti, G. Cardini, and E. L. Iorio, "Analytical performances of d-ROMs test and BAP test in canine plasma. Definition of the normal range in healthy Labrador dogs," *Veterinary Research Communications*, vol. 32, no. 2, pp. 137–143, 2008.

[53] A. Pasquini, E. Luchetti, and G. Cardini, "Evaluation of oxidative stress in hunting dogs during exercise," *Research in Veterinary Science*, vol. 89, no. 1, pp. 120–123, 2010.

[54] M. F. Egan, M. Kojima, J. H. Callicott et al., "The BDNF val66met polymorphism affects activity-dependent secretion of BDNF and human memory and hippocampal function," *Cell*, vol. 112, no. 2, pp. 257–269, 2003.

[55] A. Wu, Z. Ying, and F. Gomez-Pinilla, "Dietary omega-3 fatty acids normalize BDNF levels, reduce oxidative damage, and counteract learning disability after traumatic brain injury in rats," *Journal of Neurotrauma*, vol. 21, no. 10, pp. 1457–1467, 2004.

[56] W. Duan, J. Lee, Z. Guo, and M. P. Mattson, "Dietary restriction stimulates BDNF production in the brain and thereby protects neurons against excitotoxic injury," *Journal of Molecular Neuroscience*, vol. 16, no. 1, pp. 1–12, 2001.

[57] G. Oboh, A. O. Ademosun, A. O. Ademiluyi, O. S. Omojokun, E. E. Nwanna, and K. O. Longe, "*In vitro* studies on the antioxidant property and inhibition of α-amylase, α-glucosidase, and angiotensin I-converting enzyme by polyphenol-rich extracts from cocoa (*Theobroma cacao*) bean," *Pathology Research International*, vol. 2014, Article ID 549287, 6 pages, 2014.

[58] D. K. Gessner, A. Fiesel, E. Most et al., "Supplementation of a grape seed and grape marc meal extract decreases activities of the oxidative stress-responsive transcription factors NF-kappaB and Nrf2 in the duodenal mucosa of pigs," *Acta Veterinaria Scandinavica*, vol. 55, article 18, 2013.

[59] K. B. Pandey and S. I. Rizvi, "Plant polyphenols as dietary antioxidants in human health and disease," *Oxidative Medicine and Cellular Longevity*, vol. 2, no. 5, pp. 270–278, 2009.

[60] J. Ø. Moskaug, H. Carlsen, M. C. W. Myhrstad, and R. Blomhoff, "Polyphenols and glutathione synthesis regulation," *The American Journal of Clinical Nutrition*, vol. 81, no. 1, pp. 277S–283S, 2005.

[61] W. Yu, Y.-C. Fu, and W. Wang, "Cellular and molecular effects of resveratrol in health and disease," *Journal of Cellular Biochemistry*, vol. 113, no. 3, pp. 752–759, 2012.

3

Effect of Sweet Orange Fruit Waste Diets and Acidifier on Haematology and Serum Chemistry of Weanling Rabbits

Oluremi Martha Daudu,[1] **Rahamatu Usman Sani,**[1] **Iyetunde Ifeyori Adedibu,**[1]
Lawrence Anebi Ademu,[2] **Gideon Shaibu Bawa,**[1] **and Taiye Sunday Olugbemi**[1]

[1] *Department of Animal Science, Faculty of Agriculture, Ahmadu Bello University, Zaria 810107, Nigeria*
[2] *Department of Animal Production and Health, Federal University Wukari, 641111, Nigeria*

Correspondence should be addressed to Oluremi Martha Daudu; remidaudu@yahoo.com

Academic Editor: Antonio Ortega-Pacheco

A total of thirty-five mixed breed (35) rabbits of average weight of 700 g aged 5-6 weeks were allocated to seven treatments in a completely randomised design to investigate the effect of sweet orange fruit waste (SOFW) and acidomix acidifier on haematology and serum chemistry. The diets were 0% SOFW, 10% SOFW with 0.5% acidomix, 10% SOFW with 0.7 acidomix, 15% SOFW with 0.5% acidifier, 15% SOFW with 0.7% acidifier, 20% SOFW with 0.5% acidifier, and 20% SOFW with 0.7% acidifier. Blood samples were analyzed for haemoglobin (hb) concentration, white blood cells (WBC), red blood cells (RBC), differential WBC count (lymphocyte, basophil, eosinophil, monocyte, and neutrophil), alanine amino transferase (ALT), alkaline phosphatase (ALP), aspartate amino transferase (AST), total protein, albumin, and globulin. There was no interaction between SOFW and acidifier for the haematological and most of the serum chemistry parameters but significant difference was observed in ALT; however the values were within the normal range. SOFW had no significant effect on all haematological and serum chemistry parameters. Acidomix had significant effect ($P < 0.05$) on haemoglobin concentration; rabbits fed 0.5% acidomix diets had higher values which were within the normal range. It is therefore concluded that SOFW with acidifier up to 20% had no detrimental effect on serum chemistry and haematology.

1. Introduction

Rabbit production has a considerable potential in the developing countries for the supply of the much needed animal protein due to low capital investment and space requirement, short generation interval, rapid growth rate, high proliferation, and use of agricultural by-products Cheeke [1]. Feed is the single largest expense in livestock production which constitutes about 70% of the total cost of rabbit production Oyawoye and Nelson [2]. Maize grain is the major source of energy in rabbit feeds in Nigeria, usually accounting for over 40% of the diet [3, 4]. Rabbit production for fast meat yield is affected by inadequate and high cost of feed ingredients and brought about mainly by the stiff competition between man and monogastric animals for grain and oil seeds Agunbiade et al. [5].

A lot of research work has been conducted in Nigeria in an effort to substitute maize with cheaper and readily available ingredients in order to reduce cost and overdependence on this feedstuff for rabbit feeding. Many of these alternative feed stuffs are by-products and edible waste products from food processing, food preparation and food services industries, and bio fuel industries. Nigeria produces 3% of fresh citrus in the world and Africa produces 3,741,000 ton of different varieties of citrus fruits of which Nigeria contributes 3,240,000 ton FAO [6]. A lot of the orange harvested is wasted due to few and small capacity of the processing industries to convert the fruit to juice, concentrate, and canned fruit Hon et al. [7]. It constitutes an environmental challenge since it is not being put into productive use. The excess can be utilized for feeding of livestock such as rabbits that can handle high fibre diets.

Organic acids have been used for decades in feed preservation, protection of feed ingredients from microbial and fungal deterioration, or improving the shelf life of fermented feed Canibe et al. [8]. It also has the capacity to reduce pH and

TABLE 1: Composition of experimental diets fed to weaner rabbits.

Ingredients (Kg)	0% control	10% + 0.5% acidomix	10% + 0.7% acidomix	15% + 0.5% acidomix	15% + 0.7% acidomix	20% + 0.5% acidomix	20% + 0.7% acidomix
Maize	45.95	35.26	35.26	29.90	29.90	24.55	24.55
Soyabean meal	25.20	25.39	25.19	25.75	25.55	26.10	25.90
SOFW	—	10.00	10.00	15.00	15.00	20.00	20.00
Palm kernel cake	10.00	10.00	10.00	10.00	10.00	10.00	10.00
Rice offal	15.00	15.00	15.00	15.00	15.00	15.00	15.00
Bone meal	3.00	3.00	3.00	3.00	3.00	3.00	3.00
Salt	0.30	0.30	0.30	0.30	0.30	0.30	0.30
Acidomix AFG	—	0.50	0.70	0.50	0.70	0.50	0.70
Vitamin premix	0.25	0.25	0.25	0.25	0.25	0.25	0.25
Methionine	0.20	0.20	0.20	0.20	0.20	0.20	0.20
Lysine	0.10	0.10	0.10	0.10	0.10	0.10	0.10
Total	**100.00**	**100.00**	**100.00**	**100.00**	**100.00**	**100.00**	**100.00**
Calculated analyses							
Crude protein (%)	18.00	18.00	18.00	18.00	18.00	18.00	18.00
Ether extract (%)	4.52	5.86	5.86	6.53	6.53	7.21	7.21
Crude fibre (%)	10.15	10.46	10.46	10.62	10.62	10.78	10.78
Calcium (%)	0.89	0.89	0.89	0.89	0.89	0.89	0.89
ME (Kcal/Kg)	2604	2651	2651	2675	2675	2699	2699
Feed cost (₦/kg)	68.31	70.07	72.85	67.48	70.26	64.89	67.67

0.25 kg of premix will supply the following: vitamin A 1500 IU, vitamin D 300 IU, vitamin E 3.00, vitamin K 0.25 g, thiamine 0.2 mg, riboflavin 0.6 mg, pantothenic acid 1.00 mg, pyridoxine 0.4999 mg, niacin 4.00 mg, vitamin B12 0.002 mg, folic acid 0.10 mg, biotin 0.008 mg, choline chloride 0.05 g, antioxidant 0.012 g, manganese 0.0096 g, zinc 0.0060 g, copper 0.0006 g, iodine 0.006 g, iodine 0.00014 g, selenium 0.024, and cobalt 0.004 mg.

the feed's buffering capacity and its antimicrobial effect helps prevent the growth of bacteria and kills microorganisms. The acidifier used in the study was Acidomix AFG. It is a microgranulated feed acidifier based on formic acid (E-236), propionic acid (E-280), ammonium formate (E-295), and ammonium propionate (E-284) adsorbed to a silica carrier (E-551a).

Dried citrus pulp is susceptible to moulds due to its hygroscopic capacity particularly in humid tropical climates. These moulds produce secondary metabolites such as aflatoxins and citrinin (the latter is known to cause hemorrhagic syndrome) [9]. Contamination with pesticide residues can also occur and depends on the compound, dose used, amount of rain, time between application and harvest, and Citrus species [9]. Blood analysis determines explicit states of stress which can be management; breed of an animal, environment, and physiology of the animal. Haematological indices are generally used to determine the health condition of animals generally Kamal et al. [10]. This study aimed at determining the effect of feeding varying levels of sweet orange fruit waste meal and acidomix© diets on the haematology and serum chemistry of rabbits.

2. Materials and Methods

2.1. Experimental Site.
The experiment was conducted at the research farm unit of the Department of Animal Science, Ahmadu Bello University, Samaru, Zaria, Kaduna State. Zaria is within the Northern guinea savannah zone of Nigeria, latitude 11°12′N and longitude 7°33′E, at an altitude of 610 m above sea level.

2.2. Source and Processing of the Sweet Orange Fruit Waste (SOFW).
The sweet orange fruit waste used in the experiment consisted of discarded sweet oranges gathered from traders at the Railway station market in Kaduna State. The unpeeled oranges were washed, split-open, sun-dried, stored in polythene bags until they were milled, and incorporated into the experimental diets. Most of the seeds were removed during the drying process to reduce the limonene content of the fruit.

2.3. Experimental Diets.
The diets consisted of the sweet orange fruit waste at graded levels of 0%, 10%, 15%, and 20% and two levels of Acidomix AFG (0.5% and 0.7%) as shown in Table 1. The diets were formulated to meet the nutritional requirements for weaner rabbits.

2.4. Management of Experimental Animals and Data Collection.
A total of 35 mixed breed weanling rabbits aged 5-6 weeks with average weight of 700 g were used for the study, each treatment consisted of five rabbits. The experimental design was 2 × 2 factorial arrangement, in a completely randomized design. There were seven treatments with graded levels of the sweet orange fruit waste treated with Acidomix AFG at two levels. The animals were kept individually in cages equipped with feeding and drinking troughs; feed and

water were administered ad lib. The cages had wire screen bottoms, which allowed faeces and urine to pass into a collection grid; hence the rabbits had little contact with their voided faeces and urine. The rabbits were subjected to a two-week adjustment period before the trial commenced. The experiment lasted for 56 days.

2.5. Blood Analyses. The rabbits were fasted for 14 hours prior to blood analysis. The rabbits fasted for 14 hours prior to blood collection. During blood collection, 1 mL of blood was collected via the ear vein of the rabbits into sample bottles containing Ethylene Diamine Tetra acetic Acid (EDTA) to prevent clotting of blood for haematological analysis and 2 mL was collected in a plain bottle for serum chemistry analysis. The total red blood cell (RBC) and white blood cell (WBC) count were determined using improved haemocytometer method as described by Lamb [11]. Differential WBC count was determined by preparing blood smear stained with Wrights stain as described by Ross et al. [12]. Haemoglobin concentration was estimated using cyanomethaemoglobin method as described by Jain [13].

Blood samples collected in the plain test tubes were centrifuged at 3,000 revolutions per minute (rpm) for 10 minutes and the serum was collected and stored at −20°C until analyzed for alanine aminotransferase (ALT) and aspartate aminotransferase (AST) using Reitman and Frankel Method, alkaline phosphatase (ALP) was determined using Beckman Synchron method. Total Proteins (TP) was determined using Biuret method as described by Reinhold [14], albumin values were obtained by bromocresol green method as described by Doumas and Biggs [15], and globulin values were determined according to the method of Coles [16].

2.6. Data Analyses. Data were subjected to analysis of variance, using the General Linear Model (GLM) procedure of Statistical Analysis System [17]. Difference between treatment means was separated using Duncan multiple range test.

3. Results and Discussion

Table 2 shows the proximate composition of sweet orange fruit waste (SOFW). The dry matter was 93.46%, crude protein was 6.44%, crude fibre was 4.89%, and ash was 4.01%. The minerals were sodium 0.68%, potassium 0.92%, total phosphorus 0.11% calcium 0.62%, and magnesium 0.15%. Metabolizable energy was 4030 kcal/kg.

Table 3 shows the effect of SOFW on haematology and serum chemistry of weaner rabbits. There was no significant difference ($P > 0.05$) observed in WBC values; the values fell within the range of $5–13 \times 10^9$ as reported by Chilson [18]. There was no significant difference ($P > 0.05$) observed in RBC across the treatments' the values obtained fell within the normal range of $3.8–7.9 \times 10^6/mm^3$ as reported by Chilson [18]. There was no significant difference ($P > 0.05$) in lymphocyte count (39.7–41%), the values were within the normal range (40–80%) as reported by RAR [19]. There was no significant difference ($P > 0.05$) for eosinophil (7.9–8.5%), but the values were higher than the normal range of 0–4% as reported by Research Animal Resources [19]. The increase

TABLE 2: Proximate composition of sweet orange fruit waste.

Nutrient	Sweet orange fruit waste (SOFW)
Dry matter (%)	93.46
Crude protein (%)	6.44
Crude fibre (%)	4.89
Ether extract (%)	17.00
Ash (%)	4.01
Nitrogen free extract (%)	67.66
Neutral detergent fibre (%)	19.11
Acid detergent fibre (%)	17.75
Minerals	
Na (%)	0.68
K (%)	0.92
Total Phosphorus (%)	0.11
Ca (%)	0.62
Mg (%)	0.15
[1]Metabolizable energy (Kcal/kg)	40.30

[1]$(37 \times \%CP) + (81.8 \times \%EE) + (35.5 \times \%NFE)$; Pauzenga (1985).

TABLE 3: The effect of sweet orange fruit waste on haematology and serum chemistry of weaner rabbits.

Parameter	Levels of sweet orange fruit waste (%)				SEM
	0	10	15	20	
WBC ($\times 10^9$/L)	5.05	7.80	5.08	5.69	0.105
RBC ($\times 10^{12}$/L)	4.09	5.91	5.14	5.27	0.045
Lymphocyte (%)	39.74	40.99	40.36	40.08	0.006
Eosinophil (%)	7.89	8.11	8.17	8.51	0.022
Monocyte (%)	8.92	8.71	8.37	8.82	0.009
Basophil (%)	4.53	4.47	4.17	4.56	0.015
Neutrophil (%)	44.23	44.27	44.65	43.48	0.007
Haemoglobin (g/dL)	12.20	13.03	13.15	13.08	0.013
AST (u/L)	15.72	16.10	20.24	18.90	0.038
ALT (u/L)	29.46	31.95	33.83	33.77	0.024
ALP (u/L)	72.36	71.54	76.16	77.19	0.029
Total protein (g/L)	72.89	74.09	69.74	70.48	0.024
Albumin (g/L)	32.99	39.65	39.39	39.89	0.019
Globulin (g/L)	30.22	41.57	33.55	40.64	0.052

AST: aspartate amino transferase, ALT: alanine amino transferase, ALP: alkaline phosphatase, RBC: red blood cells, WBC: white blood cell.

in eosinophils is likely due to allergy and respiratory or gastrointestinal disease Ganong [20]. There was no significant difference ($P > 0.05$) observed in monocyte (8.37–8.92%); the values were higher than normal range of 1–4% [16]. The primary function of monocytes is their role as critical immune effector cells that respond to signals from both innate and antigen-specific immune cells. They also contribute to wound healing and immune regulation. Monocytes carry out phagocytosis to protect the organism from harmful pathogens and to remove dead, dying, or damaged cells from the blood.

TABLE 4: The effect of acidomix AFG on haematology and serum chemistry of weaner rabbits.

Parameter	Levels of acidomix (%)		SEM
	0.5	0.7	
WBC ($\times 10^9$/L)	5.52	4.81	0.01
RBC ($\times 10^{12}$/L)	5.20	5.23	0.06
Lympocyte (%)	40.22	40.57	0.01
Eosinophil (%)	8.23	8.23	0.01
Monocyte (%)	8.44	8.81	0.01
Basophil (%)	4.53	4.26	0.02
Neutrophil (%)	44.58	43.56	0.03
Haemoglobin (g/L)	13.28[a]	12.54[b]	0.02
AST (u/L)	17.39	18.68	0.05
ALT (u/L)	31.15	34.68	0.03
ALP (u/L)	70.84	80.00	0.04
Total protein (g/L)	70.96	72.51	0.03
Albumin (g/L)	38.60	38.63	0.03
Globulin (g/L)	38.79	35.00	0.07

[a,b] Means with different superscripts within a row differ significantly ($P < 0.005$), AST: aspartate amino transferase, ALT: alanine amino transferase, ALP: alkaline phosphatase, RBC: red blood cell, WBC: white blood cell.

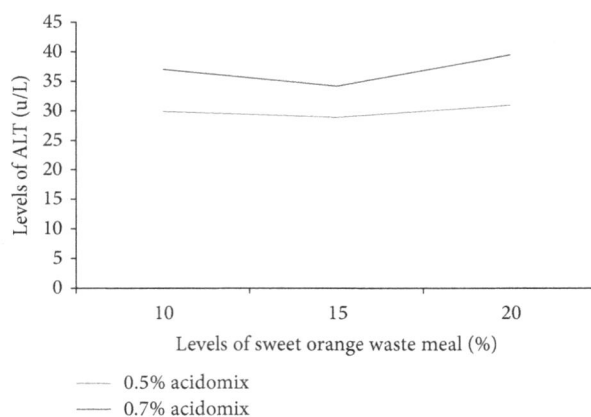

FIGURE 1: The effect of sweet orange fruit waste and acidifier on the Alanine amino transferase of weanling rabbits.

The observed increase is likely due to the presence of foreign organisms such as coccidia which needed to be eliminated from the body. There was no significant ($P > 0.05$) difference in basophil across the treatments; the values (4.17–4.56%) were within the normal range of 1–7% reported by [19]. There was no significant difference ($P > 0.05$) in neutrophil count across the treatments; the values fell within the normal range of 34–70% (http://www.medirabbit.com/). There was no significant difference ($P > 0.05$) for globulin across the treatments as reported by [18]. Slightly higher values were observed for rabbits fed 10% SOFW diet. The normal range is 25–40 g/L, reported by Chilson [18]. Globulins are carrier proteins for steroid and thyroid hormones and play a vital role in natural and acquired immunity to infection [20]. The increase in globulins observed could be attributed to the presence of an infection or due to individual differences in the rabbits fed this diet since no increase was observed for rabbits fed higher levels of SOFW diet. There was no significant difference ($P > 0.05$) for AST values; the values fell within the normal range [18]. There was no significant difference ($P > 0.05$) for ALP; the values fell within the normal range of 10–96 IU/L [18]. There was no significant difference ($P > 0.05$) observed across the treatment for total protein; the values fell within the normal range of 50–75 g/L. There was no significant difference ($P > 0.05$) observed in albumin; the values also fell within the normal range of 25–40 g/L [18].

Table 4 shows the effect of acidomix AFG on haematology and serum chemistry. There was no significant difference ($P > 0.05$) in the WBC count. The values (4.8–5.5 × 10^9) were similar to the normal range for WBC (5–13 × 10^9) as reported by Chilson [18]. There was no significant difference ($P > 0.05$) in RBC count; the values were within the range of 3.8–7.9 × 10^6/mm^3 as reported by Chilson [18]. There was

no significant difference ($P > 0.05$) in lymphocyte (40.3–40.6%) but values obtained were a bit lower than the normal range of 43–80% as reported by Chilson [18]. There was no significant difference ($P > 0.05$) in the eosinophil value (8.23%) but it was higher than the normal range of 0–2% as reported by Chilson [18]; this is an indication that the animals were possibly fighting an infection. There was no significant difference ($P > 0.05$) observed in Basophil (4.26–4.53%) but the values were higher than the normal range of 0–0.84% as reported by Chilson [18]. A combination of eosinophilia and basophilia is observed in allergic based inflammation, parasitic infestation, skin and respiratory inflammation that is allergic in nature. Postmortem reports showed presence of coccidian; this can account for increase in eosinophil and basophil [21]. There was no significant difference ($P > 0.05$) in neutrophil and it fell within the normal range of 34–70% as reported by Chilson [18]. A significant difference ($P > 0.05$) was observed across the treatments for haemoglobin (12.54–13.28 g/dL) but it fell within the normal range of 9.4–17.4 g/dL as reported by Chilson [18]. There was a significant difference ($P > 0.05$) in the AST value. Rabbits that fed 0.7% acidifier diets had higher AST level (18.68 u/L) but the values fell within the normal range of 10–98 u/L as reported by Chilson [18]. There was no significant difference ($P > 0.05$) in the value of ALT (31.15–34.68 u/L) across the treatments, but it fell below the normal range (55–260 u/L) as reported by Chilson [18]. There was no significant difference ($P > 0.05$) across the treatments for ALP; values fell within the range (10–96 u/L) as reported by Chilson [18]. There was no significant difference ($P > 0.05$) for total protein across the treatments; it lies within the normal range 25–40 g/L as reported by Chilson [18]. There was no significant difference for globulin (35–38.79 g/L) but values obtained were higher than the normal range (15–33 g/L) as reported by Chilson [18].

Figure 1 shows the effect of SOFW and acidifier on the haematology and serum chemistry of weaner rabbits. There was interaction between SOFW and acidifier; an increase was observed in ALT level for all levels of SOFW with increase in the level of acidifier. The greatest difference in slope was observed between 0.5% and 0.7% at 20% SOFW and is the strongest point of interaction. There was a significant difference ($P > 0.05$) across the treatments for ALT values; higher values were observed with the inclusion of 0.7% acidomix but the values obtained were within the range (http://www.medirabbit.com/). The increase in ALT levels could be attributed to Acidomix damaging the liver thus causing leakage of the enzyme out of the liver.

4. Conclusion

The inclusion of SOFW and acidomix in the diet of weaner rabbits did not affect haematological and serum chemistry parameters; hence it can be fed to weaner rabbits.

Conflict of Interests

The authors declare that there is no conflict of interests regarding the publication of this paper.

References

[1] P. R. Cheeke, "The potential rabbits production in production in tropical and sub-tropical agricultural system," *Journal of Animal Science*, vol. 63, pp. 1581–1586, 1986.

[2] E. O. Oyawoye and F. S. Nelson, "Optimum levels of inclusion of rice offal in the diet of young cockerels," in *Proceedings of the 26th Annual Conference of the Nigeria Society of Animal Production (NSAP '99)*, pp. 263–264, Ilorin, Nigeria, 1999.

[3] T. A. Adegbola and J. C. Okwonkwo, "Nutrient intake, digestibility and growth rate of rabbits fed varying levels of cassava leaf meal," *Nigerian Journal of Animal Production*, vol. 29, pp. 21–26, 2002.

[4] A. M. Bamgbose, S. D. Ogungbenro, E. E. Obasohan et al., "Replacement value of maize offal/cashew nut for maize in broiler diets," in *Proceedings of the 29th Annual Conference of the Nigeria Society for Animal Production*, pp. 219–221, Sokoto, Nigeria, 2004.

[5] J. A. Agunbiade, R. A. Bello, and O. A. Adeyemi, "Performance characteristics of weaner rabbits on cassava peel-based balanced diets," *Nigerian Journal for Animal Production*, vol. 29, pp. 171–175, 2002.

[6] FAO, *FAOSTAT Data*, Food and Agriculture Organisation of the United Nation, Rome, Italy, 2005.

[7] F. M. Hon, O. I. A. Oluremi, and F. O. I. Anugwa, "The effect of dried sweet orange (*Citrus sinensis*) fruit pulp meal on the growth performance of rabbits," *Pakistan Journal of Nutrition*, vol. 8, no. 8, pp. 1150–1155, 2009.

[8] N. Canibe, R. M. Engberg, and B. B. Jensen, "An overview of the effect of organic acids on gut flora and gut health," in *Proceedings of the Workshop on Alternatives to Feed Antibiotics and Coccidiostats in Pigs and Poultry (AFAC '01)*, Norfa Network, October 2001.

[9] V. Hevze, G. Trans, and P. Hassoun, "Citrus pulp, dried. Feedipedia.org. A programme by INRA, CIRAD, AFZ and FAO," 2013, http://www.feedipedia.org/node/680.

[10] M. S. Kamal, A. Khane, F. Rizvi, M. Siddique, and Sadeeq-Ur-Rehman, "Effect of cypermethrin on haematological Parameters in Rabbit," *Pakistan Veterinary Journal*, vol. 27, no. 4, pp. 171–175, 2007.

[11] G. M. Lamb, *Manual of Veterinary Laboratory Rabbit*, Techniques, Ciba-Geigy, Kenya, 1981.

[12] G. Ross, G. Christie, W. G. Hattiday, and R. M. Jones, "Determination of haematology and blood chemistry values in health six week old broiler hybrid," *Avian Pathology*, vol. 5, pp. 273–281, 1976.

[13] N. C. Jain, *Schalms Veterinary Haematology*, Eea and Febiger, Philadelphia, Pa, USA, 4th edition, 1986.

[14] J. G. Reinhold, *Standard Methods of Clinical Chemistry*, Academic Press, New York, NY, USA, 1953.

[15] B. T. Doumas and H. G. Biggs, "Determination of serum albumin," in *Standard Methods of Clinical Chemistry*, G. R. Cooper, Ed., vol. 7, p. 175, Academy Press, New York, NY, USA, 1971.

[16] E. H. Coles, *Veterinary Clinical Pathology*, W.B. Saunders Company, Philadelphia, Pa, USA, 4th edition, 1986.

[17] Statistical Analysis System, *Users Guide Statistics*, SAS institute, Cary, NC, USA, 9th edition, 2002.

[18] K. Chilson, "Complete blood count and biochemical reference values in rabbits," MediRabbits.com, 2003–2014.

[19] Research Animal Resources, "Reference Values for Laboratory Animals: Normal Haematological Values," Research Animal Resources, University of Minnesota, 2007, http://www.ahc.umn.edu/rar/index.html.

[20] W. F. Ganong, *Review of Medical Physiology*, McGraw-Hill Education, 22nd edition, 2005.

[21] "The Merck Veterinarinary Manual for Veterinary Professionals," http://www.merckmanuals.com/vet/circulatory_system/leucocyte_disorders/leukogram_abnormalities.html.

4

High Infestation by *Dawestrema cycloancistrioides* in *Arapaima gigas* Cultured in the Amazon Region, Peru

Patrick D. Mathews,[1] **Antonio F. Malheiros,**[2] **Narda D. Vasquez,**[3] **and Milton D. Chavez**[4]

[1] *Department of Parasitology, Institute of Animal Biology, University of Campinas, 13083-862 Campinas, Brazil*
[2] *Department of Biological Science, University of State of Mato Grosso, 78200-000 Cáceres, Brazil*
[3] *Department of Tropical Aquaculture, Institute of Biology, National University of the Peruvian Amazon, 765 Iquitos, Peru*
[4] *Department of Health, Safety and Environment, Enersul Limited Partnership, Calgary, Canada T2H 1M5*

Correspondence should be addressed to Patrick D. Mathews; patrickmathews83@gmail.com

Academic Editor: Antonio Ortega-Pacheco

The aim of this study was to evaluate the presence of *Dawestrema cycloancistrioides* in semi-intensive fish farming of fingerlings of *Arapaima gigas*. Between September and November 2013, 60 individuals of *A. gigas* born in captivity, were collected in three concrete ponds, from a semi-intensive fish farm in the Peruvian Amazon. For the study of sclerotized structures, parasites were fixed in a solution of ammonium picrate glycerine and mounted in Canada balsam. To visualize internal structures, parasites were fixed in hot formaldehyde solution (4%) for staining with Gomori's trichrome. The parasitic indexes calculated were prevalence, mean intensity, and mean abundance. This study identified a high infestation of a monogenean *D. cycloancistrioides* in gills of *A. gigas*. The prevalence was 100%. The mean intensity and mean abundance of the parasite were 144.9 of parasites per individual. This study confirms the necessity of constant monitoring of fish in order to reduce fish mortality.

1. Introduction

The *Arapaima gigas* is an endemic species of the Basin Amazon and is considered one of the largest freshwater fish in the world. The *A. gigas* can reach up to three meters in length and 200 kg of total weight [1] and is a much appreciated species with great acceptance in the Amazonian market being regarded as a protein source of the highest quality. However, due to its high nutritional demand for the population of the Amazon region, in recent years the natural stocks of this fish have suffered drastic reduction [2]. Farming paiche is thus a possible solution to the overexploitation of this species in many rivers of the Amazon. However, to allow the breeding, it turns out that the necessity to solve the problems regarding diseases and parasites upsurge, which are affecting this species in controlled environments as a consequence of intensive farming under inadequate management.

The dactylogyrid monogeneans are ectoparasites usually attached to the gills of fish. Like other monogeneans, dactylogyrids have a direct life cycle and can easily multiply and disperse under fish culture conditions, reaching very high intensities. These monogeneans have been linked to major losses in fish culture [3, 4]. Recently, studies in several species of farmed fishes in the Amazon region of Peru showed a high infestation by monogeneans species, indicated as the probable cause of high mortality [5–8].

Therefore, with the gradual increase of intensive and semi-intensive fish farming in the Peruvian Amazon, there is a need for constant monitoring of the fish for the diagnosis and timely control of infestations by monogeneans. In this sense, the present study aims to evaluate the monogenean infestation in *A. gigas* bred in a fish farm in the Peruvian Amazon.

2. Materials and Methods

2.1. Study Site and Animals. Between September and November 2013, the period which corresponds to the relative dry season, 60 individuals of the species *A. gigas* (20.40 ± 0.10 cm of length and weight of 76.06 ± 0.86 g), born in captivity (Figure 1), were collected in three concrete ponds, from a semi-intensive fish farm, belonging to the fish culture station Quistococha Research Center, located between the cities Iquitos and Nauta, northeast of Department of Loreto, Peru (3°48'48.9" N and 073°19'18.2" W). The relative humidity in this region varies between 80% and 100%. Annual rainfall ranged between 1500 and 3000 mm at 328 mean sea level.

2.2. Physicochemical Parameters of the Water. The parameters were measured three times daily (at 7 AM and noon and at 5 PM) with daily checks of dissolved oxygen, pH, temperature, and conductivity by means of an YSI multiparameter meter (Model MPS 556). Ammonium values, hardness, carbon dioxide, and total alkalinity were monitored weekly in the morning at 8 AM, using a complete package for analysis of freshwater (LaMotte AQ-2).

2.3. Parasitological Analysis. Following that, the fish were sacrificed by cerebral puncture and placed in individual containers. For examination of the gills, the samples were separated and placed in glass containers with a 1 : 4.000 formalin solution. After one hour, the gills were stirred in the same solution and then removed from the containers. Helminthes were allowed to settle on the bottom of the glass containers in the remaining formalin solution and subsequently collected with the aid of a small probe and a dissecting microscope (Nikon SM-30). For the study of sclerotized structures, parasites were fixed in a solution of ammonium picrate glycerine (GAP) and mounted in Canada balsam according to Thatcher [9]. Some specimens were mounted unstained in Gray and Wess' medium. To visualize internal structures, parasites were fixed in hot formaldehyde solution (4%) for staining with Gomori's trichrome. The identification of the parasites was based on the methodology of Thatcher [9] and Kritsky et al. [10].

The parasitic indexes calculated for assessing the level of infestation of parasites in the fish, prevalence (number of hosts infected divided by the total number of hosts in a sample), mean intensity (total number of parasites divided by number of hosts infected), and mean abundance (number of parasites divided by the total number of hosts in a sample) are the same as those described in Bush et al. [11]. The research was authorized by the Research Institute of the Peruvian Amazon.

3. Results

The moribund fishes collected for analysis were in emaciated condition. Due to the accumulation of mucus, the gills were pale and viscous. The necropsy of fingerlings from *A. gigas* evidenced the infestation by *Dawestrema cycloancistrioides* in the gill filaments of the fish (Figure 2). Indeed, the totality of the examined fish (60) showed a high parasitic infestation (Table 1).

In the present study, the values of the physicochemical parameters of the water from the culture ponds were dissolved oxygen (5.74 ± 0.8 mg L^{-1}), pH (6.84 ± 0.10), temperature (24 to 30°C) and conductivity (106.1 ± 14.0 μs cm^{-1}),

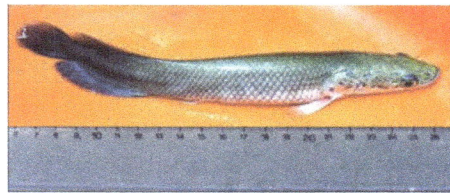

FIGURE 1: Specimen of *Arapaima gigas* collected from cultured ponds.

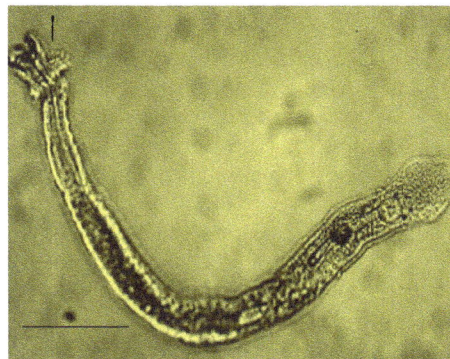

(a)

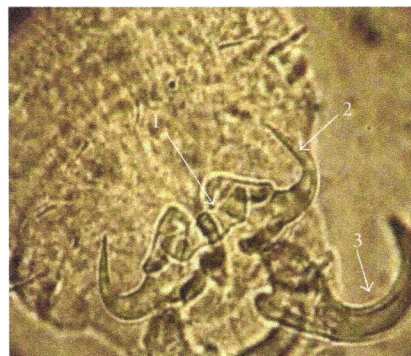

(b)

FIGURE 2: *Dawestrema cycloancistrioides* (a) total. (b) Posterior region, 1—ventral bar, 2—ventral anchor, 3—dorsal anchor. Scale bars = 10 μm.

TABLE 1: Parasitic indexes of *Dawestrema cycloancistrioides* in juveniles of paiche (*Arapaima gigas*) cultured in the Peruvian Amazon.

Parasitic indexes	*Dawestrema cycloancistrioides*
Prevalence (%)	100
Abundance	8695
Mean abundance	144.9
Mean intensity	144.9

ammonium values (0.20 ± 0.10 mg L^{-1}), hardness (20.40 ± 1.60 mg L^{-1}), carbon dioxide (3.1 ± 0.6 mg L^{-1}), and total alkalinity (16.12 ± 0.80 mg L^{-1}).

4. Discussion

In intensive fish farming, diseases outbreaks are a major concern to the farmers because in such systems fish are exposed to a high number of stressors (poor water quality, crowding, manipulation, breeding, and transport) which may negatively affect their immune system and disease resistance [12, 13]. Water temperature of the fish ponds presented a strong variation during the present study, reaching its lowest values (24°C) during the first hours of the day and the highest values (30°C) between noon and three hours later. In the same sense, in our study the concentration of ammonia, found in the ponds of cultivated *A. gigas*, was not within the expected range of values for tropical species. In this context, the fish are subjected to stress thus becoming more susceptible to infestation by parasites and reduced disease resistance [14, 15]. We suspect that the high parasitism by monogeneans was due to the imbalance in the homeostasis of fish.

Parasites that have a direct life cycle, such as monogeneans, are more frequently found in lentic environments and this type of environment favors the transmission of these parasites [3]. In regions with tropical and semitropical climates, the life cycle of monogenean can be completed in less than one day and the monogeneans proliferate rapidly [3, 9]. The climate in the region of this study is tropical humid with annual average temperature of 28.3°C and relative humidity of 85%, favoring the speed of life cycle. In the earthen ponds where fish were collected, the water circulation is almost negligible or nonexistent and the same have a high density of fish population. These drawbacks favor the contact with the monogeneans [3] and may justify the fact that the fishes have shown elevated prevalence of monogenean.

In *A. gigas* three species of monogeneans assigned to *Dawestrema* genus (*D. cycloancistrium*, *D. cycloancistrioides*, and *D. punctatum*) have been reported from natural environments and two in specimens from fish farming (*D. cycloancistrium* and *D. cycloancistrioides*) [9, 10, 16, 17], evidencing a high specificity of *Dawestrema* species parasitizing *A. gigas*. However, this specificity may be related to the fact that many of monogeneans which parasitize fish are host-specific, because they have co-evolved with their hosts [18].

In the present study, *D. cycloancistrioides* showed high parasitism along with prevalence rates of 100%. Our results agree with Hargreaves and Tucker [15], who reported similar prevalence, with mean intensity and mean abundance of 280 for specimens of *A. gigas* collected from fish farming in Brazil. In addition, Gross et al. [14] reported a prevalence of 100% from an aquarium in the United States, confirming the occurrence of this parasite in cultivated *A. gigas*.

5. Conclusion

The results of this study and studies addressing various aspects of parasites in other cultivated species confirm the necessity of constant monitoring of fish, seeking the diagnosis and timely control of infestations by monogeneans, in order to reduce fish mortality.

Conflict of Interests

The authors declare that there is no conflict of interests regarding the publication of this paper.

Acknowledgments

The authors thank Conselho Nacional de Desenvolvimento Cientifico e Tecnológico (CNPq) for a postdoctoral fellowship to Antonio F. Malheiros and Narda D. Vasquez is in receipt of a fellowship from CONCYTEC.

References

[1] E. A. Ono, R. Roubach, and M. F. Pereira, "Pirarucu production-advances in central Amazon, Brazil," *Global Aquaculture Advocate*, vol. 6, pp. 44–46, 2003.

[2] M. Casares, M. A. Arevalo, and E. Fernandez, "Notes on the husbandry of the arapaima *Arapaima gigas*, at 'Faunia', Madrid," *Zoologische Garten*, vol. 72, no. 4, pp. 238–244, 2002.

[3] J. Flores-Crespo and C. F. Flores, "Monogenean, parasites in Mexican fish: a recapitulation," *Técnica Pecuaria México*, vol. 41, no. 2, pp. 175–192, 2003.

[4] D. C. Kritsky and F. Stephens, "Haliotrema abaddon n. sp. (Monogenoidea: Dactylogyridae) from the gills of wild and maricultured West Australian dhufish *Glaucosoma hebraicum* (Teleostei: Glaucosomatidae), in Australia," *Journal of Parasitology*, vol. 87, no. 4, pp. 749–754, 2001.

[5] D. P. Mathews, J. P. D. Mathews, and O. R. Ismiño, "Massive infestation by *Gussevia undulata* (Platyhelminthes: Monogenea: Dactylogyridae) in fingerlings of *Cichla monoculus* cultured in the Peruvian Amazon," *Neotropical Helminthology*, vol. 6, no. 2, pp. 231–237, 2012.

[6] D. P. Mathews, J. P. D. Mathews, and O. R. Ismiño, "Parasitic infections in juveniles of *Prochilodus nigricans* kept in a semi-intensive fish farm in the Peruvian Amazon," *Bulletin of the European Association of Fish Pathologists*, vol. 33, no. 1, pp. 28–32, 2013.

[7] P. D. Mathews, O. Mertins, J. P. D. Mathews, and R. I. Orbe, "Massive parasitism by *Gussevia tucunarense* (Platyhelminthes: Monogenea: Dactylogyridae) in fingerlings of bujurqui-tucunare cultured in the Peruvian Amazon," *Acta Parasitologica*, vol. 58, no. 2, pp. 223–225, 2013.

[8] D. P. Mathews, A. F. Malheiros, O. R. Ismiño, and N. D. Vasquez, "*Jainus amazonensis* (Monogenea : Dactylogyridae) parasites of *Brycon cephalus* (Günther, 1869) cultured in the lowland of the Peruvian Amazon," *Croatian Journal of Fisheries*, vol. 72, no. 2, pp. 83–86, 2014.

[9] V. E. Thatcher, *Amazon Fish Parasites*, Pensoft Publishers, Moscow, Russia, 2nd edition, 2006.

[10] D. C. Kritsky, A. Boeger, and V. E. Thatcher, "Neotropical monogenea. 7. Parasites of the pirarucu, *Arapaima gigas* (Cuvier), with descriptions of two new species and redescription of *Dawestrema cycloancistrium* Price and Nowlin, 1967 (Dactylogyridae: Ancyrocephalinae)," *Proceedings of the Biological Society of Washington*, vol. 98, no. 2, pp. 321–331, 1985.

[11] A. O. Bush, K. D. Lafferty, J. M. Lotz, and A. W. Shostak, "Parasitology meets ecology on its own terms: margolis et al. revisited," *Journal of Parasitology*, vol. 83, no. 4, pp. 575–583, 1997.

[12] R. Y. Sado, Á. J. A. Bicudo, and J. E. P. Cyrino, "Dietary levamisole influenced hematological parameters of juvenile pacu, *Piaractus mesopotamicus* (Holmberg 1887)," *Journal of the World Aquaculture Society*, vol. 41, supplement 1, pp. 66–75, 2010.

[13] A. K. Jha, A. K. Pal, N. P. Sahu, S. Kumar, and S. C. Mukherjee, "Haemato-immunological responses to dietary yeast RNA, ω-3 fatty acid and β-carotene in Catla catla juveniles," *Fish and Shellfish Immunology*, vol. 23, no. 5, pp. 917–927, 2007.

[14] A. Gross, C. E. Boyd, and C. W. Wood, "Nitrogen transformations and balance in channel catfish ponds," *Aquacultural Engineering*, vol. 24, no. 1, pp. 1–14, 2000.

[15] J. A. Hargreaves and C. A. Tucker, *Managing Ammonia in Fish Ponds*, vol. 4603, Southern Regional Aquaculture Center, 2004.

[16] C. J. Bonar, S. L. Poynton, Y. F. Schulman, R. L. Rietcheck, and M. M. Garner, "Hepatic *Calyptospora* sp. (Apicomplexa) infection in a wild-born, aquarium-held clutch of juvenile arapaima *Arapaima gigas* (Osteoglossidae)," *Diseases of Aquatic Organisms*, vol. 70, no. 1-2, pp. 81–92, 2006.

[17] C. S. O. Araújo, S. M. Andrade, M. Tavares-Dias et al., "Parasitic infections in pirarucu fry, *Arapaima gigas* Schinz, 1822 (Arapaimidae) ket in a semi-intensive fish farm in Central Amazon, Brazil," *Veterinarski Arhiv*, vol. 79, no. 5, pp. 499–507, 2009.

[18] A. Šimková, O. Verneau, M. Gelnar, and S. Morand, "Specificity and specialization of congeneric monogeneans parasitizing cyprinid fish," *Evolution*, vol. 60, no. 5, pp. 1023–1037, 2006.

5

Real-Time RT-PCR for the Detection of Lyssavirus Species

A. Deubelbeiss, M.-L. Zahno, M. Zanoni, D. Bruegger, and R. Zanoni

Institute of Virology and Immunology, 3012 Berne, Switzerland

Correspondence should be addressed to R. Zanoni; zanoni@vetsuisse.unibe.ch

Academic Editor: Masanori Tohno

The causative agents of rabies are single-stranded, negative-sense RNA viruses in the genus *Lyssavirus* of Rhabdoviridae, consisting of twelve classified and three as yet unclassified species including classical rabies virus (RABV). Highly neurotropic RABV causes rapidly progressive encephalomyelitis with nearly invariable fatal outcome. Rapid and reliable diagnosis of rabies is highly relevant for public and veterinary health. Due to growing variety of the genus *Lyssavirus* observed, the development of suitable molecular assays for diagnosis and differentiation is challenging. This work focused on the establishment of a suitable real-time RT-PCR technique for rabies diagnosis as a complement to fluorescent antibody test and rabies tissue culture infection test as gold standard for diagnosis and confirmation. The real-time RT-PCR was adapted with the goal to detect the whole spectrum of lyssavirus species, for nine of which synthesized DNA fragments were used. For the detection of species, seven probes were developed. Serial dilutions of the rabies virus strain CVS-11 showed a 100-fold higher sensitivity of real-time PCR compared to heminested RT-PCR. Using a panel of thirty-one lyssaviruses representing four species, the suitability of the protocol could be shown. Phylogenetic analysis of the sequences obtained by heminested PCR allowed correct classification of all viruses used.

1. Introduction

Rabies diagnosis is based on fluorescent antibody testing (FAT) in brain smears and inoculation of brain suspension either in mouse neuroblastoma cell cultures or intracerebrally in mice as confirmatory assays with high sensitivity and specificity for postmortem diagnosis [1–3]. These techniques are well suited for rapid and reliable routine diagnosis, if brain material is available. For other diagnostic specimens sampled intra vitam in case of clinical suspicion, for example, saliva, cerebrospinal fluid, or skin biopsies, more suited molecular techniques with excellent sensitivity have been developed and validated, mostly targeting the conserved nucleoprotein gene of the lyssavirus genome, for example, [4–10]. Among these, there are protocols both for classical RT-PCR and for real-time RT-PCR, which adds speed, efficiency, contamination safety, and reliability to the technique combined with the potential to quantify the viral load [11, 12]. A major advantage offered by these molecular techniques is the characterisation of viral isolates by sequencing the given amplification products followed by phylogenetic or phylogeographic analysis [13–15]. The greatest challenge for these powerful novel techniques is the ever growing spectrum of known lyssavirus species/genotypes (GT), probably all of which having the potential to cause animal and human rabies fatalities [16, 17]. So far, 12 lyssavirus species and three as yet unclassified species have been identified [17]. The development of classical simple or (hemi)nested RT-PCR methods with particular emphasis on the diagnosis of a broad spectrum of lyssaviruses species has been published in a number of studies [18–23]. Also several real-time RT-PCR protocols suited for the broad detection or differentiation of several genotypes have been developed [9, 24–28]. The work of Wakeley et al. [25] is of particular interest for the rabies epidemiology in Europe concerning the European bat lyssaviruses types 1 and 2 [29–32] apart from classical rabies [33, 34]. This assay uses genotype (GT) specific probes and fluorophore signals for direct differentiation of GT1, GT5, and GT6 in a single-tube reaction. The protocol proposed by Nadin-Davis et al. [8] is highly suited for the detection of a broad range of classical rabies viruses.

The goal of this work was, based on a comprehensive review of the rich literature on the theme and adapting thereof, to develop, establish, and validate classical and real-time RT-PCR protocols for (intravitam) diagnosis of rabies and molecular-epidemiological characterisation of viral strains with the main emphasis on the growing number of known species/genotypes.

2. Materials and Methods

2.1. Samples

2.1.1. Cell Culture Supernatant of Viral Strains. All operations with potentially infectious material apart from centrifugation in closed tubes were performed in a class II biological safety cabinet. Frozen cell culture supernatants of rabies virus strains propagated previously on BHK-21 cells (baby hamster kidney cells, ATCC, Manassas, USA) were thawed, centrifuged at 2,000 g for 10 min at 4°C, and filtrated using the Millex-HA 450 nm Filter (Millipore, Cork, Ireland).

2.1.2. Brain Suspension. Approximately 1 g of cerebellum, medulla oblongata, and hippocampus from unfixed, freshly obtained brain material was homogenized to a 20% brain suspension using a mortar and pestle, after addition of approximately 1 g of quartz sand (Merck KGaA, Darmstadt, Germany) and 5 mL of Modified Eagle Medium with Earle's salts with 2.2 g/L NaHCO$_3$ (Bioswisstec AG, Schaffhausen, Switzerland) supplemented with 5% penicillin 10,000 IU/mL (Bioswisstec AG, Schaffhausen, Switzerland) and 20% foetal calf serum (FCS; PAA Laboratories GmbH, Pasching, Austria). The suspension was then decanted into a 5 mL tube (5 mL Polystyrene Round-Bottom Tube; BD Biosciences, Erembodegem, Belgium) to let it sediment for 1 hour at 4°C and subsequently centrifuged at 1,400 g for 10 min and filtrated as above. Frozen brain suspensions from former mouse inoculation tests [39] were handled like frozen cell culture supernatant.

2.1.3. Saliva and Oral Swabs. 500 µL of RNA Storage Solution (Ambion, Foster City, USA) was added to 100–200 µL of fresh or previously frozen saliva samples or swabs, which were subsequently vortexed (Vortex Genie 2, TEWIS Laborbedarf AG, Berne, Switzerland) for 1 min and centrifuged in a Biofuge Pico (Heraeus Holding GmbH, Hanau, Germany) at 5,000 rpm for 10 min.

2.1.4. Cerebrospinal Fluid. Cerebrospinal fluid (CSF) samples were diluted 1 : 2 to 1 : 4 with RNA Storage Solution (Ambion, Foster City, USA).

2.1.5. Skin Biopsies. Skin biopsies were shaved, cut into small pieces with a sterile pair of scissors, and further processed as described for brain suspension.

2.2. Viral Strains and Propagation in Cell Culture. A panel of 31 lyssaviruses (including 4 species) was used to test the diagnostic performance of our PCR (Table 1). Stocks of viral strains were produced in neuroblastoma cells (MNA 42/13) as described for the rabies tissue culture infection test (RTCIT, described below). The maintenance medium

used for the first passage was Dulbecco's MEM supplemented with 0.5% neomycin 50 IU/mL (Bioswisstec AG, Schaffhausen, Switzerland), 5% tryptose phosphate (BioConcept Ltd. Amimed, Allschwil, Switzerland), 1% nonessential amino acids (Bioswisstec AG, Schaffhausen, Switzerland), 3% foetal calf serum, and 1% L-Glutamine 200 mM (Bioswisstec AG, Schaffhausen, Switzerland) to which 1% Diethylaminoethyl-Dextran (DEAE-Dextran; Sigma-Aldrich Corporation, St. Louis, USA) was added. Dulbecco's MEM with 10% foetal calf serum was used for the 3 consecutive passages. Staining of the cells was performed after each passage using Rabies DFA Reagent (Millipore, Livingston, UK) as a conjugate.

2.3. FAT and RTCIT. The standard fluorescent antibody test (FAT) was performed with brain tissue samples as previously described [40]. Rabies tissue culture infection test (RTCIT) using four consecutive passages on murine neuroblastoma cells [41–43] was applied to clinical specimens like brain specimens, liquor, saliva, or skin biopsies.

2.4. Primers, Probes, and Synthetic DNA. Primers, probes, and synthetic DNA were obtained from Microsynth (Microsynth GmbH, Balgach, Switzerland). The location of suitable N-directed primers and probes for heminested RT-PCR and real-time RT-PCR, respectively, was chosen and evaluated based on published work [8, 18, 22, 25]. Using multiple sequence alignment (ClustalX 2.0.3 program [44–46]) of the N gene region of the available lyssavirus species RABV (33 sequences), LBV (4 sequences), MOKV (5 sequences), DUVV (4 sequences), EBLV-1 (17 sequences), EBLV-2 (14 sequences), ABLV, Aravan, Khujand, Irkut, and West Caucasian bat (each one) from GenBank (National Center for Biotechnology Information and National Library of Medicine, Rockville Pike, USA), variable positions of primers and probes were adjusted with wobble positions for a potentially broader match. Alternatively, primers with single wobbles or substitutions were mixed. Several probes for real-time RT-PCR for broadening the spectrum of detectable species were designed in this work (Table 2). As internal control for conventional RT-PCR, amplification of GAPDH (glyceraldehyde 3-phosphate dehydrogenase) was used [37]. As internal inhibition control for real-time RT-PCR, primers and probes for the amplification of Sendai virus (ATCC, Manassas, USA [38]), which was added to the samples before RNA isolation, were used (Table 2).

Synthetic DNA with a length of 125 bases encompassing positions 48–172 according to the Pasteur virus genome (X03673) of the following lyssavirus species were obtained from Microsynth: Aravan virus (ARAV) EF614259, Khujand virus (KHUV) EF614261, Bokeloh bat lyssavirus (BBLV) JF311903, Australian bat lyssavirus (ABLV) AF418014, Irkut virus (IRKV) EF614260, Lagos bat virus (LBV) EU293110, Mokola virus (MOKV) 293117, Shimoni bat virus (SHIV) GU170201, and West Caucasian bat virus (WCBV) EF614258.

2.5. RNA Extraction. RNA was isolated from 140 µL of sample supernatant using the QIAamp Viral RNA Mini Kit

TABLE 1: Rabies viruses used.

Species	Designation	Host species	Origin, year of isolation/receipt[a]	Material	Accession number[b]
EBLV-1	Bat Stade	Bat (*E. serotinus*)	Germany (Stade), 1970	Mouse brain suspension	KF831524/KF831550
EBLV-1	Bat Hamburg RV 9	Bat (*E. serotinus*)	Germany (Hamburg), 1968	Mouse brain suspension	KF831526/KF831552
EBLV-2	Bat Finland RV 8	Human, bat exposure	Finland, 1986	Mouse brain suspension	KF831528/KF831553
EBLV-1	Bat Holland RV 31	Bat	Netherlands, 1988[a]	Mouse brain suspension	KF831525/KF831551
RABV	Dog Tunisia	Dog	Tunisia, 1986	BHK-21 cell culture supernatant	KF831519/KF831545
EBLV-1	Bat Spain RV 119	Bat	Spain, 1989[a]	BHK-21 cell culture supernatant	KF831527
RABV	Bat Florida	Yellow bat	USA (Florida), 1986[a]	BHK-21 cell culture supernatant	KF831522/KF831548
EBLV-1	Bat Denmark	Bat (*E. serotinus*)	Denmark, 1986[a]	BHK-21 cell culture supernatant	KF831523/KF831549
RABV	Raccoon dog Poland	Raccoon dog	Poland, 1985	Mouse brain suspension	KF831518/KF831544
RABV	Raccoon Florida	Raccoon	USA (Florida), 1986	BHK-21 cell culture supernatant	KF831521/KF831547
RABV	Bat Chile RV 108	Bat	Chile, 1988[a]	Mouse brain suspension	KF831520/KF831546
RABV	Jackal Zimbabwe	Jackal	Zimbabwe, 1990[a]	Mouse brain suspension	KF831529/KF831554
RABV	Cattle Zimbabwe	Cattle	Zimbabwe, 1990[a]	Mouse brain suspension	KF831555
RABV	Canada Red Fox	Red Fox	Canada (Ontario), 1986[a]	Mouse brain suspension	KF831530/KF831556
RABV	LEP	Human	USA (Georgia), 1939	BHK-21 cell culture supernatant	KF831531/KF831557
RABV	HEP	Human	USA, 1939	BHK-21 cell culture supernatant	KF831532/KF831568
RABV	Dog Nepal Nr. 96	Dog	Nepal, 1989[a]	BHK-21 cell culture supernatant	KF831534/KF831559
RABV	Sri Lanka dog 121	Dog	Sri Lanka, 1986	BHK-21 cell culture supernatant	KF831535/KF831572
RABV	Eurofox 912/87	Fox	Switzerland, 1987	BHK-21 cell culture supernatant	KF831538/KF831562
DUVV	Duvenhage RV6	Human	South Africa, 1988[a]	BHK-21 cell culture supernatant	KF831533/KF831558
RABV	NYC 58	Laboratory strain	USA, 1987[a]	Mouse brain suspension	KF831540/KF831563
RABV	Dog Lima	Dog	Peru (Lima), 1985[a]	Mouse brain suspension	KF831540/KF831564
EBLV-1	Bat Bremerhaven RV11	Bat	Germany (Bremerhaven), 1989[a]	BHK-21 cell culture supernatant	KF831541/KF831565
EBLV-1	Bat B24	Bat	Europe, 1986[a]	Mouse brain suspension	KF831536/KF831560
RABV	Skunk Canada	Striped skunk	Canada (Ontario), 1986	BHK-21 cell culture supernatant	KF831537/KF831561
RABV	SAD Bern	ERA*	USA, 1935 (received 1976)	BHK-21 cell culture supernatant	KF831542/KF831566
RABV	CSSR/A-virus	Rodent, laboratory strain	CSSR (Prague), 1987[a]	BHK-21 cell culture supernatant	KF831543/KF831567
RABV	Challenge virus standard (CVS-11) ATCC VR 959	Laboratory strain	France (CNEVA), 1995[a]	BHK-21 cell culture supernatant	GU992321
EBLV-2	TW 18l4/92	Bat (*M. daubentonii*)	Switzerland (Plaffeien), 1992	Na 42/13 cell culture supernatant	KF831569
EBLV-2	TW 1392/93	Bat (*M. daubentonii*)	Switzerland (Versoix), 1993	Na 42/13 cell culture supernatant	KF831570
EBLV-2	TW 118/02	Bat (*M. daubentonii*)	Switzerland (Geneva), 2002	Na 42/13 cell culture supernatant	KF831571

Lyssaviruses of 4 different species were tested.
[a]Year of receipt at the Swiss rabies center.
[b]Accession numbers of 220 bp and 543 bp N fragments, respectively, sequenced in this work.
*Reference [36].

TABLE 2: Primers and probes.

Method	Name	Sequence	Length	Position[a]	Product	Reference
	JW12-F	ATGTAACACCYCTACAATG	19	55–73		Panning et al., 2010 [22]
hnRT-PCR	JW6ASI-R1	CAATTGGCACACATTTTGTG	20	660–641	606 bp	
	JW6AS2-R1	CAGTTAGCGCACATCTTATG	20	660–641	606 bp	
	JW10ASI-R2	GTCATCAATGTGTGATGTTC	20	636–617	582 bp	
	JW10AS2-R2	GTCATTAGAGTATGGTGCTC	20	636–617	582 bp	
Cloning RT-PCR	TWclon-F	ACGCTTAACRACMAAACCAG	20	1–20		This work
	TWclon-R	TGKATGAARTAAGAGTGWGGRAC	23	933–911	933 bp	
Control[1]	GAPDH-F	GGCAAGTTCCATGGCACAGT	20	58–72[b]		Ravazzolo et al., 2006 [37]
	GAPDH-R	ACGTACTCAGCACCAGCATCAC	22	161–182[b]	125 bp	
	RABVD1-F	ATGTAACACCYCTACAATG	19	55–73		Nadin-Davis et al., 2009 [8]
	RABVD1-R	GCMGGRTAYTTRTAYTCATA	20	165–146	111 bp	Nadin-Davis et al., 2009 [8]
	RABVD1-P	5′-FAM-CCGAYAAGATTGTATTYAARGTCAAKAATCAGGT-BHQ1-3′	34	78–111		Nadin-Davis et al., 2009 [8]
	LysGT5-P	5′-YY-AACARGGTTGTTTTYAAGGTCCATAA-BHQ1-3′	26	80–105		Wakeley et al., 2005 [25]
	LysGT6-P	5′-Cy5-ACARAATTGTCTTCAARGTCCATAATCAG-BHQ2-3′	29	81–109		Wakeley et al., 2005 [25]
Real-time RT-PCR	ivvWCBV-P	5′-FAM-TCGGATATCACTTCGGGTTTGAGAGTCA-BHQ1-3′	28	141–114		This work
	ivvMok-P	5′-YY-TTGTGTTCAAGGTGAAYAAYCAAGT-BHQ1-3′	25	87–111		This work
	ivvABLV2n-P	5′Cy5-ATTGTCTTTAAGGTCAACAATCAGTT-BHQ2-3′	26	86–111		This work
	ivvLBV-P	5′-FAM-ATTGTTTTCAAAGTYCAYAATCAGGTMGTGTC-BHQ1-3′	32	86–117		This work
	ivvKhujand-P	5′-YY-ACAGAATTGTCTTYAAAGTYMAKAATCA-BHQ1-3′	28	81–108		This work
	ivvSBLV2-P	5′-Cy5-TCWGAGATTATRTCTGGCTTCAAAGACAC-BHQ2-3′	29	141–113		This work
Control[1]	Sendai-F	GTCATGGATGGGCAGGAGTC	20	8553–8572[b]		Kaiser, 2001 [38]
	Sendai-R	CGTTGAAGAGCCTTACCCAGA	21	8788–8768[b]	236 bp	
	Sendai-P	5′-FAM-CAAAATTAGGAACGGAGGATTGTCCCCTC-Tamra-3′	29	8720–8748[b]		

Changed bases referring to the reference are underlined. Wobbled positions are as follows: Y = C/T; X/N = G/A/T/C, W = A/T, S = C/G, R = A/G, M = A/C, K = G/T, H = A/C/T, and B = C/G/T.

[a] Rabies primer and probe positions are given according to the Pasteur virus genome (accession number X03673).

[b] Positions of the GAPDH-primers refer to the GenBank sequence AJ431207; positions of the Sendai-primers refer to the GenBank sequence M30202.

[1] Controls for classical and real-time RT-PCR.

FAM: 6-carboxyfluorescein reporter dye, BHQ-1: Black Hole Quencher-1, YY: Yakima Yellow, Cy5: Cyanine 5, BHQ-2: Black Hole Quencher-2, and Tamra: carboxy-tetramethyl-rhodamine.

(QIAGEN, Germantown, USA) according to the manufacturer's instructions, except the usage of RNA Storage Solution (Ambion, Foster City, USA) for elution. Extracted RNA was stored at −20°C until use.

2.6. Heminested RT-PCR. Heminested RT-PCR was performed as previously described [22] using the OneStep RT-PCR Kit. Briefly, for the first round $3 \mu L$ of extracted RNA was amplified in the RT-PCR mix prepared according to manufacturer's instructions, supplemented with $0.6 \mu M$ of each primer (JW12-F, JW6AS1-R1, and JW6AS2-R1; Table 2) and 5 U RNase inhibitor (RNasin Plus, 40 U/μL; Promega, Madison, USA), with the following cycling conditions: 50°C for 30 min and 95° for 15 min for reverse transcription and subsequent activation of the polymerase, followed by 10 cycles of 95°C for 20 s, 60°C for 30 s (1°C decrease/cycle), followed by 72°C for 30 s and 35 cycles of 95°C for 20 s, 52°C for 30 s, followed by 72°C for 30 s. For the second round, the Taq DNA Polymerase Kit (QIAGEN, Germantown, USA) was used with $2 \mu L$ of the first round product, $2.5 \mu L$ 10x PCR buffer, 1.2 mM final dNTP concentration (Invitrogen, Foster City, USA), $0.4 \mu M$ of heminested primers (JW12-F, JW10AS1-R2, and JW10AS2-R2; Table 2), 0.5 U of Taq DNA polymerase, and $19.35 \mu L$ Nuclease Free Water (Ambion, Foster City, USA). Cycling conditions were as follows: 95°C for 5 min followed by 35 cycles of 94°C for 20 s, 52°C for 20 s, followed by 72°C for 30 s. Amplifications were performed in a 2720 Thermal Cycler. Internal controls using GAPDH primers, as described in the one-round PCR, were run in parallel in the first round.

2.7. Gel Electrophoresis for Sequencing. Gel electrophoresis was performed using a 1.5% TAE agarose gel (agarose LE, analytical grade; Promega, Madison, USA) stained with ethidium bromide (Eurobio, Courtaboeuf, France). For sequencing, the desired band was excised under UV light [47].

2.8. Real-Time RT-PCR (NDWD). Real-time RT-PCR (NDWD) adapted from Nadin-Davis et al. and Wakeley et al. [8, 25] was performed using the QuantiTect Probe RT-PCR Kit (QIAGEN, Germantown, USA). The $25 \mu L$ reaction volume consisted of $9.5 \mu L$ RNase-free water, or $9 \mu L$ in the multiplex mix, $12.5 \mu L$ 2x QuantiTect RT-PCR Master Mix, $0.25 \mu L$ of the RABVD1 forward and reverse primer ($0.4 \mu M$ final concentration each), $0.25 \mu L$ of the probes RABVD1, LysGT5, and LysGT6 together in the multiplex mix or $0.25 \mu L$ of the probes ivvWCBV-P, ivvMok-P, ivvABLV2n-P, ivvLBV-P, ivvKhujand-P, and ivvSBLV2-P (Table 2) alone in a mix (all $0.2 \mu M$ final concentration), $0.25 \mu L$ of QuantiTect RT Mix, and $2 \mu L$ of sample RNA. Additionally, for the internal Sendai virus control, $5 \mu L$ of sample RNA was added to a mix containing $6.625 \mu L$ of RNase-free water, $12.5 \mu L$ 2x QuantiTect RT-PCR Master Mix, $0.625 \mu L$ of Sendai forward primer, reverse primer, and probe mix (Sendai-F, Sendai-R, and Sendai-P, $8 \mu M$; Table 2), and $0.25 \mu L$ of QuantiTect RT Mix. The reactions were carried out in MicroAmp Fast Optical 96-Well Reaction Plates with Barcode 0.1 mL (Applied Biosystems, Foster City, USA) in a

7500 Fast Real-Time PCR System v1.3.1 (Applied Biosystems, Foster City, USA) using the following cycling conditions: 1 cycle of 50°C for 30 min and 95°C for 15 min followed by 45 cycles of 95°C for 15 sec and 50°C for 1 min. Amplification curve analysis was performed using the 7500 Software v2.0.6 (Applied Biosystems, Foster City, USA).

2.9. Cloning for Analytical Sensitivity Analysis. For cloning, a segment of viral genome covering a part of the N gene (positions 1–933 according to the Pasteur virus genome accession number X03673) of CVS-11 was generated using primers designed for this purpose (TWclon-F and TWclon-R, Table 2). Amplification was performed using the OneStep RT-PCR Kit with the master mix consisting of $29.25 \mu L$ of RNase-free water, $10 \mu L$ 5x QIAGEN OneStep RT-PCR buffer, 0.4 mM of each dNTP, $0.6 \mu M$ of the cloning primers, 10 U RNasin (40 U/μL), and $2 \mu L$ of QIAGEN OneStep RT-PCR Enzyme mixed with $5 \mu L$ of extracted RNA to a total volume of $50 \mu L$. Amplifications were performed in a Veriti 96-Well Thermal Cycler (Applied Biosystems, Foster City, USA) using the following cycling conditions: 30 min at 50°C, followed by 15 min at 95°C and 40 repetitive cycles of 1 min at 94°C, 1 min with a temperature gradient from 56°C to 46°C in steps of 2°C, and 1 min at 72°C. Elongation at 72°C was extended for 10 additional minutes in the last cycle. After gel electrophoresis excised PCR fragments with a length of 933 bp were eluted with the QIAquick Gel Extraction Kit (QIAGEN, Germantown, USA) and cloned into the pCR-II-TOPO vector using the TOPO TA Cloning Kit (Invitrogen, Foster City, USA) according to the manufacturer's instructions.

2.10. Sequencing. Sequencing reactions were performed by Microsynth AG, Balgach, Switzerland. For this purpose, reaction mixtures containing 22.5 ng DNA per 100 bp, 30 pmol of each primer used for the amplification (Table 2), and DEPC treated water (Ambion, Foster City, USA) to a final volume of $15 \mu L$ were prepared. Sequences were edited using the SeqMan II v5.01 Software (DNASTAR, Madison, USA) and subsequently evaluated using the Clone Manager 9 software (Scientific & Educational Software, Cary, USA).

2.11. Phylogenetic Reconstruction. The 543 bp nucleotide sequences of the nucleoprotein gene obtained from the heminested PCR reaction, together with additional sequences retrieved from GenBank, were saved in Fasta file format. The sequences were then aligned using the ClustalX 2.0.3 Software and the GeneDoc Software v2.5.0 [48]. Phylogenetic trees were constructed with the MEGA5 software using Kimura 2-parameter distances [35].

3. Results

3.1. Cell Culture. Thirty-one lyssaviruses (19x RABV, 7x EBLV-1, 4x EBLV-2, and 1x DUVV) were analysed in RTCIT. All isolates were viable in murine neuroblastoma cells and could be visualized using Rabies DFA Reagent as a conjugate.

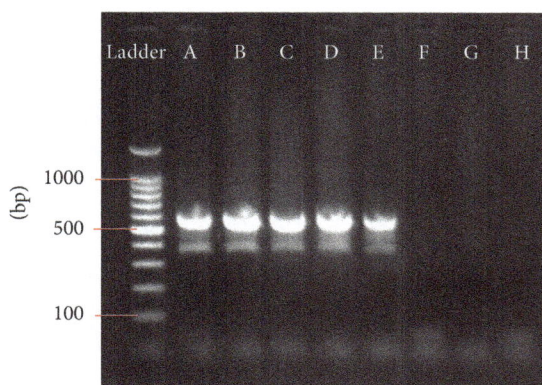

FIGURE 1: Amplification of a CVS-11 serial dilution using hnRT-PCR. Ethidium bromide stained gel after amplification of the CVS-11 strain using dilutions from 10^{-1} to 10^{-8} (A–H). The amplification product of 582 bp is clearly visible up to a dilution of 10^{-5} (lane E). Ladder = standard for determination of amplification product size.

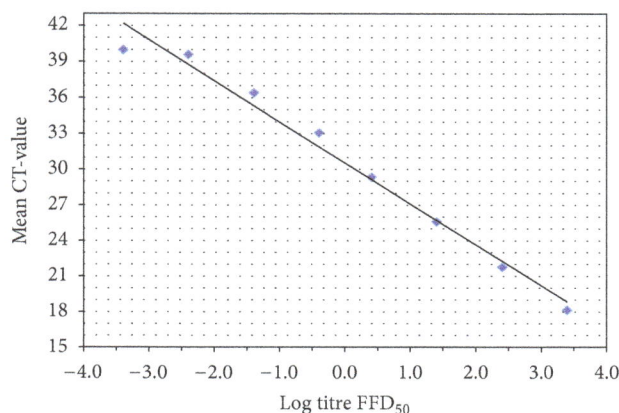

FIGURE 2: Efficiency of the real-time RT-PCR (NDWD). The linear regression of the CT-values (ordinate) and the titres of serially diluted CVS-11 (abscissa) exhibited a slope coefficient of −3.46 corresponding to an efficiency of 94.5% ($E = 10^{(-1/\text{slope coefficient})} - 1$).

3.2. Sensitivity of PCR Methods.

For the comparison with infectious titres, RNA of the classical rabies virus strain CVS-11 was extracted from cell culture supernatants (BHK-21 cells or neuroblastoma cells MNA 42/13) and serially diluted from 10^{-1} to 10^{-8}. The infectious titre was determined according to the Spearman-Karber formula [49, 50] in fluorescent focus forming doses 50% (FFD_{50}). In the heminested RT-PCR (hnRT-PCR), the amplification product of 582 bp was visible up to a dilution of 10^{-5} corresponding to a detection limit of 0.4 FFD_{50} ($10^{-0.4}$ FFD_{50}; Figure 1). In the real-time RT-PCR (NDWD) the serial dilution was performed in triplicate. The limit of detection was defined as the last dilution at which at least 2 out of 3 replicates were positive. Using this definition, CVS-11 was detectable up to a dilution of 10^{-7} (once at a dilution of 10^{-8}). The amplification plot showed regular intervals of the curves with CT-values from 18.1 (dilution 10^{-1}) to 40.0 (dilution 10^{-7}). Relating to infectious titre real-time RT-PCR reached a detection limit of 0.003 FFD_{50} ($10^{-2.6}$) for CVS-11.

The efficiency of the real-time RT-PCR (NDWD) was determined using linear regression of the CT-values and the titres of the samples (Figure 2). On the basis of the slope coefficient, the efficiency can be inversely derived as $E = 10^{(-1/\text{slope coefficient})} - 1$. The efficiency for CVS-11 was 94.5% with a slope coefficient of −3.46.

3.3. Analytical Sensitivity.

The limit of detection in terms of DNA copy numbers was determined using 10-fold serial dilutions of a cloned 933 bp segment of N of CVS-11 containing 10^6 to 10^0 DNA copies/PCR reaction. In the hnPCR, the limit of detection was 100 DNA copies/3 μL of starting material of the CVS-11 plasmid. In the real-time PCR (NDWD), the 10-fold serial dilution of the CVS-plasmid was tested in triplicate. The limit of detection was 10 DNA copies/2 μL of the CVS-11 plasmid with CT-values between 38.6 and 47.5. The efficiency was at 82.8% with a slope coefficient of −3.82 (not shown). The intra-assay repeatability of the real-time PCR (NDWD)

proved to be excellent with very low coefficients of variation up to 10^2 DNA copies (0.18–1.37%) with and outlier at 10^1 copies (12.05%; Table 3).

3.4. Diagnostic Broadness of PCR Methods.

A total of 31 lyssaviruses (19 identified as classical RABV, 7 as EBLV-1, 4 as EBLV-2, and 1 as DUVV) were used to test the diagnostic performance of the PCR (Table 1). All viruses used were detected with the expected band size in the hnRT-PCR technique (Table 4). The specificity of the amplified product was confirmed as RABV, EBLV-1, EBLV-2, or DUVV by sequencing in each case. Host GAPDH (glyceraldehyde 3-phosphate dehydrogenase) was detected in all of the cell culture supernatants and mouse brain suspensions as internal control, indicating that sample material was present and RNA isolation, reverse transcription, and amplification were not inhibited. All samples were also tested positive by the real-time RT-PCR assay (Table 4). Sendai virus as internal control for inhibition was run in parallel using the same cycling conditions. In the real-time RT-PCR (NDWD) with an annealing temperature of 50°C, some samples were detected with more than one probe. With the exception of the sample derived from a raccoon dog from Poland, the probe for the homologous genotype always yielded the lowest CT-value. In this exceptional case, the probe for the detection of genotype 6 was slightly lower than the one for genotype 1 (15.0 versus 16.1; Table 4). Comparison of these two probes with the sequence of the rabies variant in question showed 1 and 2 mismatches with the RABVD1-P and LysGT6-P probe, respectively (Figure 3). Duvenhage virus, also designated as genotype 4, was detectable with the probe adapted for genotype 6 in spite of 3 mismatches (LysGT6-P). The probe LysGT6-P was able to detect synthetic DNA fragments of BBLV, ARAV, and IRKV, although containing one or two mismatches, respectively. The synthetic DNA fragments of KHUV, ABLV, LBV, MOKV, SHIBV, and WCBV, which exhibited from four (ABLV/KHUV) up to ten (WCBV) mismatches to the best fitting probe for GT1,

Table 3: Serial dilutions of the CVS-11 plasmid in real-time PCR (NDWD).

Dilution	Copy numbers/2 μL	CT-value 1	CT-value 2	CT-value 3	Mean $\pm$ SD	CV (%)
10^{-1}	10^6	22.6	22.0	22.4	22.3 $\pm$ 0.31	1.37
10^{-2}	10^5	25.1	25.2	25.3	25.2 $\pm$ 0.10	0.40
10^{-3}	10^4	29.1	28.8	28.7	28.9 $\pm$ 0.21	0.72
10^{-4}	10^3	32.9	32.9	32.8	32.9 $\pm$ 0.06	0.18
10^{-5}	10^2	36.4	36.2	35.9	36.2 $\pm$ 0.25	0.70
10^{-6}	10^1	47.5	38.6	39.0	41.7 $\pm$ 5.03	12.05
10^{-7}	10^0	—	—	—	—	—

SD: standard deviation; CV: coefficient of variation.

Table 4: PCR-results of rabies viruses tested.

	Sample	Species	hnRT-PCR	Real-time RT-PCR (NDWD) CT-value[a] FAM (GT1)	YY (GT5)	Cy5 (GT6)
1	Bat Stade (1970)	EBLV-1	+		14.7	17.3
2	Bat Hamburg RV 9 (1968)	EBLV-1	+	20.2	14.8	16.4
3	Bat Finland RV 8 (1986)	EBLV-2	+			15.1
4	Bat Holland RV 31	EBLV-1	+	20.2	14.7	16.8
5	Dog Tunisia (1986)	RABV	+	24.6	27.2	33.2
6	Bat Spain RV 119	EBLV-1	+	33.4	27.6	31.6
7	Bat Florida	RABV	+	24.2	41.6	
8	Bat Denmark	EBLV-1	+	26.5	21.1	22.4
9	Raccoon dog Poland (1985)	RABV	+	16.1		15.0
10	Raccoon Florida (1986)	RABV	+	25.8		
11	Bat Chile RV 108	RABV	+	14.4		
12	Jackal Zimbabwe	RABV	+	14.6		
13	Cattle Zimbabwe	RABV	+	18.0		
14	Canada Red Fox	RABV	+	17.9		
15	LEP (Flury, 1939)	RABV	+	17.7		
16	HEP (Flury)	RABV	+	28.5		
17	Dog Nepal Nr. 96	RABV	+	21.7		
18	Sri Lanka dog 121 (1986)	RABV	+	23.2		
19	Eurofox 912/87	RABV	+	28.3		
20	Duvenhage RV6	DUVV	+			27.0
21	NYC 58	RABV	+	16.5		
22	Dog Lima	RABV	+	20.0		
23	Bat Bremerhaven RV11	EBLV-1	+		27.0	
24	Bat B24	EBLV-1	+		16.9	20.6
25	Skunk Canada	RABV	+	23.2		
26	SAD Bern, 1935	RABV	+	18.8		
27	CSSR/A-virus	RABV	+	18.5		
28	Challenge virus standard (CVS-11) ATCC VR 959	RABV	+	19.8		
29	TW 1814/92	EBLV-2	+			
30	TW 1392/93	EBLV-2	+			
31	TW 118/02	EBLV-2	+			

[a]Only for samples with positive reaction.
FAM: 6-carboxyfluorescein reporter dye, to detect RABV (GT1); YY: Yakima Yellow, to detect EBLV-1 (GT5); Cy5: Cyanine 5, to detect EBLV-2 (GT6); ND: not done.

RABVD1-P   5′-78 ccgayaagattgtattyaargtcaakaatcaggt 111-3′   LysGT6-P   5′-81 acaraattgtcttcaargtccataatcag 109-3′
RABV raccoon dog   ....c.........c..a...c.t........   RABV raccoon dog   ..ag....a.....a............

(a)   (b)

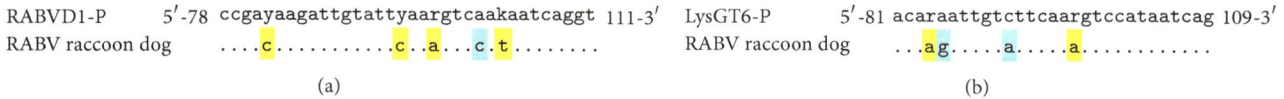

Figure 3: Alignment of probes RABVD1-P (a) and LysGT6-P (b) with a RABV strain isolated from a raccoon dog from Poland. Matches in nondegenerated positions are displayed as dots. Matches in wobbled positions are highlighted in yellow. Mismatches are highlighted in turquoise.

GT6, or GT5, respectively, were all detected with the corresponding species-specific new probe (Table 2). $10^{5.2}$ copies of the synthetic DNA were detected at CT-values of 27.9–33.5 for ABLV, MOKV, SHIBV, and WCBV (not shown). The efficiency of detection of KHUV, which showed an atypical amplification plot at the highest number of $10^{10.2}$ copies of the synthetic DNA, and that of LBV was lower with CT-values of 40.0 and 40.5 at a copy number of $10^{5.2}$, respectively (not shown). Multiplexing of combinations of these probes (ivvLBV-P (FAM: 6-carboxyfluorescein), ivvKhujand-P (YY: Yakima Yellow), and ivvSBLV2-P (Cy5: Cyanine 5), as well as ivvWCBV-P (FAM), ivvMok-P (YY), and ivvABLV2n-P (Cy5)) as for the species 1, 5, and 6 was not successful.

3.5. Sequencing of Amplification Products and Phylogenetic Analysis. The 543 bp amplification products of the nucleoprotein gene obtained in the heminested PCR reactions were sequenced (Table 1) and analysed phylogenetically with additional sequences retrieved from GenBank representing all known lyssaviruses. The similarity of the 543 bp nucleotide sequences of the nucleoprotein gene (positions 74–616 according to the Pasteur virus genome) among the lyssaviruses included ranged from 64.6% to 90.1% (Hamming distance). Similarity at the amino acid level was 68.0–95%. The resulting phylogenetic tree obtained by the neighbor-joining method implemented in the MEGA5 software is presented in Figure 4. All known genotypes were resolved with high bootstrap confidence with our samples grouping expectedly.

3.6. Clinical Specimens. Clinical specimens like brain suspensions (1x human, 12x mouse), skin biopsies from the nape of the neck (3x human, 1x mouse), saliva (4x human), and cerebrospinal fluids (6x human) were used for the establishment of the assays. Both hnRT-PCR and real-time RT-PCR (NDWD) were shown to work properly on all these samples without significant inhibition using GAPDH as internal control for conventional RT-PCR and Sendai virus for real-time RT-PCR (NDWD), which was mixed to the samples before RNA isolation. Skin biopsies taken from the neck and lip of a mouse (white Swiss mouse at an age of 3 weeks) euthanized 2 weeks after intracerebral infection with SAD Bern virus 20 years ago were positive with the hnRT-PCR and real-time PCR (NDWD). Skin biopsies taken from other locations on the head were positive with the real-time PCR (NDWD) and weakly positive in hnRT-PCR whereas samples taken around the vibrissae were weakly positive in real-time PCR (NDWD) only. Sequencing of amplification

products excluded a contamination with the positive CVS-11 control (not shown).

Brain suspension from an imported human rabies case in 2012 was already strongly positive after one round of the hnRT-PCR. Phylogenetic analysis of the 543 bp nucleotide fragment revealed its close relationship to the classical rabies virus strains circulating in the insectivorous Mexican free-tailed bat, *Tadarida brasiliensis*, a species common in the southern United States and Mexico. This allowed identification of the origin of the patient's infection, who had travelled extensively and did not report any previous biting incident [51, 52].

4. Discussion

Based on a large amount of published work, we were able to establish and quantitatively characterise RT-PCR protocols for the detection of lyssaviruses in clinical samples. Well suited real-time protocols [8, 25] for the detection of classical rabies virus and the genotypes 5 and 6 (EBLV-1 and EBLV-2) were adapted and extended for the detection of at least 13 lyssavirus species. To this goal, 6 species-specific probes (KHUV, ABLV, LBV, MOKV, SHIBV, and WCBV) were designed and verified on synthetic DNA fragments encompassing the targeted sequence of the lyssaviral nucleoprotein gene. Multiplexing the probes in a single-tube reaction as described for the genotypes 1, 5, and 6 was not possible with the newly designed probes, probably due to false priming and/or interference within the mix of reagents and synthetic target sequence [53]. As far as evaluated with the multiplexed probes for the genotypes 1, 5, and 6 using 31 viral isolates, which were all detectable with high sensitivity, direct differentiation of targeted genotypes on the base of the quantitative reaction (CT-values) was mostly possible. Furthermore, a single probe for genotype 6 (species EBLV-2) was able to detect up to 7 genotypes/species. We consider this type of cross hybridization as an advantage of the technique using degenerate primers and probes in terms of a broad detectability of lyssavirus rather than a lack of accuracy of discrimination. In an approach using SYBR Green qPCR with similarly degenerate primers spanning the same part of N as in this work [28], the detection of all lyssavirus species known at that time was achieved. Using several genotype-specific probes in a TaqMan real-time protocol, we were able to add more intrinsic confidence to the specificity of the analysis [54]. Quantitative characterisation of the assay using the probe for genotypes 1, 5, and 6 on CVS-11 showed excellent sensitivity and repeatability with a detection limit of as low as an infectious dose of 0.003 FFD_{50} combined

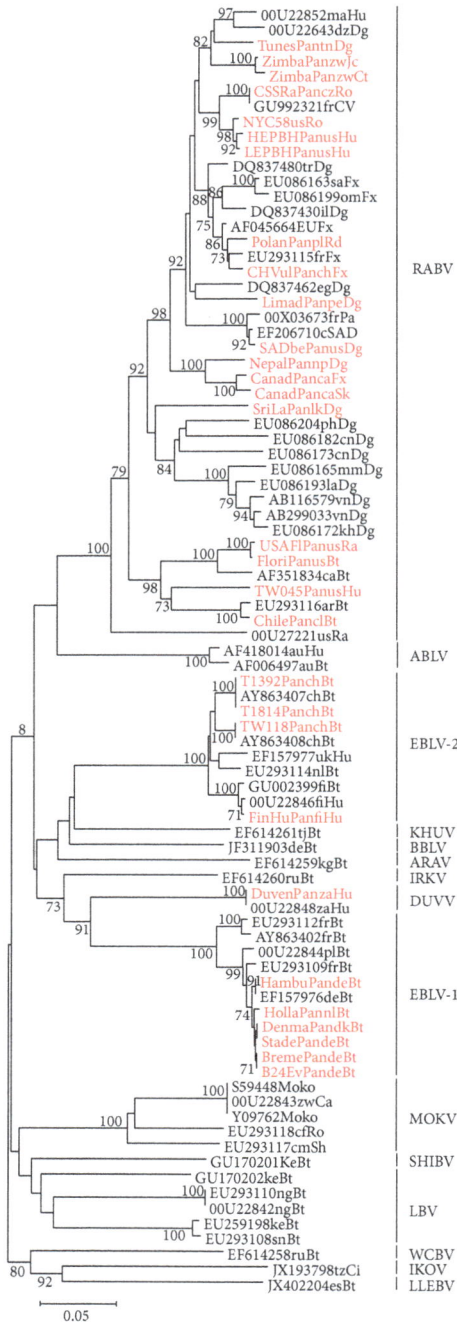

FIGURE 4: Phylogenetic tree with 543 bp fragments of N. Phylogenetic tree obtained with MEGA5 software [35]. The length of branches (horizontal lines) corresponds to phylogenetic distance between different sequences (scale bar in substitutions per site). Numbers proximal to nodes indicate bootstrap confidence of subjacent groups. Lyssavirus strains used in this study are depicted in red. Sequences are given with GenBank or own designation followed by the two-letter country code and a two-letter code for the source species as follows: Bt, bat; Ca, cat; Ci, African civet; Dg, dog; Fx, fox; Hu, human; Jc, jackal; Ra, raccoon; Rd, raccoon dog; Ro, rodent; Sh, shrew; Sk, skunk, except for Pa, cSAD, and CV, which are standing for Pasteur strain, Street Alabama Dufferin strain, and challenge virus standard, respectively. The currently used abbreviations for species are shown next to the tree. RABV, rabies virus; ABLV, Australian bat lyssavirus; WCBV, West Caucasian bat virus; IKOV, Ikoma virus; LLEBV, Lleida bat lyssavirus; MOKV, Mokola virus; SHIBV, Shimoni bat virus; LBV, Lagos bat virus; KHUV, Khujand virus; BBLV, Bokeloh bat lyssavirus; ARAV, Aravan virus; DUVV, Duvenhage virus; EBLV, European bat lyssavirus; IRKV, Irkut virus.

with an analytical sensitivity of 10 DNA copies at efficiencies of 94.5% and 82.8%, respectively. Considering the amount of degeneration in both primers and probes, the efficiencies determined must be considered satisfactory. As far as the absolute detection limit in terms of target copies is concerned, the usage of plasmid DNA rather than RNA must be kept in mind. Since reverse transcription cannot be assumed as 100% efficient and reproducible [55], the limit for RNA might be somewhat lower.

For further characterisation of samples with a positive reaction in real-time RT-PCR, excellent simple and (hemi)nested RT-PCR protocols are available. With the protocol used for this work [22], all 31 viral strains used could be amplified and sequenced, confirming the diagnostic broadness of the assay. Phylogenetic analysis of these partial nucleotide sequences belonging to genotypes 1, 4, 5, and 6 along with known sequences confirmed the suitability of this relatively conserved genomic region for molecular-epidemiological characterisation of lyssaviruses circulating worldwide [56–58]. This was also confirmed in the context of a human rabies case imported to Switzerland in 2012, which could be attributed unequivocally to an exposure to a bat of the species *Tadarida brasiliensis* in California, USA.

5. Conclusion

In this work we could show and validate the suitability of an adapted and further developed real-time RT-PCR protocol for the rapid, efficient, and highly sensitive intravitam diagnosis of a wide spectrum of lyssavirus species followed by rapid molecular-epidemiological characterisation of viral isolates respective to origin of the virus and source of exposure, using heminested RT-PCR. This new tool is also particularly promising for active surveillance of European bat lyssaviruses using oral swabs in live-captured bats.

Conflict of Interests

The authors declare that there is no conflict of interests regarding the publication of this paper.

Acknowledgments

The authors wish to acknowledge the critical review of the paper of PD Dr. Philippe Plattet. The help of Audrey Megali for her advice in the molecular techniques is greatly acknowledged.

References

[1] *Laboratory Techniques in Rabies*, World Health Organization, Geneva, Switzerland, 4th edition, 1996.

[2] WHO, "WHO expert consultation on rabies," Second Report, WHO, Geneva, Switzerland, 2013.

[3] O. I. E. Rabies, *Manual of Standards for Diagnostic Tests and Vaccines for Terrestrial Animals*, World Health Organization, Paris, France, 2013.

[4] D. Sacramento, H. Bourhy, and N. Tordo, "PCR technique as an alternative method for diagnosis and molecular epidemiology of rabies virus," *Molecular and Cellular Probes*, vol. 5, no. 3, pp. 229–240, 1991.

[5] H. Bourhy, P. Sureau, and J. A. Montano Hirose, *Méthodes de Laboratoire pour le Diagnostic de la Rage*, Institut Pasteur, Paris, France, 1990.

[6] E. Picard-Meyer, V. Bruyère, J. Barrat, E. Tissot, M. J. Barrat, and F. Cliquet, "Development of a hemi-nested RT-PCR method for the specific determination of European Bat Lyssavirus 1: comparison with other rabies diagnostic methods," *Vaccine*, vol. 22, no. 15-16, pp. 1921–1929, 2004.

[7] T. Nagaraj, J. P. Vasanth, A. Desai, A. Kamat, S. N. Madhusudana, and V. Ravi, "Ante mortem diagnosis of human rabies using saliva samples: comparison of real time and conventional RT-PCR techniques," *Journal of Clinical Virology*, vol. 36, no. 1, pp. 17–23, 2006.

[8] S. A. Nadin-Davis, M. Sheen, and A. I. Wandeler, "Development of real-time reverse transcriptase polymerase chain reaction methods for human rabies diagnosis," *Journal of Medical Virology*, vol. 81, no. 8, pp. 1484–1497, 2009.

[9] S. Wacharapluesadee and T. Hemachudha, "Ante- and postmortem diagnosis of rabies using nucleic acid-amplification tests," *Expert Review of Molecular Diagnostics*, vol. 10, no. 2, pp. 207–218, 2010.

[10] M. Fischer, K. Wernike, C. M. Freuling et al., "A step forward in molecular diagnostics of lyssaviruses—results of a ring trial among European laboratories," *PLoS ONE*, vol. 8, no. 3, Article ID e58372, 2013.

[11] C. Freuling, A. Vos, N. Johnson et al., "Experimental infection of serotine bats (*Eptesicus serotinus*) with European bat lyssavirus type 1a," *Journal of General Virology*, vol. 90, no. 10, pp. 2493–2502, 2009.

[12] K. Schutsky, D. Curtis, E. K. Bongiorno et al., "Intramuscular inoculation of mice with the live-attenuated recombinant rabies virus TriGAS results in a transient infection of the draining lymph nodes and a robust, long-lasting protective immune response against rabies," *Journal of Virology*, vol. 87, no. 3, pp. 1834–1841, 2013.

[13] H. Bourhy, J.-M. Reynes, E. J. Dunham et al., "The origin and phylogeography of dog rabies virus," *Journal of General Virology*, vol. 89, no. 11, pp. 2673–2681, 2008.

[14] D. T. S. Hayman, N. Johnson, D. L. Horton et al., "Evolutionary history of rabies in Ghana," *PLoS Neglected Tropical Diseases*, vol. 5, no. 4, Article ID e1001, 2011.

[15] S. A. Nadin-Davis and L. A. Real, "Molecular phylogenetics of the lyssaviruses-insights from a coalescent approach," *Advances in Virus Research*, vol. 79, pp. 203–238, 2011.

[16] C. A. Hanlon and J. E. Childs, "Epidemiology," in *Rabies: Scientific Basis of Disease and its Management*, A. C. Jackson, Ed., pp. 61–121, Academic Press, New York, NY, USA, 2013.

[17] S. A. Nadin-Davis, "Molecular epidemiology," in *Rabies: Scientific Basis of Disease and Its Management*, A. C. Jackson, Ed., pp. 123–177, Academic press, Amsterdam, The Netherlands, 2013.

[18] P. R. Heaton, P. Johnstone, L. M. McElhinney, R. Cowley, E. O'Sullivan, and J. E. Whitby, "Heminested PCR assay for detection of six genotypes of rabies and rabies-related viruses," *Journal of Clinical Microbiology*, vol. 35, no. 11, pp. 2762–2766, 1997.

[19] H. Bourhy, "Lyssaviruses—special emphasis on rabies virus," in *Diagnostic Virology Protocols*, J. R. Stephenson and A. Warnes, Eds., vol. 12 of *Methods in Molecular Medicine*, pp. 129–142, Humana Press, Totowa, NJ, USA, 1998.

[20] F. Cliquet and E. Picard-Meyer, "Rabies and rabies-related viruses: a modern perspective on an ancient disease," *Revue Scientifique et Technique de L'Office International des Epizooties*, vol. 23, no. 2, pp. 625–642, 2004.

[21] S. Vázquez-Morón, A. Avellón, and J. E. Echevarría, "RT-PCR for detection of all seven genotypes of *Lyssavirus* genus," *Journal of Virological Methods*, vol. 135, no. 2, pp. 281–287, 2006.

[22] M. Panning, S. Baumgarte, S. Pfefferle, T. Maier, A. Martens, and C. Drosten, "Comparative analysis of rabies virus reverse transcription-PCR and virus isolation using samples from a patient infected with rabies virus," *Journal of Clinical Microbiology*, vol. 48, no. 8, pp. 2960–2962, 2010.

[23] P. de Benedictis, C. de Battisti, L. Dacheux et al., "Lyssavirus detection and typing using pyrosequencing," *Journal of Clinical Microbiology*, vol. 49, no. 5, pp. 1932–1938, 2011.

[24] E. M. Black, J. P. Lowings, J. Smith, P. R. Heaton, and L. M. McElhinney, "A rapid RT-PCR method to differentiate six established genotypes of rabies and rabies-related viruses using TaqMan (TM) technology," *Journal of Virological Methods*, vol. 105, pp. 25–35, 2002.

[25] P. R. Wakeley, N. Johnson, L. M. McElhinney, D. Marston, J. Sawyer, and A. R. Fooks, "Development of a real-time, TaqMan reverse transcription-PCR assay for detection and differentiation of lyssavirus genotypes 1, 5, and 6," *Journal of Clinical Microbiology*, vol. 43, no. 6, pp. 2786–2792, 2005.

[26] J. Coertse, J. Weyer, L. H. Nel, and W. Markotter, "Improved PCR methods for detection of african rabies and rabies-related lyssaviruses," *Journal of Clinical Microbiology*, vol. 48, no. 11, pp. 3949–3955, 2010.

[27] B. Hoffmann, C. M. Freuling, P. R. Wakeley et al., "Improved safety for molecular diagnosis of classical rabies viruses by use of a TaqMan real-time reverse transcription-PCR "double check" strategy," *Journal of Clinical Microbiology*, vol. 48, no. 11, pp. 3970–3978, 2010.

[28] D. T. S. Hayman, A. C. Banyard, P. R. Wakeley et al., "A universal real-time assay for the detection of *Lyssaviruses*," *Journal of Virological Methods*, vol. 177, no. 1, pp. 87–93, 2011.

[29] T. Müller, N. Johnson, C. M. Freuling, A. R. Fooks, T. Selhorst, and A. Vos, "Epidemiology of bat rabies in Germany," *Archives of Virology*, vol. 152, no. 2, pp. 273–288, 2007.

[30] A. C. Banyard, N. Johnson, K. Voller et al., "Repeated detection of European bat lyssavirus type 2 in dead bats found at a single roost site in the UK," *Archives of Virology*, vol. 154, no. 11, pp. 1847–1850, 2009.

[31] A. Megali, G. Yannic, M.-L. Zahno et al., "Surveillance for European bat lyssavirus in Swiss bats," *Archives of Virology*, vol. 155, no. 10, pp. 1655–1662, 2010.

[32] W. W. Müller, "Review of reported rabies case data in Europe to the WHO Collaborating Centre, Tübingen, from 1977 to 1988," *Rabies Bulletin Europe*, vol. 4, pp. 16–19, 1977.

[33] C. Freuling, T. Selhorst, A. Kliemt, and T. Müller, "Rabies surveillance in Europe, 2004–2007," *Rabies Bulletin Europe*, vol. 31, no. 4, pp. 7–8, 2004.

[34] P. Demetriou and J. Moynagh, "The European Union strategy for external cooperation with neighbouring countries on rabies control," *Rabies Bulletin Europe*, vol. 35, no. 1, pp. 5–7, 2011.

[35] K. Tamura, D. Peterson, N. Peterson, G. Stecher, M. Nei, and S. Kumar, "MEGA5: molecular evolutionary genetics analysis using maximum likelihood, evolutionary distance, and maximum parsimony methods," *Molecular Biology and Evolution*, vol. 28, no. 10, pp. 2731–2739, 2011.

[36] M. K. Abelseth, "An attenuated rabies vaccine for domestic animals produced in tissue culture," *Canadian Veterinary Journal*, vol. 5, no. 11, pp. 279–286, 1964.

[37] A. P. Ravazzolo, C. Nenci, H.-R. Vogt et al., "Viral load, organ distribution, histopathological lesions, and cytokine mRNA expression in goats infected with a molecular clone of the caprine arthritis encephalitis virus," *Virology*, vol. 350, no. 1, pp. 116–127, 2006.

[38] D. Kaiser, *Entwicklung und Evaluation eines RT-TaqMan-PCR-Testverfahrens zum Nachweis des BVD-Virus [Ph.D. dissertation]*, Universität Bern, 2001.

[39] H. Koprowski, "The mouse inoculation test," in *Laboratory Techniques in Rabies*, M. M. Kaplan and H. Koprowski, Eds., pp. 85–93, World Health Organization, Geneva, Switzerland, 1973.

[40] D. J. Dean and M. K. Abelseth, "The fluorescent antibody test," in *Laboratory Techniques in Rabies*, M. M. Kaplan and H. Koprowski, Eds., pp. 73–83, World Health Organization, Geneva, Switzerland, 1973.

[41] A. Gerhardt, *Teilvalidierung einer Zellkulturmethode als Alternative zum Tierversuch für den Nachweis von Tollwutvirus aus Hirnmaterial [dissertation thesis]*, Veterinärmedizinische Universität Wien, Universität Bern, 1995.

[42] R. J. Rudd and C. V. Trimarchi, "Development and evaluation of an in vitro virus isolation procedure as a replacement for the mouse inoculation test in rabies diagnosis," *Journal of Clinical Microbiology*, vol. 27, no. 11, pp. 2522–2528, 1989.

[43] P. Stöhr, K. Stöhr, H. Kiupel, and E. Karge, "Immunofluorescence investigations of rabies field viruses in comparison of several fluorescein-labelled antisera," *Tierärztliche Umschau*, vol. 47, pp. 813–818, 1992.

[44] J. D. Thompson, T. J. Gibson, F. Plewniak, F. Jeanmougin, and D. G. Higgins, "The CLUSTAL X windows interface: flexible strategies for multiple sequence alignment aided by quality analysis tools," *Nucleic Acids Research*, vol. 25, no. 24, pp. 4876–4882, 1997.

[45] D. G. Higgins and P. M. Sharp, "CLUSTAL: a package for performing multiple sequence alignment on a microcomputer," *Gene*, vol. 73, no. 1, pp. 237–244, 1988.

[46] M. A. Larkin, G. Blackshields, N. P. Brown et al., "Clustal W and clustal X version 2.0," *Bioinformatics*, vol. 23, no. 21, pp. 2947–2948, 2007.

[47] T. Maniatis, E. F. Fritsch, and J. Sambrook, *Molecular Cloning: A Laboratory Manual*, Cold Spring Harbor Laboratory, Cold Spring Harbor, NY, USA, 1982.

[48] K. B. Nicholas, H. B. J. Nicholas, and D. W. Deerfield II, "GeneDoc: analysis and visualization of genetic variation," *Embnew News*, vol. 4, article 14, 1997.

[49] G. Kaerber, "Beitrag zur kollektiven Behandlung pharmakologischer Reihenversuche," *Archiv for Experimentelle Pathologie und Pharmakologie*, vol. 162, pp. 480–487, 1931.

[50] C. Spearman, "The method of "right or wrong cases" (constant stimuli) without Gauss's formulae," *British Journal of Psychology*, vol. 2, pp. 227–242, 1908.

[51] A. N. Deubelbeiss, C. Trachsel, E. B. Bachli et al., "Imported human rabies in Switzerland, 2012: a diagnostic conundrum," *Journal of Clinical Virology*, vol. 57, no. 2, pp. 178–181, 2013.

[52] S. Farley, S. Zarate, E. Jenssen et al., "U.S-acquired human rabies with symptom onset and diagnosis abroad, 2012," *Morbidity and Mortality Weekly Report*, vol. 61, no. 39, pp. 777–781, 2012.

[53] A. Apte and S. Daniel, *PCR Primer Design*, Cold Spring Harbor Protocols, 2009.

[54] C. J. Smith and A. M. Osborn, "Advantages and limitations of quantitative PCR (Q-PCR)-based approaches in microbial ecology," *FEMS Microbiology Ecology*, vol. 67, no. 1, pp. 6–20, 2009.

[55] R. Sanders, D. J. Mason, C. A. Foy, and J. F. Huggett, "Evaluation of digital PCR for absolute RNA quantification," *PLoS ONE*, vol. 8, no. 9, Article ID e75296, 2013.

[56] E. C. Holmes, C. H. Woelk, R. Kassis, and H. Bourhy, "Genetic constraints and the adaptive evolution of rabies virus in nature," *Virology*, vol. 292, no. 2, pp. 247–257, 2002.

[57] A. J. Foord, H. G. Heine, L. I. Pritchard et al., "Molecular diagnosis of lyssaviruses and sequence comparison of Australian bat lyssavirus samples," *Australian Veterinary Journal*, vol. 84, no. 7, pp. 225–230, 2006.

[58] T. Scott, R. Hassel, and L. Nel, "Rabies in kudu (*Tragelaphus strepsiceros*)," *Berliner und Munchener Tierarztliche Wochenschrift*, vol. 125, no. 5-6, pp. 236–241, 2012.

6

Influence of a Diester Glucocorticoid Spray on the Cortisol Level and the CCR4$^+$ CD4$^+$ Lymphocytes in Dogs with Atopic Dermatitis: Open Study

Masato Fujimura and Hironobu Ishimaru

Fujimura Animal Allergy Hospital, Aomatanihigashi 5-10-26, Minou-shi, Osaka 562-0022, Japan

Correspondence should be addressed to Masato Fujimura; hope3413@gmail.com

Academic Editor: Fulvia Bovera

This study investigated the influence of 0.00584% hydrocortisone aceponate spray (HCA; Cortavance Virbac SA, Carros, France) on blood serum cortisol levels and peripheral blood CCR4$^+$ CD4$^+$ T-lymphocyte levels in dogs with atopic dermatitis. Patients were randomly divided into group I ($N = 8$) and group II ($N = 8$). The dogs in group I were sprayed with HCA on the affected skin once a day for three weeks. The dogs in group II were treated once a day for 3 days followed by no treatment for 4 days for a total of three weeks. For the dogs in group I and group II the CADESI-03 scores before and after use of HCA showed significant reduction ($P < 0.01$). The postcortisol level after the use of HCA in group I showed 36.0% decrease and showed significant suppression ($P < 0.01$). By comparison, the use of HCA on group II did not show decrease in postcortisol levels. There was a tendency of suppression for hypothalamus—pituitary gland—adrenal gland system, but it was not serious influence. In addition, there was no influence on peripheral blood CCR4$^+$ CD4$^+$ lymphocytes percentage in dogs in group I after treatment with HCA.

1. Introduction

Canine atopic dermatitis is an intractable chronic skin disease, and management requires a combination of many treatments [1]. Treatment generally involves the use of an antifungal drug, an antibiotic, a shampoo therapy, a humidity retention treatment, an anti-inflammatory drug, and/or hyposensitization. The most frequently used therapy is a corticosteroid. Unfortunately there are not many practical guidelines for use of steroid therapy [2] in veterinary medicine, and there are only a few reports about the side effects. The prolongation of steroid treatment can cause atrophy of the skin, ulceration, hair loss, and skin calcification [3], but the adverse reaction we are concerned about most is the influence on hypothalamus—pituitary gland—adrenal gland system [4, 5].

0.00584% hydrocortisone aceponate spray (HCA; Cortavance Virbac SA, Carros, France) is different from a conventional steroid, due to the fact that the absence of a halogen at C6, C9, and C21 is associated with better local and systemic tolerance [6, 7]. Double esterification of C21 and C17 enhances penetration of the stratum corneum and ensures specific metabolism in the lower dermis. These actions minimize the effects on hair follicles, dermal fibroblasts, and blood vessels, decreasing the likelihood of local cutaneous and systemic adverse effects [6, 7].

The effectiveness of HCA for treatment of inflammation is proved in former studies [8–10]. The purpose of this study is to confirm the influence of HCA on the patient by measuring the clinical score, the cortisol levels by the ACTH stimulation test, and the CCR4$^+$ CD4$^+$ lymphocytes percentage in blood both before and after use of HCA in randomized clinical study.

2. Materials and Methods

2.1. Animals. All dogs were diagnosed with canine atopic dermatitis and had severe itch; they were seen at one hospital (Fujimura Animal Allergy Hospital, Osaka, Japan). The study was conducted from June to November, 2011, with the owners' consent.

2.2. Diagnosis of CAD (Canine Atopic Dermatitis). The diagnosis of CAD was made by ruling out other causes of the itch. All dogs received flea control and appropriate treatment for scabies mites. If bacterial pyoderma and yeast (*Malassezia dermatitis*) were diagnosed by cytology, it was treated mainly by shampoo therapy. All dogs underwent an elimination diet using "hypoallergenic" foods (Hill's prescription diet z/d Canine Ultra: Hill's Pet Nutrition, Topeka, KS, USA; or Royal Canin Veterinary Diet Sensitivity Control: Royal Canin, Aimargue, France; or Iams Veterinary Formulas FP: Cincinnati, Ohio, USA) for at least 8 weeks. The diagnosis of CAD was based on compatible history and clinical signs of Favrot's criteria [11]. Intradermal allergy testing was performed with 24 selected antigens (Greer Pharmacy, Lenoir, NC, USA; or Torii Pharmaceutical Co., Ltd., Tokyo, Japan).

2.3. Test Method and Cases. Sixteen dogs diagnosed with CAD were distributed into two groups randomly. In group I, four of the eight dogs had positive reactions to house dust mite mix (*Dermatophagoides farinae and D. pteronyssinus*) and the other four showed no reactions to intradermal test and were diagnosed as having atopic like dermatitis. In group II, five dogs had positive reactions to house dust mite mix and the other three were diagnosed with atopic like dermatitis. Owners were instructed to apply to the dog two pumps of HCA spray per 100 cm^2 of affected skin. HCA spray was mainly applied to axilla and inguina, not to the face. They were instructed not to spray more than 1/3 of the whole body. The clinical evaluation and blood tests were performed on day 0 and day 21. Owners of dogs in group I sprayed HCA on the affected skin once a day for three weeks. Owners of dogs in group II sprayed HCA on the affected skin (all owners use a 7-day cycle of 3 days of spray plus 4 days of no spray, for a total of 3 weeks). Owners were instructed to apply the spray once daily to affected skin only from 10 cm away at a dose rate of two sprays per 100 cm^2 of affected skin [8].

2.4. CADESI-03: Canine Atopic Dermatitis Extent and Severity Index. CADESI-03 was used to assess lesion severity. The severity of erythema, lichenification, excoriations, and alopecia was assessed at 62 body sites using a scale from 0–5 (0 = none, 1 = mild, 2-3 = moderate, and 4-5 = severe) [12]. The same investigator performed all assessments on open labelled study.

2.5. Blood Biochemical Test. Blood sample was collected from the jugular vein, and the peripheral blood was used for each inspection. The following inspection was performed before and after use of HCA.

2.5.1. Cortisol Level by the ACTH Stimulation Examination. Cortrosyn (tetracosactide acetate, 0.25 mg/2 mL, Daiichi Sankyo, Tokyo) 5 ug/kg was injected intravenously [13]. The serum was collected before and 1 hour after injection; cortisol level was measured using fluorescence polarization immunoassay (the CLEIA method) in commercial laboratory (Doubutu kensa, Osaka).

2.5.2. Blood Immunologic Test (CCR4⁺ CD4⁺ Lymphocytes: CCR4⁺ Cells in Peripheral CD4⁺ T-Lymphocytes). A sample of peripheral blood was collected in EDTA before and after use of HCA. The sample was saved by refrigeration and transported to a commercial laboratory (Animal Allergy Clinical Laboratories, Inc., Kanagawa). The CCR4⁺ CD4⁺ T lymphocytes were detected by flow cytometry following methods previously reported [14, 15].

2.6. Statistical Analysis (Wilcoxon Signed-Rank Test). Statistical analysis was performed by paired *t*-tests and Wilcoxon signed-rank test. Statistical significance was defined as $P < 0.05$.

3. Results

3.1. CADESI-03: Canine Atopic Dermatitis Extent and Severity Index. In group I, the mean and SD of the total CADESI-03 score before and after the use of HCA was 294.8 ± 175.0 and 208.8 ± 138.4, respectively. A total score rate of decrease was 29.2%, and it was significantly different after use of HCA ($P < 0.01$). In group II, the mean and SD of the total CADESI-03 score before and after the use of HCA was 393.3 ± 171.4 and 335.4 ± 157.0, respectively. A total score rate of decrease was 14.8%, and it was significantly different after use of HCA ($P < 0.01$). Even though, CADESI-03 scores of group I and II are different, both groups showed decrease in the score which were significantly different. It represents the efficacy of HCA on both treatment methods.

3.2. Cortisol Level by the ACTH Stimulation Examination. In group I, prior to the use of HCA, the mean and SD of the cortisol levels were $3.7 \pm 2.4 \mu g/dL$ (standard range 1.0–7.7 $\mu g/dL$) pre-ACTH and $13.9 \pm 4.3 \mu g/dL$ (standard range 1.0–18.0 $\mu g/dL$) post-ACTH, Figure 1. The mean and SD of cortisol levels after use of HCA were $1.4 \pm 1.2 \mu g/dL$ pre-ACTH and $8.9 \pm 3.6 \mu g/dL$ post-ACTH, Figure 2.

In group II, the mean and SD of cortisol levels after use of HCA were $2.8 \pm 1.7 \mu g/dL$ pre-ACTH and $13.6 \pm 3.0 \mu g/dL$ post-ACTH, Figure 3.

In group I, the decrease in cortisol levels post-ACTH before and after use of HCA was 36.0% and showed significant difference ($P < 0.01$). The post-ACTH cortisol level before use of HCA in group I and the postcortisol level after use of HCA in group II showed no significant difference ($P > 0.05$). From these results, limitation use of the spray might recover the postcortisol value of after use of the spray.

3.3. Blood Immunologic Test (CCR4⁺ CD4⁺ Lymphocytes: CCR4⁺ Cells in Peripheral CD4⁺ T-Lymphocytes). In group I, the mean and SD of CCR4⁺ CD4⁺ lymphocytes percentage before the use of HCA was $37.8 \pm 10.8\%$. After the use of the spray the percentage was $39.6 \pm 14.4\%$, Figure 4. CCR4⁺ CD4⁺ lymphocytes percentage did not fall below 28.7%, a cut-off level [15]. The CCR4⁺ CD4⁺ lymphocytes percentage before and after use of HCA did not show significant difference ($P > 0.05$).

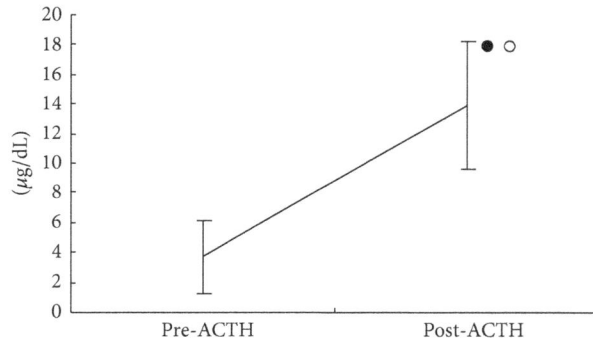

● Postcortisol level mean after use of HCA spray in group I, statistically significant difference ($P < 0.01$)

○ Postcortisol level mean after use of HCA spray in groups I and II, no statistically significant difference ($P > 0.05$). A decrease in the suppression of post-ACTH cortisol level was confirmed in group II. A decrease in CADESI-03 is confirmed in groups I and II

FIGURE 1: Three weeks use of HCA spray on dogs with CAD, group I ($n = 8$), cortisol level of pre-ACTH and post-ACTH before use of HCA spray, pre-ACTH cortisol level mean ± SD; 3.7 ± 2.4 μg/dL and post-ACTH cortisol level mean ± SD; 13.9 ± 4.3 μg/dL.

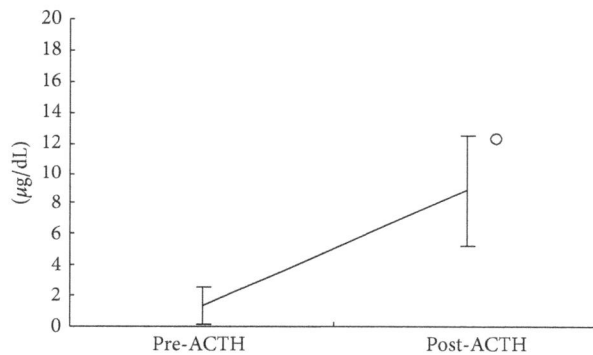

● Postcortisol level mean after use of HCA spray in group I, statistically significant difference ($P < 0.01$)

○ Postcortisol level mean after use of HCA spray in groups I and II, no statistically significant difference ($P > 0.05$). A decrease in the suppression of post-ACTH cortisol level was confirmed in group II. A decrease in CADESI-03 is confirmed in groups I and II

FIGURE 3: Group II ($n = 8$), cortisol level pre-ACTH and post-ACTH after use of HCA spray for 21 days (use days-limited cases), pre-ACTH cortisol level mean ± SD; 2.8 ± 1.7 μg/dL and post-ACTH cortisol level mean ± SD; 13.6 ± 3.0 μg/dL.

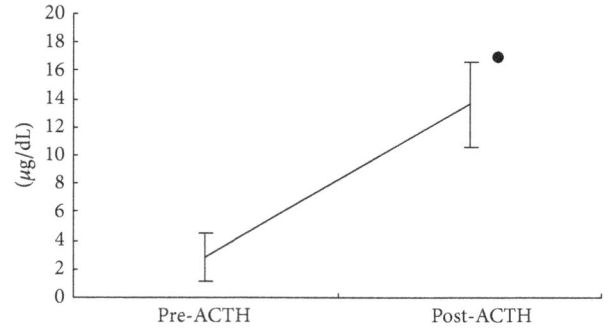

● Postcortisol level mean after use of HCA spray in group I, statistically significant difference ($P < 0.01$)

○ Postcortisol level mean after use of HCA spray in groups I and II, no statistically significant difference ($P > 0.05$). A decrease in the suppression of post-ACTH cortisol level was confirmed in group II. A decrease in CADESI-03 is confirmed in groups I and II

FIGURE 2: Group I ($n = 8$), cortisol level pre-ACTH and post-ACTH after use of HCA spray for 21 days, pre-ACTH cortisol level mean ± SD; 1.4 ± 1.2 μg/dL and post-ACTH cortisol level mean ± SD; 8.9 ± 3.6 μg/dL.

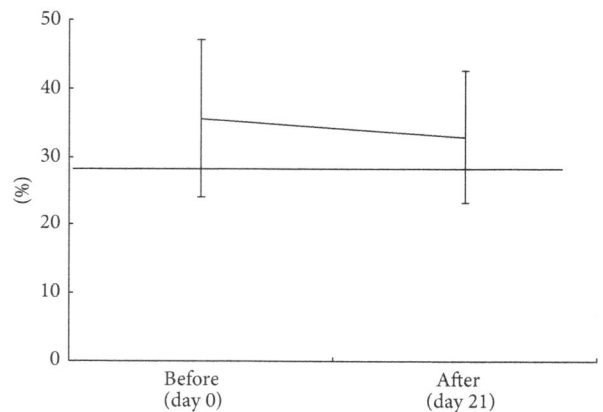

FIGURE 4: Three weeks use of HCA spray on dogs with CAD, $CCR4^+CD4^+$ lymphocytes percentage before and after use of HCA spray for 21 days, before (day 0) $CCR4^+CD4^+$ mean ± SD; 37.8 ± 10.8% and after (day 21) $CCR4^+CD4^+$ mean ± SD; 39.6 ± 14.4%. Statistically no significant difference was found ($P > 0.05$), Crossbar; <28.7 cut-off value.

show a difference in the percent decrease but the reason was unclear.

One report of the use HCA described the skin atrophy as an adverse effect [9]. In the report of Bizikova and others, they confirm mild skin atrophy to be visible in eight of ten dogs in the axillary and inguinal region at the end of the second week of the spray application [9]. Such reduction in dermal thickness was associated with atrophy of dermal collagen and partial atrophy of adnexa with decreased numbers of hair follicles in the anagen phase of the hair cycle. Hair loss was identified in one dog out of the 16 dogs treated. Atrophy was not observed in the report of Nutall and others. It is inspected

4. Discussion

After 21 days of HCA use, the total score of CADESI-03 decreased by 29.2% in group I and 14.8% in group II. Dogs in both groups showed significant difference after use of the spray. It represents an effectiveness of HCA which resembles a result in the report of Nutall and others [10], which showed 57.1% decrease in the CADESI-03 on day 28. Our results that the effect of HCA is equal to oral cyclosporine [10]. The advantage of the use of HCA in comparison to the use of oral or parenteral steroids may avoid some systemic adverse effect suppression of the hypothalamic-pituitary-adrenal axis [4, 5] which can be seen occasionally with the administration of systemic steroids. In the report of Bizikova and others [9], the HCA suppressed histamine related intradermal test reactivity distal to the site of application seven days after use of HCA once daily. These data suggest HCA might be absorbed systemically from the skin surface causing anti-inflammatory effect on other remote nontreated regions. Another hypothesis is that the dog might lick sprayed region creating systemic administration which would cause anti-inflammatory effect on the other side of the skin. It was very unique, and this report was the study that understood enough the characteristic of this drug, but it was supplemented by the lack of data. Therefore, in this study, blood cortisol level and CCR4$^+$ CD4$^+$ lymphocytes percentage were measured to make up for these lacks. This study showed 36.0% decrease in postcortisol value compared with before and after use of HCA and it showed significant difference (<0.01). On the other hand, CCR4$^+$ CD4$^+$ lymphocytes percentage did not move and showed no effect to it. These results suggest weak suppression of the hypothalamus pituitary gland; adrenal gland axis might be caused by use of HCA. These data support the first hypothesis of Bizikova and others, which is that HCA might be absorbed from the treated skin with activity and it can be said that there was not enough degradation of HCA. However, influence was in the tolerated level, and it can be avoided by limited use of the spray. And there was little influence of the recurrence of the clinical score even if it reduce the frequency of use.

Comparing with the result of past study, use of the HCA showed little influence than other dosage routes [16–20]. For example, the injection of the steroid dosage, oral, showed more suppression to cortisol than that of the spray. In this study, it showed no influence on peripheral blood CCR4$^+$ CD4$^+$ lymphocytes percentage in group I.

Because a Langerhans cell present antigen to a T-cell in the skin epidermis, these T-cells migrate the main route of the expose to the live body of the sensitization antigen of the CAD to lesion skin. In other words peripheral blood CCR4$^+$ CD4$^+$ lymphocytes percentage detects the migration degree of these T-cells and it can also judge the allergic strength of the live body or an immunoreactive state [13, 14]. There was no significant difference in CCR4$^+$ CD4$^+$ lymphocytes percentage before and after the use of HCA in this study. It meant that HCA shows extremely little influence to systemic immunoreaction. The Bizikova and others [9] also performed skin biopsy 24 hours after intradermal test challenge, and intraepidermal histologic measurement of the treatment side showed reduction in the total leukocyte, eosinophile, and CD3$^+$ lymphocytes. From two studies, HCA spray infiltrated very small amount systemically, but the main area of the effect is limited to the skin epidermis and restrained inflammation and the cell-mediated immunity in that part, so the influence on systemic immunoreaction might be extremely little.

5. Conclusion

HCA spray is a promising next generation anti-inflammatory steroidal therapeutic drug. The use of HCA spray should be compared with other steroid ointments and sprays. It is thought that the use of HCA spray is likely to help the transition from the use of an oral steroid, helping to minimize the development of iatrogenic Cushing disease.

Conflict of Interests

The study was financed by Virbac, Japan, which had no influence on the study design or on data evaluation.

References

[1] T. Olivry, D. J. DeBoer, C. Favrot et al., "Treatment of canine atopic dermatitis: 2010 clinical practice guidelines from the International Task Force on Canine Atopic Dermatitis," *Veterinary Dermatology*, vol. 21, no. 3, pp. 233–248, 2010.

[2] J. C. Angus, "Canine pruritus-practical guide to management," in *Proceedings of the North American Veterinary Conference-Small Animal and Exotics*, pp. 351–354, 2008.

[3] M. Nakamura, Y. Kawamura, M. Minegishi, Y. Momoi, and T. Iwasaki, "Hypercalcemia in a dog with resolution of iatrogenic Cushing's syndrome," *Journal of Veterinary Medical Science*, vol. 66, no. 3, pp. 329–331, 2004.

[4] H. B. Ridgway and K. A. Moriello, "Iatrogenic Cushing's syndrome in a dog from owner's topical corticosteroid," *Archives of Dermatology*, vol. 129, no. 3, article 379, 1993.

[5] N. Komiyama, S. Tsumagari, S. Ohba, K. Takagi, S. Satoh, and M. Takeishi, "Hypophyseal-adrenocortical function in experimental iatrogenic canine Cushing's syndrome," *The Journal of Veterinary Medical Science*, vol. 53, no. 2, pp. 351–353, 1991.

[6] B. Brazzini and N. Pimpinelli, "New and established topical corticosteroids in dermatology: clinical pharmacology and therapeutic use," *American Journal of Clinical Dermatology*, vol. 3, no. 1, pp. 47–58, 2002.

[7] C. Schackert, H. C. Korting, and M. Schäfer-Korting, "Qualitative and quantitative assessment of the benefit-risk ratio of medium potency topical corticosteroids in vitro and in vivo: characterisation of drugs with an increased benefit-risk ratio," *BioDrugs*, vol. 13, no. 4, pp. 267–277, 2000.

[8] T. Nuttall, R. Mueller, E. Bensignor et al., "Efficacy of a 0.0584% hydrocortisone aceponate spray in the management of canine atopic dermatitis: a randomised, double blind, placebo-controlled trial," *Veterinary Dermatology*, vol. 20, no. 3, pp. 191–198, 2009.

[9] P. Bizikova, K. E. Linder, J. Paps, and T. Olivry, "Effect of a novel topical diester glucocorticoid spray on immediate- and late-phase cutaneous allergic reactions in Maltese-beagle atopic dogs: a placebo-controlled study," *Veterinary Dermatology*, vol. 21, no. 1, pp. 70–79, 2010.

[10] T. J. Nuttall, N. A. McEwan, E. Bensignor, L. Cornegliani, C. Löwenstein, and C. A. Rème, " Comparable efficacy of a topical 0.0584% hydrocortisone aceponate spray and oral ciclosporin in treating canine atopic dermatitis," *Veterinary Dermatology*, vol. 20, no. 3, pp. 191–198, 2009.

[11] C. Favrot, J. Steffan, W. Seewald, and F. Picco, "A prospective study on the clinical features of chronic canine atopic dermatitis

and its diagnosis," *Veterinary Dermatology*, vol. 21, no. 1, pp. 23–31, 2010.

[12] T. Olivry, R. Marsella, T. Iwasaki et al., "Validation of CADESI-03, a severity scale for clinical trials enrolling dogs with atopic dermatitis," *Veterinary Dermatology*, vol. 18, no. 2, pp. 78–86, 2007.

[13] E. C. Feldman and R. W. Nelson, *Canine and Feline Endocrinology and Reproduction*, Saunders, Philadelphia, Pa, USA, 3rd edition, 2003.

[14] S. Maeda, K. Ohmori, N. Yasuda et al., "Increase of CC chemokine receptor 4-positive cells in the peripheral CD4$^+$ cells in dogs with atopic dermatitis or experimentally sensitized to Japanese cedar pollen," *Clinical & Experimental Allergy*, vol. 34, no. 9, pp. 1467–1473, 2004.

[15] N. Yasuda, K. Masuda, and S. Maeda, "CC chemokine receptor 4-positive CD4$^+$ lymphocytes in peripheral blood increases during maturation in healthy beagles," *Journal of Veterinary Medical Science*, vol. 70, no. 9, pp. 989–992, 2008.

[16] C. B. Chastain and C. L. Graham, "Adrenocortical suppression in dogs on daily and alternate day prednisone administration," *American Journal of Veterinary Research*, vol. 40, no. 7, pp. 936–941, 1979.

[17] G. E. Moore and M. Hoenig, "Duration of pituitary and adrenocortical suppression after long-term administration of anti-inflammatory doses of prednisone in dogs," *American Journal of Veterinary Research*, vol. 53, no. 5, pp. 716–720, 1992.

[18] R. J. Kemppainen, M. D. Lorenz, and F. N. Thompson, "Adrenocortical suppression in the dog given a single intramuscular dose of prednisone or triamcinolone acetonide," *The American Journal of Veterinary Research*, vol. 43, no. 2, pp. 204–206, 1982.

[19] C. J. Reeder, C. E. Griffin, N. L. Polissar, B. Neradilek, and R. D. Armstrong, "Comparative adrenocortical suppression in dogs with otitis externa following topical otic administration of four different glucocorticoid-containing medications," *Veterinary Therapeutics*, vol. 9, no. 2, pp. 111–121, 2008.

[20] R. D. Zenoble and R. J. Kemppainen, "Adrenocortical suppression by topically applied corticosteroids in healthy dogs," *Journal of the American Veterinary Medical Association*, vol. 191, no. 6, pp. 685–688, 1987.

7

Subcutaneous Implants of Buprenorphine-Cholesterol-Triglyceride Powder in Mice

L. DeTolla,[1] R. Sanchez,[2] E. Khan,[2] B. Tyler,[3] and M. Guarnieri[3]

[1] Departments of Pathology, Medicine, Epidemiology and Public Health and the Program of Comparative Medicine,
School of Medicine, University of Maryland, Baltimore, MD, USA
[2] Program of Comparative Medicine, School of Medicine, University of Maryland, Baltimore, MD, USA
[3] Johns Hopkins School of Medicine Department of Neurological Surgery, 1550 Orleans Street CRB-264, Baltimore, MD 21231, USA

Correspondence should be addressed to M. Guarnieri; mguarnieri@comcast.net

Academic Editor: Vito Laudadio

Subcutaneous drug implants are convenient systems for the long-term delivery of drugs in animals. Lipid carriers are logical tools because they generally allow for higher doses and low toxicity. The present study used an US Food and Drug Administration Target Animal Safety test system to evaluate the safety of a subcutaneous implant of a cholesterol-triglyceride-buprenorphine powder in 120 BALB/c mice. Mice were evaluated in 4- and 12-day trials with 1- and 5-fold doses of the intended 3 mg/kg dose of drug. One male mouse treated with three 3 mg/kg doses and surgery on days 0, 4, and 8 died on day 9. The cause of death was not determined. In the surviving 119 mice there was no evidence of skin reaction at the site of the implant. Compared to control animals treated with saline, weight measurements, clinical pathology, histopathology, and clinical observations were unremarkable. These results demonstrate that the lipid carrier is substantially safe. Cholesterol-triglyceride-drug powders may provide a valuable research tool for studies of analgesic and inflammatory drug implants in veterinary medicine.

1. Introduction

Guidelines for the care and use of laboratory animals uniformly recommend the use of analgesia in any procedure with a potential for pain [1]. Yet, the use of analgesics in research remains low [2, 3]. One factor that may account for the modest utilization of analgesia is the management challenge involved with intraperitoneal (IP) and subcutaneous (SC) injections of mice and rats at the 6–8-hour intervals necessary to maintain effective blood concentrations of drug [4]. In addition, it has been considered that repeated IP or SC injections in surgically traumatized rodents may induce stress responses and depress weight gain [5, 6]. Several strategies are being investigated to address this problem.

The practicality and duration of slow-release oral preparations for 11-hour morphine therapy in laboratory rats have been described [7]. Food- and water-based analgesia has been explored by several investigators [8–10]. Grant and colleagues demonstrated that liposomal morphine implants

could deliver long-acting analgesia to mice [11]. More recently, Smith, Krugner-Higby, and colleagues have published a series of studies demonstrating the 2-3-day activity of lipid encapsulated morphine derivatives in laboratory animal models of pain [12–14]. Foley and colleagues described the 2-3-day efficacy of a proprietary sustained release polymer-based buprenorphine preparation in rats [15]. Carbone and coworkers described the efficacy of a similar formulation in two strains of mice [16].

In 2006, our laboratory began to investigate extended release opiate preparations for pain therapy in rodent brain and spine tumor models. We selected buprenorphine as a model drug because of the range of evidence for its safety and efficacy in laboratory medicine [17, 18]. Reports of morbidity and mortality in animal studies have been rare. Buprenorphine has a wide therapeutic index in animals. Compared to morphine, the mean effective dose (ED50) is 20-fold lower and the mean lethal dose (LD50) is significantly higher [19, 20].

Toxicity reports associated with SC cholesterol implants are rare. Lipid encapsulation generally has allowed for higher doses, decreased toxicity, and prolonged activity of opiate therapy [21, 22]. We studied a cholesterol-triglyceride-buprenorphine SC delivery system described by Pontani and Misra [23]. In a separate 4-month observational study Misra and Pontani provided initial evidence that the delivery system was safe in rats. They observed no evidence of inflammation or edema in rats implanted with 50 mg lipid-drug pellets [24].

To further validate the safety of lipid encapsulated buprenorphine, we consulted the Center for Veterinary Medicine (CVM) at the US Food and Drug Administration regarding the necessary methods for establishing the safety of new veterinary drugs. The CVM provides target animal safety (TAS) guidelines for evaluating drug toxicity in target animals [25]. Similar guidelines are used by European regulatory authorities [26]. We developed a TAS protocol including clinical observations, blood chemistry, hematology, and histopathology studies to examine the safety of a long-acting cholesterol-triglyceride-buprenorphine preparation in surgically treated mice. Studies in our laboratories have shown that the dissolution of SC cholesterol pellets depends on the location of the implant and excipients used to make the pellet [27]. We therefore examined the safety of the cholesterol-triglyceride-buprenorphine unpelleted drug powder in a SC space.

The present report describes body weight, hematology, clinical pathology, histopathology, and cage side observation measurements collected in this TAS study. These results provide additional evidence for the safety of cholesterol-based drug implants and for the safety of extended-release buprenorphine analgesia in mice.

2. Materials and Methods

2.1. Animals. TAS studies were approved by the University of Maryland Medical School Institutional Animal Care and Use Committee (IACUC). The University of Maryland, Program of Comparative Medicine, Baltimore, MD, was used for the safety study. Pharmacokinetic studies of serially collected blood samples were conducted at the Johns Hopkins University School of Medicine under a protocol approved by the Johns Hopkins IACUC. Male and female BALB/c (6–8 weeks old weighing 20–22 g) were obtained from Charles River Laboratories (Wilmington MA). The mice were inspected for general health conditions before being housed at a density of 4-5 mice per cage in 750 Lab Product cages (Lab Product, Seaford, DE) with 7087 Soft Cob bedding (Harlan, Madison, WI) and allowed free access to 2018 Teklad Irradiated Global Rodent Diet chow (Harlan, Madison, WI) and Baltimore City water. A total of 120 mice were used in the safety study. A total of 18 mice were used for pharmacokinetic study of buprenorphine blood concentrations.

2.2. Study Design. The study design was based on Target Animal Safety (TAS) protocol guidance to determine the safety of a generic drug [28]. The bioequivalent target range was selected from published reports demonstrating that buprenorphine blood levels greater than 0.5 ng/mL produce positive tail-flick responses in mice [29], thermal latency in dogs [30], and responses in human volunteers [31]. In a series of dose-finding studies, male and female mice were injected with increasing doses of the drug powder containing up to 25 mg/kg buprenorphine. A dose of 3 mg/kg, which afforded blood levels of more than 1 ng buprenorphine/mL for at least 2 days, was selected for the TAS study.

For the pharmacokinetic studies, mice were housed three per cage and cages were changed daily. During the TAS studies, mice were housed one per cage. The experimental unit was the cage for statistical purposes. Safety studies were conducted with 1- and 5-fold excesses of the intended dose. The study period was 4 days, 1 day more than the 3-day elimination period. Ten male and ten female mice per group were used in the first TAS study comparing a 0x (control), 1x, and 5x dose (15 mg/kg) challenge. Ten male and ten female mice per group were used in the second TAS study comparing 0x, 1x, and 5x doses repeated at three 4-day intervals. By agreement with the CVM, the control was 3 to 15 microliters of saline. Parameters evaluated in the 4- and 12-day trials included body weight, hematology, clinical chemistry, clinical observations, and gross and histopathology. According to the trial protocol, if no differences were observed in outcome measurements from animals in the control and 5x dose groups, tissues from animals in the 1x dose groups would not be further evaluated. The hypothesis tested was that the data for these parameters would be different in mice with 0x and 5x doses of cholesterol-buprenorphine drug powder.

2.3. Trial Structure

2.3.1. Single 0, 1, and 5x Dose, 4-Day Trial. In the 4-day trial, 10 mice per group of each sex were anesthetized, subjected to a surgical procedure, and dosed on day 0 with a single control, 1x, 5x dose (15 mg/kg) of drug powder or 15 uL of saline.

2.3.2. Repeat, Three 0, 1, and 5x Doses, 12-Day Trial. In the 12-day dose-repeat trial, 10 mice per group of each sex were anesthetized, subjected to a surgical procedure, and dosed with a 1x and 5x dose (15 mg/kg) of drug or 15 uL of saline on days 0, 4, and 8.

Cages were changed daily to prevent the animals from redosing by coprophagy. Mice in the single dose and repeat dose trials were evaluated by daily clinical observations for signs of distress. At the midpoint of the two trials, day 2 or day 6, half of the mice were weighed, euthanized, and then exsanguinated to collect blood for hematology and clinical chemistry. At the endpoint of each trial, day 4 of day 12, the remaining mice were euthanized to measure body weight, hematology, clinical chemistries, and histopathology.

2.4. Test Article Details. The cholesterol-buprenorphine drug powder was supplied by Animalgesic Laboratories Inc. (Millersville, MD). The drug powder contained USP (United States Pharmacopeia) grade buprenorphine HCl (Noramco, Wilmington, DE), cholesterol, and glycerol tristearate, (Sigma, St. Louis, MO). Drug preparations were verified for purity and content by AAI Pharma (Wilmington, NC).

2.5. Drug Delivery. Dental pipets were used to deliver 3 mg aliquots of drug powder into a dorsal subcutaneous space created by a surgical procedure (described below). The drug powder was loaded into disposable 30 mm long capped dental pipets by Ora Tech (Riverton UT). The drug-filled pipets were fitted with a nylon plunger to secure the powder prior to injection in the mouse (Figure 1). At the time of surgery, the pipet cap was aseptically removed and the tip of the dental pipet was inserted into the SC space. The nylon plunger was depressed to deposit the powder into the SC space. Five drug loaded pipets were used for the 5x dose groups. To allow for histopathology evaluation of the skin at the implant site, the pipet tips were placed approximately 10 mm under the skin away from the surgical incision.

2.6. Buprenorphine Blood Level Measurements. Serial blood samples were obtained by facial bleeding of the superficial temporal vein [32]. Samples were taken at noon, 23–25-hour intervals after the drug was implanted. Plasma samples were used for buprenorphine measurements by ELISA. Samples of 5–20 μL of plasma were analyzed in triplicate using a Buprenorphine One-step ELISA kit (International Diagnostic Systems, St. Joseph, MI). The manufacturer validated the kit for clinical drug studies with high-performance liquid chromatography-electrospray mass spectrometry (HPLC-ES-MS) procedure. All known cross-reactivities are reported by the manufacturer at <0.06%, with the exception of nor-buprenorphine, which cross-reacts at 1.1%. Standards curves were prepared with five buprenorphine solutions: 0, 0.01, 0.05, 0.1, 0.5, and 1.0 ng/20 μL. Absorbance was recorded at 450 nm (reference wavelength: 650 nm) using a Perkin Elmer Victor3 model 1420 microplate reader with Wallac 1420 data manager software.

2.7. Surgical Procedure. The surgical procedure used was based on the procedure used to implant Alzet miniosmotic pumps in mice and rats. A video of the procedure, which is briefly described below, is available at the Alzet website [33].

Each mouse was weighed prior to surgery to record baseline weights. Anesthesia was provided with isoflurane. Mice were induced with 4% isoflurane (Vetone, Boise, ID) inhalant anesthesia until deep sedation was established and then reduced to 2.5–3% dose of isoflurane maintenance. Approximately 1 cm square of mid dorsal skin was shaved and aseptically prepared by three alternating scrubs of betadine scrub and 70% isopropyl alcohol. Each mouse was transferred to a procedural table that was covered with a sterile table drape that is fluid resistant. The mouse was draped with sterile quarter drapes to outline the surgical approach site. Using sterile instruments, forceps (McCullough forceps, cross serrated jaws, 1.5 mm tip) were used to lift the aseptic skin from the lumbosacral region (dorsal aspect) and a pair of scissors (delicate operating scissors, straight, sharp-sharp, and 30 mm blade length) was used to make a 4-5 mm incision through the skin only. Bleeding, if any, was controlled with

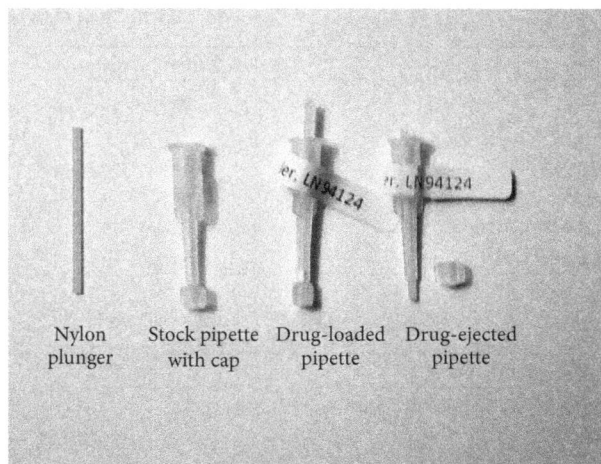

FIGURE 1: Pipets for drug powder delivery.

sterile gauze and light pressure. Keeping skin lifted with the forceps, a sterile pair of forceps (Halstead mosquito, straight) was used to separate the skin from the underlying muscular layer and to create approximately a 2 × 4 cm subcutaneous pocket. Using aseptic surgical techniques, the test article (1x, 5x drug powder, or saline) was injected into the lumbosacral region (dorsal aspect). The skin was then apposed using 5–0, reverse cutting, coated Vicryl sutures (Ethicon). After surgery was completed, the isoflurane was turned off and the animal was continuously monitored by the surgeon or veterinary technician until the animal's reflexes (monitored by toe pinch) returned.

All mice in the study were treated to this surgical procedure.

2.8. Clinical Observations. Cage conditions, motor activity, ocular findings, and the appearance of the fur were observed twice daily at about 10 am and 5 pm by a research staff. Observation forms were designed for the entry of "yes/no" scores and numerical grading of signs and symptoms including respiration, tremors, motor activity, ocular findings, nasal findings, and appearance in the morning observation period. The pm observations included ocular signs, motor activity, signs of distress, and appearance. The surgical site was observed for signs of bleeding, erythema, edema, and signs of infection: pus. Space was available for comments. The same forms were used for both TAS studies: the single 5x dose 4-day observation period and the three repeated 5x doses 12-day observation period.

2.9. Clinical Laboratory Tests. Blood chemistry, hematology, and histopathology were performed at the Johns Hopkins Phenotyping Core [34]. Hematology tests were performed on a Hemavet 950 Hematology System (Drew Scientific, Waterbury, CT). Values obtained included white blood cell, neutrophil, lymphocyte, monocyte, eosinophil, basophile, red blood cell, and platelet counts and hemoglobin concentration, hematocrit, mean corpuscular volume, mean corpuscular hemoglobin, mean corpuscular hemoglobin

TABLE 1: Summary of experimental design: histopathology phase.

Test or control article	Total weight administered	Number of doses	Days on test	Number of animals
Saline	0.005 mL	1	4	5♂, 5♀
Long acting drug powder	3 mg	1	4	5♂, 5♀
Long acting drug powder	15 mg	1	4	5♂, 5♀
Saline	0.015 mL	3	12	5♂, 5♀
Long acting drug powder	9 mg	3	12	5♂, 5♀
Long acting drug powder	45 mg	3	12	5♂, 5♀

TABLE 2: Tissues evaluated by microscopy.

Adrenal gland	Large intestine, colon	Small intestine, jejunum
Bone with bone marrow, femur	Liver	Small intestine, ileum
	Lung	Spinal cord with spine
Brain (cerebrum, midbrain, cerebellum, and medulla/pons)	Lymph nodes[a]	Spleen
Epididymis (males)	Mammary glands (females)	Stomach
Eyes (with optic Nerves)	Ovaries (females)	Ventral skin
Gall bladder	Pancreas	Dorsal skin surrounding implant(s)
Heart	Parathyroid gland	Testis (males)
Kidneys	Skeletal muscle, biceps femoris	Thyroid (with parathyroid)[b]
Large Intestine, cecum	Small intestine, duodenum	Urinary bladder

[a]Lymph nodes included submandibular superficial cervical collected with salivary glands from the neck; mesenteric and pancreaticoduodenal collected with mesentery and pancreas.
[b]Parathyroid glands were evaluated when present in the plane of section of the thyroid gland.

concentration, red cell distribution width, and mean platelet volume. A VetACE Clinical Chemistry system (AlfaWassermann, West Caldwell NJ) was used to measure blood chemistry profiles: cholesterol (Chol), triglycerides (Tri), uric acid (UA), total bilirubin (TBill), glucose (Glu), total protein (Tpr), calcium (Ca), urea nitrogen (BUN), creatinine (Creat), albumin (Alb), high density lipoproteins (HDL), direct bilirubin (DBill) and the enzymes creatine kinase (CK), lactic dehydrogenase (LDH), alkaline phosphatase (ALP), amylase (Amy), gamma glutamyl transferase (GGT), alanine amino transferase (ALT), and aspartate amino transferase (ASP).

2.10. Euthanasia. Mice were weighed and then asphyxiated with carbon dioxide followed by 1 min lack of respiration. The heart was exposed. Mice were exsanguinated via cardiac puncture to obtain approximately 0.8 mL of blood for hematology and clinical chemistry testing. Mice were then placed in 10% neutral buffered formalin.

2.11. Body Weights. Mice were weighed in procedure rooms with a calibrated Sartorius Acculab Precision Scale (Goetting, Germany) before they were assigned to a treatment group and within 24 hours before they were injected with one or more doses of drug powder or control suspensions on day 0. Mice scheduled for euthanasia weighed on an electronic Ohaus microbalance (Parsippany, NJ) then euthanized with carbon dioxide.

2.12. Histopathology. Histopathology was performed on endpoint mice listed in Table 1. These were 30 mice in the 4-day

single dose and control challenges and 30 mice in the 12-day repeat dose challenges. Heart, kidneys, liver, and spleen were collected. More than 30 tissues were examined for a total of 13 slides per mouse. The tissue list is summarized in Table 2.

One male mouse in the 12-day repeat 9 mg/kg dose trial found dead on day 10 was not perfused. Because of extensive tissue autolysis and postmortem rigor, necropsy was not indicated. In the remaining mice after fixation and trimming, the tissues were processed, embedded in paraffin, sectioned, mounted on glass slides, and stained with hematoxylin and eosin (H&E). These slides were evaluated by light microscopy. Tissues listed in Table 2 were evaluated.

2.13. Statistics. Analyses of treatment group blood levels were made using GraphPad Prism Software Version 5.04 (La Jolla CA). Microsoft Excel v2007 was used to generate average and standard deviation (St Dev) data of hematology and clinical chemistry values.

3. Results

3.1. Blood Concentrations of Drug. As shown in Table 3, plasma concentrations of buprenorphine in mice given 3 mg/kg (1x) dose of drug averaged 45 ng/mL 6 hours after a SC drug powder implant. Approximately 2 and 6 ng of drug per mL plasma were present through day 3 in male and female mice, respectively. There was no detectable drug present by day 6 in either sex.

3.2. Clinical Observations. Approximately 3,300 clinical observation entries were recorded for the mice in the 4-day

TABLE 3: Buprenorphine drug concentrations in male and female Balb/c mice, 3 mg/kg dose of buprenorphine drug powder.

Day	Male ($n = 3$)		Female ($n = 3$)	
	Average ng/mL	St Dev	Average ng/mL	St Dev
0	0.0	0.0	0.0	0.0
0.25	45.2	0.5	44.9	3.7
1	42.9	6.6	41.6	3.7
2	20.8	5.8	27.2	3.2
3	2.1	2.1	5.8	3.2
4	0.0	0.0	2.8	3.4
6	0.0	0.0	0.0	0.0

TABLE 4: Weight change in male and female mice, 3 and 15 mg/kg dose of buprenorphine drug powder.

Day	Female mice ($n = 5$)			Male mice ($n = 5$)		
	Control	1x dose	5x dose	Control	1x dose	5x dose
	Avg ± St Dev	Avg ± St Dev	Avg ± St Dev	Avg ± St Dev	Avg ± St Dev	Avg ± St Dev
0	18.0 ± 0.5	17.9 ± 0.4	18.6 ± 0.7	21.3 ± 1.0	21.7 ± 0.9	19.3 ± 1.0
4	17.6 ± 0.8	16.6 ± 0.5	17.5 ± 0.5	21.4 ± 1.3	19.8 ± 2.3	18.6 ± 1.2

trial, and 9,900 entries were recorded for the mice in the 12-day trial. In the 4-day trial, 6 female and two male mice in the 1x dose group exhibited mild erythema and edema at the surgical site on day 1. These signs were not apparent on days two and three of the trial and were not seen in the subsequent 12-day trial. On average mice in the 5x dose groups showed slower movement compared to controls. They also showed more ocular findings of squinting and closed eyes. However, these movement and ocular findings did not reach statistical significance compared to controls.

One male mouse in the 12-day trial died one day following the third cycle of anesthesia, surgery, and 3 mg/kg drug powder. The carcass was not subject to necroscopy due to a clinical impression that advanced autolysis had set in. Previous observation including weight measurements provided no information to indicate distress.

3.3. Body Weight. In the 4-day TAS trial drug-treated female and male mice given a 3 mg/kg dose lost an average of 7% and 9% body weight by day 4, respectively. Weight losses were similar in the female and male mice given the 15 mg/kg dose, 6% and 4%, respectively. The weight losses were not significantly different from weight losses in the surgically treated control mice. Similar results were observed in the 12-day trial (Table 4).

3.4. Clinical Pathology. There were no differences between hematology and clinical chemistry blood values in the drug and control groups in the 4-day and the 12-day trials in the mice receiving the 1x or 5x doses of the drug powder.

3.5. Histopathology. The histopathology examination of the tissues from the male and female mice was unremarkable. The surgical sites appeared competent. There was no sign of infection. Because an effort was made to deposit the drug powder under the skin at least 10 mm away from the incision

site, it is possible to conclude that skin above the powder was normal. In the 12-day trials where mice were injected with three 5x doses of powder at 4-day intervals for a total of 45 mg of drug powder, residual drug powder was frequently observed. There was no edema or inflammation associated the thin powder layer.

4. Discussion

The present report describes the morbidity and mortality encountered in a TAS trial of a SC extended release cholesterol-triglyceride-buprenorphine powder. A sensitive and specific ELISA analysis demonstrated that a single 3 mg/kg dose of drug implanted at the time of surgery afforded average plasma concentrations of drug of 45 ng/mL in 6 hours and 20 ng/mL or more for two days (Table 3). These concentrations have been consistently associated with effective pain therapy in animal and humans studies [18] and specifically with the use of buprenorphine analgesic in mice [35]. In the present study, the high concentration of drug measured 6 hours after implant indicates that the lipid carrier system rapidly released the drug. This suggests that the analgesic effects of the drug may overlap the anesthetic recovery period. Whether there is a continuum of pain management should be determined by pharmacokinetic measurements at earlier postimplant times and with the use of different anesthetics.

Pain assessments are required in TAS studies of drug implants. It is generally considered that signs of severe pain can be readily detected by experienced laboratory animal scientists, but signs of mild to moderate pain and pain that breaks through analgesia can be difficult to detect [36]. The system for the visual assessment of pain used in the present work was similar to the scoring system used by Clark and colleagues to assess pain in mice treated with liposome encapsulated oxymorphone in mice [12]. We observed no signs of severe pain. The implant appeared to be well tolerated by the mice. One death occurred in the 3 mg/kg dose group at day 9 in a male mouse that had three cycles of anesthesia and surgery in 8 days. The cause of death was not determined. There was no evidence from the clinical pathology and histopathology evaluations of the remaining male and female mice in this dose group of toxicity from the drug implant.

Several recent reports indicate that visual assessment system used in the present study to monitor pain may be limited. Mouse grimace scores appear to be highly sensitive indicators of postsurgical pain [37, 38]. Adamson and coworkers demonstrated that mouse pain scores were low when an observer was in the room. Video recording of behavior during light and dark cycles showed mild yet significant differences [12]. A separate limitation of the present study for the detection of mild pain is that subtle signs of pain can be inferred in rodents in relation to their behavior toward normal cage-mates. However, TAS studies required single housing of animals.

Drug-polymer implants have been investigated for long-term analgesia [15, 31]. Biocompatible ethylene vinyl acetate copolymers can be designed to provide weeks to months of linear drug release [39]. These polymers are removed when empty and are not optimal for routine use in laboratory medicine. Biodegradable copolymers are designed for safe drug release and adsorption. However, drug release from these polymers can be anomalous [40]. Long-term inflammatory reactions have been observed [41]. Significant skin reactions have been reported in mice and rats treated with polymer-bound buprenorphine [15, 16]. In contrast, the biodegradable lipid carrier system used in this study showed no evidence of skin toxicity, even in studies that used three implants at fivefold the intended dose. Further research is needed to determine if the cholesterol carrier is biocompatible in other strains and species and whether the absence of dermal reactions can be confirmed in long-term histopathology studies.

Buprenorphine decreases intestinal motility [19]. Nausea is commonly observed in mice and rats treated with oral or parenteral buprenorphine therapy [42]. Several investigators reported that the nausea can induce pica in rats held on corncob or hardwood bedding [43, 44]. In other reports, with appropriate husbandry, the opiate-induced nausea appears to be mild and transient [45].

All mice treated with the buprenorphine cholesterol-triglyceride drug powder lost weight. Weight loss was not significant compared to controls, and mice appeared to return to baseline weights by day 4. More research is needed to determine if the weight loss is greater in adult mice with slower growth curves.

5. Conclusion

The compelling needs for improved veterinary drug products support further research on chronic release drug systems. Lipid-based delivery vehicles appear to be good candidates because they are safe and biodegradable [23]. The safety profile of the extended-release cholesterol-triglyceride-buprenorphine powder described in this report confirms

previous studies of long-acting preparations of micellar morphine in mice [11], liposome encapsulated oxymorphone in mice [12], and liposome-encapsulated oxymorphone in rats [13, 14]. Carbohydrate and polymer delivery systems also offer attractive candidates for further research. Regardless of the composition of the delivery system itself, one cannot assume that SC drug-bound delivery vehicles are safe. Target animal safety studies and long-term histopathology studies of the SC space are warranted for each drug-bound vehicle.

Disclosure

Animalgesic Labs modified and commercialized the powder described in this paper. The modified product is currently offered for sale as Animalgesics for Mice. M. Guarnieri holds a significant financial interest in Animalgesic Labs.

Conflict of Interests

The authors declare that there is no conflict of interests regarding the publication of this paper.

Acknowledgments

Funding for this research was supplied by The Maryland Biotechnology Center Biotechnology Development Awards, Maryland Industrial Partnerships (MIPS), and by Animalgesic Labs. M. Guarnieri owns a significant financial interest in Animalgesic Labs.

References

[1] Institute for Laboratory Animal Research, *Guide for the Care and Use of Laboratory Animals*, National Academy Press, Washington, DC, USA, 2011.

[2] T. W. Adamson, L. V. Kendall, S. Goss et al., "Assessment of carprofen and buprenorphine on recovery of mice after surgical removal of the mammary fat pad," *Journal of the American Association for Laboratory Animal Science*, vol. 49, no. 5, pp. 610–616, 2010.

[3] E. L. Stokes, P. A. Flecknell, and C. A. Richardson, "Reported analgesic and anaesthetic administration to rodents undergoing experimental surgical procedures," *Laboratory Animals*, vol. 43, no. 2, pp. 149–154, 2009.

[4] N. M. Gades, P. J. Danneman, S. K. Wixson, and E. A. Tolley, "The magnitude and duration of the analgesic effect of morphine, butorphanol , and buprenorphine in rats and mice," *Contemporary Topics in Laboratory Animal Science*, vol. 39, no. 2, pp. 8–13, 2000.

[5] A. Bomzon, "Are repeated doses of buprenorphine detrimental to postoperative recovery after laparotomy in rats?" *Comparative Medicine*, vol. 56, no. 2, pp. 114–118, 2006.

[6] M. W. H. Schaap, J. J. Uilenreef, M. D. Mitsogiannis, J. G. Van't Klooster, S. S. Arndt, and L. J. Hellebrekers, "Optimizing the dosing interval of buprenorphine in a multimodal postoperative analgesic strategy in the rat: minimizing side-effects without affecting weight gain and food intake," *Laboratory Animals*, vol. 46, no. 4, pp. 287–292, 2012.

[7] M. C. Leach, H. E. Bailey, A. L. Dickinson, J. V. Roughan, and P. A. Flecknell, "A preliminary investigation into the practicality

of use and duration of action of slow-release preparations of morphine and hydromorphone in laboratory rats," *Laboratory Animals*, vol. 44, no. 1, pp. 59–65, 2010.

[8] M. C. Leach, A. R. Forrester, and P. A. Flecknell, "Influence of preferred foodstuffs on the antinociceptive effects of orally administered buprenorphine in laboratory rats," *Laboratory Animals*, vol. 44, no. 1, pp. 54–58, 2010.

[9] O. Kalliokoski, K. R. Jacobsen, J. Hau, and K. S. P. Abelson, "Serum concentrations of buprenorphine after oral and parenteral administration in male mice," *Veterinary Journal*, vol. 187, no. 2, pp. 251–254, 2011.

[10] A. C. Thompson, M. B. Kristal, A. Sallaj, A. Acheson, L. B. Martin, and T. Martin, "Analgesic efficacy of orally administered buprenorphine in rats: methodologic considerations," *Comparative Medicine*, vol. 54, no. 3, pp. 293–300, 2004.

[11] G. J. Grant, K. Vermeulen, M. I. Zakowski, M. Stenner, H. Turndorf, and L. Langerman, "Prolonged analgesia and decreased toxicity with liposomal morphine in a mouse model," *Anesthesia & Analgesia*, vol. 79, no. 4, pp. 706–709, 1994.

[12] M. D. Clark, L. Krugner-Higby, L. J. Smith, T. D. Heath, K. L. Clark, and D. Olson, "Evaluation of liposome-encapsulated oxymorphone hydrochloride in mice after splenectomy," *Comparative Medicine*, vol. 54, no. 5, pp. 558–563, 2004.

[13] J. R. Schmidt, L. Krugner-Higby, T. D. Heath, R. Sullivan, and L. J. Smith, "Epidural administration of liposome-encapsulated hydromorphone provides extended analgesia in a rodent model of stifle arthritis," *Journal of the American Association for Laboratory Animal Science*, vol. 50, no. 4, pp. 507–512, 2011.

[14] L. J. Smith, J. R. Valenzuela, L. A. Krugner-Higby, C. Brown, and T. D. Heath, "A single dose of liposome-encapsulated hydromorphone provides extended analgesia in a rat model of neuropathic pain," *Comparative Medicine*, vol. 56, no. 6, pp. 487–492, 2006.

[15] P. L. Foley, H. Liang, and A. R. Crichlow, "Evaluation of a sustained-release formulation of buprenorphine for analgesia in rats," *Journal of the American Association for Laboratory Animal Science*, vol. 50, no. 2, pp. 198–204, 2011.

[16] E. T. Carbone, K. E. Lindstrom, S. Diep, and L. Carbone, "Duration of action of sustained-release buprenorphine in 2 strains of mice," *Journal of the American Association for Laboratory Animal Science: JAALAS*, vol. 51, no. 6, pp. 815–819, 2012.

[17] J. V. Roughan and P. A. Flecknell, "Buprenorphine: a reappraisal of its antinociceptive effects and therapeutic use in alleviating post-operative pain in animals," *Laboratory Animals*, vol. 36, no. 3, pp. 322–343, 2002.

[18] M. Guarnieri, C. Brayton, L. Detolla, N. Forbes-Mcbean, R. Sarabia-Estrada, and P. Zadnik, "Safety and efficacy of buprenorphine for analgesia in laboratory mice and rats," *Lab Animal*, vol. 41, no. 11, pp. 337–343, 2012.

[19] A. Cowan, J. C. Doxey, and E. J. R. Harry, "The animal pharmacology of buprenorphine, an oripavine analgesic agent," *British Journal of Pharmacology*, vol. 60, no. 4, pp. 547–554, 1977.

[20] A. Cowan, "Buprenorphine: the basic pharmacology revisited," *Journal of Addiction Medicine*, vol. 1, no. 2, pp. 68–72, 2007.

[21] C. R. Bethune, C. M. Bernards, T. Bui-Nguyen, D. D. Shen, and R. J. Y. Ho, "The role of drug-lipid interactions on the disposition of liposome-formulated opioid analgesics in vitro and in vivo," *Anesthesia and Analgesia*, vol. 93, no. 4, pp. 928–933, 2001.

[22] D. K. Mishra, V. Dhote, P. Bhatnagar, and P. K. Mishra, "Engineering solid lipid nanoparticles for improved drug delivery: promises and challenges of translational research," *Drug Delivery and Translational Research*, vol. 2, no. 4, pp. 238–253, 2012.

[23] R. B. Pontani and A. L. Misra, "A long-acting buprenorphine delivery system," *Pharmacology Biochemistry and Behavior*, vol. 18, no. 3, pp. 471–474, 1983.

[24] A. L. Misra and R. B. Pontani, "An improved long-acting delivery system for narcotic antagonists," *Journal of Pharmacy and Pharmacology*, vol. 30, no. 5, pp. 325–326, 1978.

[25] Guidance for Industry (GFI#61), "FDA Approval of Animal Drugs for Minor Uses and for Minor Species, Target Animal Safety and Effectiveness Protocol Development and Submission," May 2008, http://www.fda.gov/downloads/AnimalVeterinary/GuidanceComplianceEnforcement/GuidanceforIndustry/UCM241787.pdf.

[26] European Medicines Agency Veterinary Medicines and Inspections, "Guidelines of target animal safety for pharmaceuticals," VICH Topic GL43, European Medicines Agency Veterinary Medicines and Inspections, 2006.

[27] M. Guarnieri, B. Tyler, L. Detolla, M. Zhao, and B. Kobrin, "Subcutaneous implants for long-acting drug therapy in laboratory animals may generate unintended drug reservoirs," *Journal of Pharmacy and Bioallied Sciences*, vol. 6, no. 1, pp. 38–42, 2014.

[28] Guidance for Industry 185, *Target Animal Safety for Veterinary Pharmaceutical Products, VICH GL43*, US Department of Health and Human Services Food and Drug Administration Center for Veterinary Medicine, 2009.

[29] I. Park, D. Kim, J. Song et al., "Buprederm, a new transdermal delivery system of buprenorphine: pharmacokinetic, efficacy and skin irritancy studies," *Pharmaceutical Research*, vol. 25, no. 5, pp. 1052–1062, 2008.

[30] K. Pieper, T. Schuster, O. Levionnois, U. Matis, and A. Bergadano, "Antinociceptive efficacy and plasma concentrations of transdermal buprenorphine in dogs," *Veterinary Journal*, vol. 187, no. 3, pp. 335–341, 2011.

[31] S. C. Sigmon, D. E. Moody, E. S. Nuwayser, and G. E. Bigelow, "An injection depot formulation of buprenorphine: extended biodelivery and effects," *Addiction*, vol. 101, no. 3, pp. 420–432, 2006.

[32] N. Forbes, C. Brayton, S. Grindle, S. Shepherd, B. Tyler, and M. Guarnieri, "Serial bleeding in mice: morbidity and mortality rates with superficial temporal vein phlebotomy," *Lab Animal*, vol. 39, pp. 236–240, 2010.

[33] Alzet Osmotic Pump Implantation, http://www.alzet.com/.

[34] http://www.hopkinsmedicine.org/mcp/PHENOCORE/.

[35] N. Schildhaus, E. Trink, C. Polson et al., "Thermal latency studies in opiate-treated mice," *Journal of Pharmacy and Bioallied Sciences*, vol. 6, no. 1, pp. 43–47, 2014.

[36] J. V. Roughan and P. A. Flecknell, "Effects of surgery and analgesic administration on spontaneous behaviour in singly housed rats," *Research in Veterinary Science*, vol. 69, no. 3, pp. 283–288, 2000.

[37] M. C. Leach, K. Klaus, A. L. Miller, M. S. di Perrotolo, S. G. Sotocinal, and P. A. Flecknell, "The assessment of post-vasectomy pain in mice using behaviour and the mouse grimace scale," *PloS ONE*, vol. 7, no. 4, Article ID e35656, 2012.

[38] L. C. Matsumiya, R. E. Sorge, S. G. Sotocinal et al., "Using the mouse grimace scale to reevaluate the efficacy of postoperative analgesics in laboratory mice," *Journal of the American Association for Laboratory Animal Science*, vol. 51, no. 1, pp. 42–49, 2012.

[39] S. R. Kleppner, R. Patel, J. McDonough, and L. C. Costantini, "In-vitro and in-vivo characterization of a buprenorphine delivery system," *Journal of Pharmacy and Pharmacology*, vol. 58, no. 3, pp. 295–302, 2006.

[40] R. Dinarvand, M. M. Alimorad, M. Amanlou, and H. Akbari, "In vitro release of clomipramine HCL and buprenorphine HCL from poly adipic anhydride (PAA) and poly trimethylene carbonate (PTMC) blends," *Journal of Biomedical Materials Research A*, vol. 75, no. 1, pp. 185–191, 2005.

[41] A. Della Puppa, M. Rossetto, P. Ciccarino et al., "The first 3 months after BCNU wafers implantation in high-grade glioma patients: clinical and radiological considerations on a clinical series," *Acta Neurochirurgica*, vol. 152, no. 11, pp. 1923–1931, 2010.

[42] C. C. Horn, B. A. Kimball, H. Wang et al., "Why can't rodents vomit? A comparative behavioral, anatomical, and physiological study," *PLoS ONE*, vol. 8, no. 6, pp. 1–16, 2013.

[43] L. St A Stewart and W. J. Martin, "Evaluation of postoperative analgesia in a rat model of incisional pain," *Contemporary Topics in Laboratory Animal Science*, vol. 42, no. 1, pp. 28–34, 2003.

[44] J. Clark J.A., P. H. Myers, M. F. Goelz, J. E. Thigpen, and D. B. Forsythe, "Pica behavior associated with buprenorphine administration in the rat," *Laboratory Animal Science*, vol. 47, no. 3, pp. 300–303, 1997.

[45] P. Jablonski, B. O. Howden, and K. Baxter, "Influence of buprenorphine analgesia on post-operative recovery in two strains of rats," *Laboratory Animals*, vol. 35, no. 3, pp. 213–222, 2001.

8

Morphometric Identification, Gross and Histopathological Lesions of *Eimeria* Species in Japanese Quails (*Coturnix coturnix japonica*) in Zaria, Nigeria

H. A. Umar,[1] I. A. Lawal,[1] O. O. Okubanjo,[1] and A. M. Wakawa[2]

[1] *Department of Veterinary Parasitology and Entomology, Faculty of Veterinary Medicine, Ahmadu Bello University, Zaria 2222, Nigeria*
[2] *Department of Avian Medicine, Faculty of Veterinary Medicine, Ahmadu Bello University, Zaria 2222, Nigeria*

Correspondence should be addressed to H. A. Umar; halilu_umar@yahoo.co.uk

Academic Editor: Vito Laudadio

The objective of the study was to identify the species, gross and histopathological lesions of *Eimeria* in Japanese quails in Zaria. A total of 400 fresh faecal samples were collected and 10 quail birds were purchased from a quail farm. The faecal samples were processed using simple floatation technique. Oocysts shape indices of sporulated oocysts were determined. The intestines were observed for gross lesions and segments were analyzed using Giemsa stain and Haematoxylin and Eosin stain and then observed microscopically for the developmental stages of the parasite. Four species of *Eimeria* were identified in the study. *Eimeria bateri* of shape index of 1.36 conformed to the guidelines used while the other three *Eimeria* species with shape indices of 1.48, 1.03, and 1.40 were not confirmed. The main gross lesion seen was nonhaemorrhagic ballooning of the caeca. Intestinal scrapping smear revealed a developmental stage of the parasite (merozoites) in the jejunum. Histopathology also revealed a developmental stage (schizont) of the parasite in the caecum and desquamation of the epithelial lining with areas of necrosis. Further study is required using molecular techniques to properly identify the unknown species of *Eimeria* that were detected in the study.

1. Introduction

Quails are most susceptible to various diseases such as coccidiosis which is recognized as a serious parasitic disease problem limiting quail industry [1]. Quail production has become important in Nigeria. Descriptions of *Eimeria* date from the beginning of the last century, and ever since means for an appropriate characterization and identification of the species have been discussed. Several parameters can be used [2] and new methods have been developed [3–6]. Various species of *Eimeria* have been isolated from the different species of quails such as *E. tsunodai*, *E. uzura*, and *E. bateri* described from Japanese quails [7] and *E. lophortygis* and *E. okanaganensis* described from California quails, while *E. crusti* and *E. oreortygis* are described from mountain quail [8], *E. conturnicis* and *E. bateri* are described from grey quail [9], *E. colini* and *E. lettyae* are described from bob white quail [10],

and also *E. tahamensis* is described from Arabian quail [11]. The natural infection of *Eimeria* in quails is characterized as subclinical because of the mild and nonspecific clinical signs. Nevertheless, coccidiosis is considered as an important disease because the endogenous stages of the parasites and a high number of oocysts in feces are associated with intestinal lesions [7]. Therefore, the objective of the study was to identify the species and report the gross and histopathological lesions of *Eimeria* in Japanese quails in Zaria, Nigeria.

2. Materials and Methods

2.1. Study Area. This study was carried out in Zaria located in Kaduna State, located within latitudes $11°7'$ to $11°12'$ N and longitude $07°41'$ E. It is a medium sized city with an estimated population of 408,198 [12]. It is divided administratively into Zaria and Sabon Gari LGAs [13]. It has an estimated land area

TABLE 1: Morphological characteristics and speciation of *Eimeria* in Japanese quail.

| Species | Oocyst size (μ) | | | Shape index | Morphology | Polar granule | Oocyst wall | Confirmed species |
	Length (Mean ± StE.)	Width (Mean ± StE.)	Range					
(a) *Eimeria* spp.	22.20 ± 0.58	16.38 ± 0.42	(18.20–25.48) (14.56–18.20)	1.36	Subspherical	Present	Double	*Eimeria bateri*
(b) *Eimeria* spp.	22.36 ± 1.67	15.08 ± 0.95	(14.56–25.48) (10.92–18.20)	1.48	Ovoid	Absent	Double	Unknown
(c) *Eimeria* spp.	16.64 ± 1.08	16.12 ± 0.74	(14.56–21.84) (14.56–18.20)	1.03	Ellipsoidal	Absent	Double	Unknown
(d) *Eimeria* spp.	20.57 ± 0.40	14.74 ± 0.56	(18.20–21.84) (10.92–21.84)	1.40	Subspherical	Absent	Double	Unknown

of about 300 square kilometers and it is approximated that about 40–75% of its working population derive their principal means of livelihood from agriculture [14]. Zaria which is located in the North Guinea Savannah zone of Nigeria has an annual ambient temperature, ranging between 18.0 ± 3.7°C and 31.8 ± 3.2°C. The harmattan season (the cold-dry period of the year) lasts from November to February, while the hot-dry season lasts from March to May and the rainy season lasts from June to October [15, 16].

2.2. Sample Collection, Handling, and Processing. Forty fresh faecal samples were collected using polythene bags. Ten live quail birds were also gotten from the farm. The samples were labeled and transported to the Helminthology Laboratory in the Department of Veterinary Parasitology and Entomology, Faculty of Veterinary Medicine, Ahmadu Bello University, Zaria. In the laboratory samples not examined immediately were refrigerated at 4°C to maintain the integrity of the oocyst [17].

2.3. Laboratory Examination. The faecal samples were examined for the presence of coccidia oocysts using the simple floatation technique as described by Urquhart et al. [18].

Oocyst positive samples were diluted into 2.5% aqueous potassium dichromate ($K_2Cr_2O_7$) and kept in Petri dishes for sporulation at room temperature. After sporulation, oocysts were recovered by centrifugation with saturated sugar solution as described by Duszynski and Wilber [17] and used in subsequent analysis.

The shape indices (length/width) of the sporulated oocysts were determined by using the method for species identification as described by Harper and Penzorn [19].

The calculated oocysts shape index values were then compared with the standard diagnostic guide provided by Teixeira et al. [20] to determine the species encountered in the study.

2.4. Necropsy. The birds were euthanized and this was accomplished in accordance with guide for the care and use of laboratory animals [21].

Segments of the small intestine (duodenum, jejunum, and ileum) and large intestine (caeca) were taken for gross and histopathological studies.

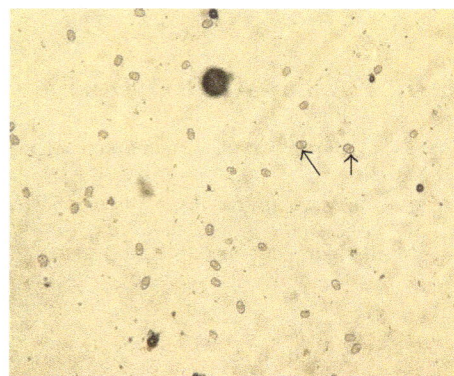

FIGURE 1: Numerous unsporulated *Eimeria* oocyst from quails using simple floatation technique (×10).

The segments were examined macroscopically for gross lesions. Intestinal scraping smear was carried out to detect the presence of developmental stages of the parasite within the intestine using Giemsa stain as described by Dubey [22].

Histological examination was carried out to confirm the presence of the developmental stages of the parasites and pathological lesions within the small and large intestine using Haematoxylin and Eosin stain as described by Mitchell et al. [23].

2.5. Statistical Analysis. Oocysts measurements were analyzed using the software Excel (Microsoft) for mean and standard deviation.

3. Results

3.1. Oocyst Speciation. Table 1 shows the oocyst dimensions and morphological characteristics of different *Eimeria* species identified in the study. The *Eimeria* species encountered in the study were *Eimeria bateri* (Figure 2) and three other *Eimeria* species (Figures 3, 4, and 5) not covered by the diagnostic guidelines.

3.2. Gross and Histopathological Lesions. The fresh faecal sample was positive for *Eimeria* oocysts (Figure 1). The main gross pathology seen was the ballooning of the caeca which

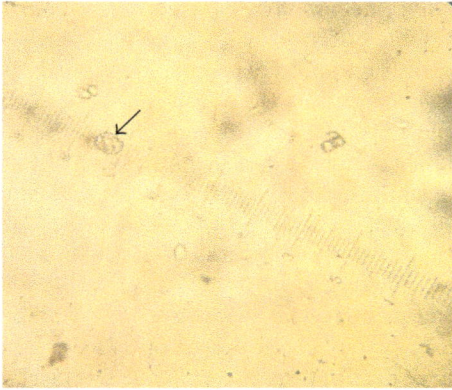

FIGURE 2: Subspherical *Eimeria bateri* oocyst with a polar granule using ocular micrometer (×40).

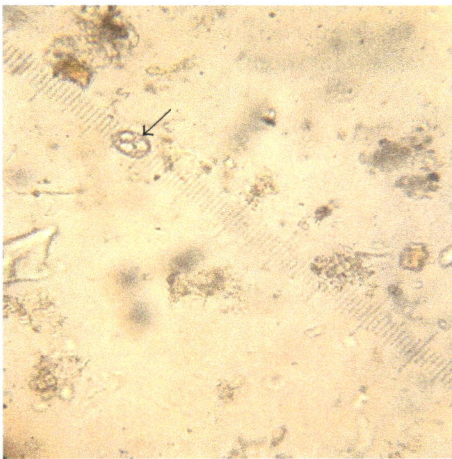

FIGURE 3: Ovoid *Eimeria* oocyst using ocular micrometer (×40).

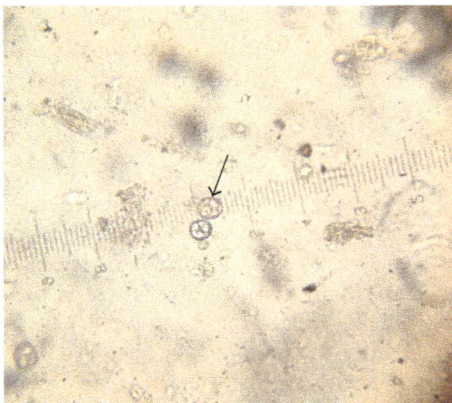

FIGURE 4: Ellipsoidal *Eimeria* oocyst using an ocular micrometer (×40).

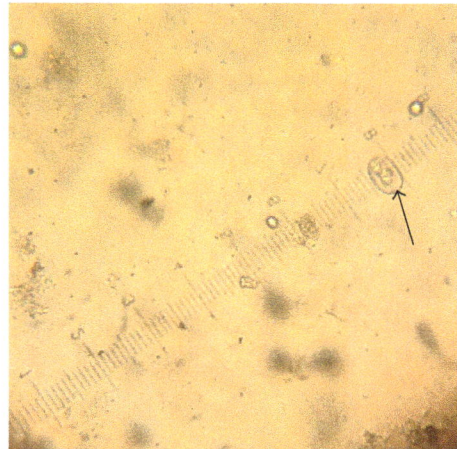

FIGURE 5: Subspherical *Eimeria* oocyst with no polar granule using ocular micrometer (×40).

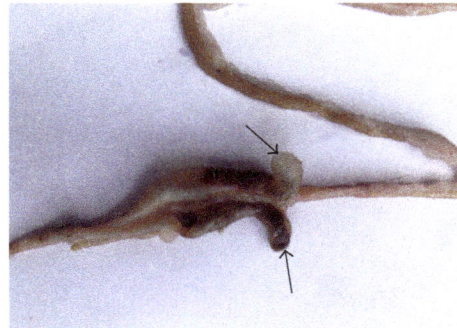

FIGURE 6: Ballooning of the caeca of a Japanese quail naturally infected with *Eimeria bateri*.

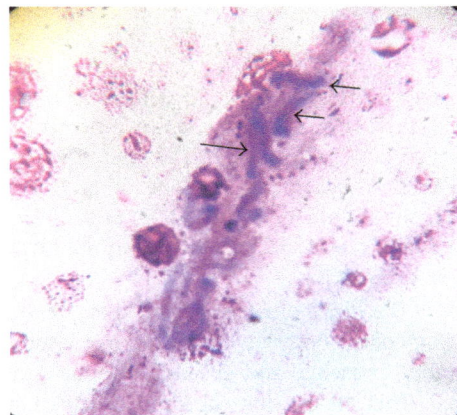

FIGURE 7: Jejunum of Japanese quail showing the developmental stage (merozoite) of *Eimeria* spp. in the epithelium using Giemsa stain (×100) oil immersion.

contains no bloody exudate in the lumen (Figure 6). Histopathologically, desquamation of intestinal mucosa was observed (Figure 9) and caecal necrosis (Figure 8). Developmental stages of the parasite especially the merozoites and schizont were seen in the intestinal epithelium (Figures 7, 8, and 9).

4. Discussion

Quails are considered a branch of the modern poultry industry in Nigeria. The study showed that there were coccidia oocysts in the farm sampled from. In our study the identification of *Eimeria* species was done using the oocysts

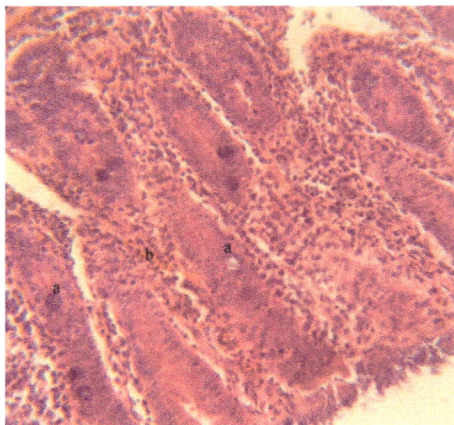

FIGURE 8: Histological section of the caecum showing the (a) developmental stage (schizont) of *Eimeria* spp. and (b) area of necrosis H&E (×40).

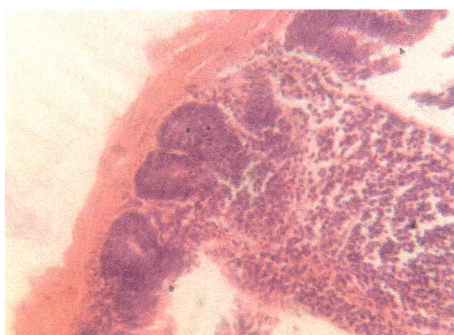

FIGURE 9: Histological section of duodenum showing the (a) developmental stage (schizonts) of *Eimeria* spp. and (b) desquamation of the epithelium H&E (×40).

morphometric technique. Four *Eimeria* species were identified from Japanese quails in the study. *Eimeria bateri* with shape index of 1.36 conformed to the guidelines of Teixeira et al. [20] and Mohammad [24]. The other three *Eimeria* species with shape indices of 1.48, 1.03, and 1.40 could not speciate as they do not conform to any of the given species by the above authors.

In spite of the shortcomings identified above, differences in morphology of the oocyst which were ovoid, subspherical, and ellipsoidal, presence and absence of polar granule can be observed. This means that other unidentified species of *Eimeria* exist in Zaria. Discrimination of *Eimeria* species using this technique has sort of limitations to be used as a single tool for diagnosis, meaning that results obtained with this method should be carefully interpreted [25, 26]. This is because the measurements of the oocysts may undergo variations due to changes in metabolism of the parasites or birds and even in the value of the shape morphometric indices of the oocysts that may overlap leading to misleading conclusions regarding the species [27]. Despite the limitations of morphometric techniques, there are some reports that indicated that oocyst morphometry could also

be a sensitive method for the discrimination of *Eimeria* species of poultry in field trials as it shows high degree of agreement with the molecular methods [28–31]. The use of molecular techniques is the most specific and rapid way of diagnosing *Eimeria* infection especially when it involves several species occurring concurrently [32–34]. However, in developing countries like Nigeria very few laboratories have the facilities and personnel to carry out these molecular techniques for routine diagnosis of coccidiosis. The study also showed that the gross lesions associated with *Eimeria* infection in Japanese quails were limited to mainly ballooning of the caeca. The only clinical signs observed were diarrhea. The reports of previous works seem to be at variance with the present observation as regards the pathogenicity of *Eimeria* in quails. Mazurkiewicz et al. [35] reported a wide range of clinical signs such as lack of appetite, ruffled feathers, uncoordinated movements, inhibition of laying, and loss of weight in naturally infected young and mature quails reared at the laboratory. In young Japanese quailsinfected with *Eimeria bateri*, mild loss of weight, anorexia, and softening of feces were observed and were considered mild and easy to overcome [36]. Tsunoda and Muraki [37] also reported low pathogenicity in Japanese quails experimentally infected with 1×10^5 oocysts of *Eimeria uzura* with signs limited to diarrhea and anemia with no mortality was reported. However, Ruff et al. [38] used pure and mixed cultures of *E. uzura* to infect quails and reported mortality, lower weight gain, and poor reproductive performance. Several factors such as environment, differences in the parasite strain, and management system may be responsible for the discrepancies in the observation of the various works. The findings from this study show that merozoites are the main endogenous stages of the parasites found in the small intestine and schizonts in the large intestine. The absence of other pathogenic stages such as the gametocytes means that the pathology of the infected quails will be mild. Histopathological lesions were located in the villi. These observations resemble those of Norton and Peirce [36], Mazurkiewicz et al. [35], and Tsutsumi [9] as regards the site of infection. Desquamation of epithelial lining and caecal necrosis were also observed in the study.

In conclusion, four *Eimeria* species were identified in the study, only *Eimeria bateri* speciated as it conformed to the guideline used. Due to the limitations of speciation using the oocysts morphometry technique, there is the need for further studies to be carried out using molecular techniques to properly identify the unknown species of *Eimeria* which were detected in the study. The study also showed that the gross and histopathological changes in intestinal tract pointed to the serious effect of *Eimeria* species in quails. This observation has an important value since there is a paucity of information on the pathogenicity of *Eimeria* spp. in quails.

Conflict of Interests

The authors declare that there is no conflict of interests regarding the publication of this paper.

References

[1] S. Seok, J. Park, S. Cho, M. Baek, H. Lee, and D. Kim, "Coccidian (*Eimeria spp*) in small intestine of Japanese quail (*Coturnix coturnix japonica*)," *Korean Journal of Laboratory Animal Science*, vol. 19, no. 2, pp. 90–91, 2003.

[2] P. L. Long and L. P. Joyner, "Problems in the identification of species of Eimeria," *Journal of Protozoology*, vol. 31, no. 4, pp. 535–541, 1984.

[3] J. Kucera and M. Reznický, "Differentiation of species of *Eimeria* from the fowl using a computerized image-analysis system.," *Folia Parasitologica*, vol. 38, no. 2, pp. 107–113, 1991.

[4] A. Daugschies, S. Imarom, and W. Bollwahn, "Differentiation of porcine *Eimeria* spp. by morphologic algorithms," *Veterinary Parasitology*, vol. 81, no. 3, pp. 201–210, 1999.

[5] A. Gruber and S. Fernandez, "Recentes avanços na biologia molecular de protozoários do gênero *Eimeria*," in *II Simpósio Internacional sobre coccidiose aviária*, pp. 9–21, Foz do Iguaçu, Brazil, 1999.

[6] M. J. S. Pereira, A. H. Fonseca, and C. W. G. Lopes, "Regressão linear na caracterização de variações morfométricas em coccidia," *Revista Brasileira de Parasitologia Veterinária*, vol. 10, pp. 75–78, 2001.

[7] M. Teixeira and C. W. G. Lopes, "Species of the genus *Eimeria* (Apicomplexa : Eimeriidae) from Japanese quails (*Coturnix japonica*) in Brazil and *Eimeria fluminensis* for the preoccupied *Eimeria minima* of this quail," *Revista Brasileira de Ciências Veterinárias*, vol. 9, pp. 53–56, 2002.

[8] D. W. Duszynski and R. J. Gutiérrez, "The coccidia of quail in the United States," *Journal of Wild Diseases*, vol. 17, no. 3, pp. 371–379, 1981.

[9] Y. Tsutsumi, "*Eimeria tsunodai* sp. nov. (protozoa: Eimeriidae). A caecal coccidium of Japanese quails (*Coturnix coturnix japonica*)," *The Japanese journal of veterinary science*, vol. 34, no. 1, pp. 1–9, 1972.

[10] M. D. Ruff, "Life cycle and biology of *Eimeria lettyae* sp. n. (Protozoa: Eimeriidae) from the Northern bobwhite, *Colinus virginianus* (L.)," *Journal of Wildlife Diseases*, vol. 21, no. 4, pp. 361–370, 1985.

[11] M. A. Amoudi, "*Eimeria tahamensis* N. sp. (Apicomplexa: Eimeriidae) from the Arabian quail (*Coturnix delegorguei arabica*)," *Journal of Protozoology*, vol. 34, no. 4, pp. 455–456, 1987.

[12] National Population Commission (NPC), "Location of Zaria," in *The Latitude and Longitude of Zaria Zone in Kaduna State, Nigeria*, pp. 26–35, 2006.

[13] Ministry of Economic Development, *Kaduna State Statistical Year Book*, Statistics Division, Ministry of Economic Development, Kaduna, Nigeria, 1996.

[14] Ahmadu Bello University, *Zaria Master Plan*, Department of Urban and Regional Planning, ABU Zaria, Zaria, Nigeria, 2000.

[15] J. O. Ayo, J. A. Obidi, and P. I. Rekwot, "Effects of heat stress on the well-being, fertility and hatchability of chicken in the Northern Guinea Savannah zone of Nigeria: a review," *ISRN Veterinary Science*, vol. 2011, Article ID 838606, 10 pages, 2011.

[16] T. Dzenda, J. O. Ayo, C. A. M. Lakpini, and A. B. Adelaiye, "Seasonal, sex and live weight variations in feed and water consumptions of adult captive African Giant rats (*Cricetomys gambianus*, Waterhouse-1840) kept individually in cages," *Journal of Animal Physiology and Animal Nutrition*, vol. 97, no. 3, pp. 465–474, 2013.

[17] D. W. Duszynski and P. G. Wilber, "A guideline for the preparation of species descriptions in the Eimeriidae," *Journal of Parasitology*, vol. 83, no. 2, pp. 333–336, 1997.

[18] G. M. Urquhart, J. Armour, J. L. Dunkan, A. M. Dunn, and F. W. Jennings, *Veterinary Parasitology*, Longman, Essex, UK, 1987.

[19] C. K. Harper and B. L. Penzhorn, "Occurrence and diversity of coccidia in indigenous, Saanen and crossbred goats in South Africa," *Veterinary Parasitology*, vol. 82, no. 1, pp. 1–9, 1999.

[20] M. Teixeira, F. W. L. Teixeira, and C. W. G. Lopes, "Coccidiosis in Japanese quails (*Coturnix japonica*) characterization of a naturally occurring infection in a commercial rearing farm," *Revista Brasileira de Ciência Avícola*, vol. 6, no. 2, pp. 129–134, 2004.

[21] National Research Council, *Guide for the Care and Use of Laboratory Animals*, The National Academies Press, Washington, DC, USA, 1996.

[22] J. P. Dubey, *Toxoplasmosis of Animals and Humans*, CRC Press, Boca Raton, Fla, USA, 2nd edition, 2009.

[23] R. S. Mitchell, V. Kumar, A. K. Abbas, and N. Fausto, *Robbins Basic Pathology*, chapter 11, Saunders, Philadelphia, Pa, USA, 2003.

[24] N. H. Mohammad, "A study on the pathological and diagnosis of Eimeria species infection in Japanese quail," *Basrah Journal of Veterinary Research*, vol. 11, no. 1, pp. 318–333, 2012.

[25] W. G. Woods, G. Richards, K. G. Whithear, G. R. Anderson, W. K. Jorgenses, and R. B. Gasser, "High-resolution electrophoretic procedures for the identification of five *Eimeria* species from chickens and detection of population variation," *Electrophoresis*, vol. 21, pp. 3558–3563, 2000.

[26] G. J. López, J. Figuerola, and R. Soriguer, "Time of day, age and feeding habits influence coccidian oocyst shedding in wild passerines," *International Journal for Parasitology*, vol. 37, no. 5, pp. 559–564, 2007.

[27] X. M. Sun, W. Pang, T. Jia et al., "Prevalence of Eimeria species in broilers with subclinical signs from fifty farms," *Avian Diseases*, vol. 53, no. 2, pp. 301–305, 2009.

[28] A. T. Terra, P. S. Costa, P. C. Figueiredo, and E. C. Q. Carvalho, "Frequency of species of the genus *Eimeria* in broilers slaughtered industrially in the municipality of Monte Algre do Sul, State of Sao Paulo," *Revista Brasileira de Parasitologia Veterinaria*, vol. 10, no. 2, pp. 87–90, 2001.

[29] F. C. Luchese, M. Perin, R. S. Aita, V. D. Mottin, M. B. Molento, and S. G. Monteiro, "Prevalence of *Eimeria* species in industrial and alternative bred chicken," *Brazilian Journal of Veterinary Research and Animal Science*, vol. 44, no. 2, pp. 81–86, 2007.

[30] A. Haug, A.-G. Gjevre, P. Thebo, J. G. Mattsson, and M. Kaldhusdal, "Coccidial infections in commercial broilers: epidemiological aspects and comparison of *Eimeria* species identification by morphometric and polymerase chain reaction techniques," *Avian Pathology*, vol. 37, no. 2, pp. 161–170, 2008.

[31] F. S. Carvalho, A. A. Wenceslau, M. Teixeira, J. A. Matos Carneiro, A. D. B. Melo, and G. R. Albuquerque, "Diagnosis of *Eimeria* species using traditional and molecular methods in field studies," *Veterinary Parasitology*, vol. 176, no. 2-3, pp. 95–100, 2011.

[32] S. Fernandez, A. H. Pagotto, M. M. Furtado, Â. M. Katsuyama, A. M. B. N. Madeira, and A. Gruber, "A multiplex PCR assay for the simultaneous detection and discrimination of the seven *Eimeria* species that infect domestic fowl," *Parasitology*, vol. 127, no. 4, pp. 317–325, 2003.

[33] A. Haug, P. Thebo, and J. G. Mattsson, "A simplified protocol for molecular identification of *Eimeria* species in field samples," *Veterinary Parasitology*, vol. 146, no. 1-2, pp. 35–45, 2007.

[34] V. Vrba, D. P. Blake, and M. Poplstein, "Quantitative real-time PCR assays for detection and quantification of all seven *Eimeria* species that infect the chicken," *Veterinary Parasitology*, vol. 174, no. 3-4, pp. 183–190, 2010.

[35] M. Mazurkiewicz, D. Podlewska, and Z. Wachnik, "Kokcydioza u przepiórek japonskich," *Medycyna Weterynaryjna*, vol. 23, pp. 536–537, 1967.

[36] C. C. Norton and M. A. Peirce, "The life cycle of *Eimeria bateri* (Protozoa, Eimeriidae) in the Japanese quail *Coturnix coturnix japonicum*," *The Journal of Protozoology*, vol. 18, no. 1, pp. 57–62, 1971.

[37] K. Tsunoda and Y. Muraki, "A new coccidium of Japanese quails: *Eimeria uzura* sp. nov," *The Japanese Journal of Veterinary Science*, vol. 33, no. 5, pp. 227–235, 1971.

[38] M. D. Ruff, J. M. Fagan, and J. W. Dick, "Pathogenicity of coccidia in Japanese quail (*Coturnix coturnix japonica*)," *Poultry Science*, vol. 63, no. 1, pp. 55–60, 1984.

9

A Limited Sampling, Simple, and Useful Method for Determination of Glomerular Filtration Rate in Cats by Using a New Accurate HPLC Method to Measure Iohexol Plasmatic Concentrations

Meucci Valentina, Guidi Grazia, Melanie Pierre, Breghi Gloria, and Lippi Ilaria

Department of Veterinary Clinics, University of Pisa, San Piero a Grado, Via Livornese Lato Monte, 56122 Pisa, Italy

Correspondence should be addressed to Meucci Valentina; valentinam@vet.unipi.it

Academic Editor: Antonio Ortega-Pacheco

Glomerular filtration rate (GFR) is still a highly underutilized tool in cats because available methods are not easy to be performed in clinical practice. Iohexol (IOX) has been shown to be a useful and reliable marker of GFR both in animals and in humans. The aim of the present study was to develop a rapid and reliable method for measuring IOX in feline plasma and to evaluate the accuracy of limited sampling models to establish a low-cost and clinically suitable GFR test. IOX concentrations were determined by using a new HPLC-UV method. GFR was assessed as plasma clearance of IOX, which was calculated by dividing dose administered by area under the curve of plasmatic concentration *versus* time (AUC), and indexed to body weight (BW). Correlation and agreement analysis between the GFR values obtained by a seven-point clearance method and the GFR values determined by the application of simplified sample combinations indicated that the 3-blood sample clearance model (5, 30, and 60 min) was the best simplified method because it provided an accurate GFR value in only one hour. The reported method is a simple and accurate way of GFR determination, which may be easily used in a clinical setting.

1. Introduction

Chronic kidney disease (CKD) is one of the most common disorders in cats, especially in older ones for which it represents a major cause of illness and death [1, 2]. Plasma creatinine (PCr) and urea (PU), the most used parameters for assessing renal function in veterinary practice, cannot be used in the early diagnosis of renal failure because they start to rise too late, when the 75% of functioning nephrons are lost [3, 4], and are also affected by several extra renal factors [5]. Glomerular filtration rate (GFR), directly related to the functional renal mass, is considered the most sensitive and early marker of kidney failure [6]. At present, in veterinary medicine, GFR can be assessed by using different methods, which have both advantages and disadvantages. Many methods have several disadvantages including the labour intense nature, risks caused by anaesthesia, cost of the test substance, assay of the substance used, or need for specialized

licensing and equipment. The traditional gold standard for measurement of GFR (urinary clearance of inulin) is not suitable in a clinical setting [7, 8]. These methods are labor intensive and require the placement of an indwelling urinary catheter with associated risk of sedation and of causing lower urinary tract infection. Over the past two decades, many alternative methods for determining GFR have been shown to provide acceptable measurements of renal function in cats [9]. Unfortunately, most of these methods are not routinely available for use by veterinary practitioners in a clinical setting due to lack of drug availability (inulin, exogenous creatinine) or the need for special licensing and equipment (radiolabeled compounds) [10–13]. Plasma clearance of iohexol (IOX) has been shown to provide a reliable estimate of GFR in cats [9, 14–16]. More recently, limited sampling strategies were also investigated in order to estimate GFR by the use of colorimetric assays or correction formula

[17–19]. In feline patients, the use of three-sample and one-sample procedures through plasma clearance of iodixanol showed a close correlation with multisample inulin method in both clinically healthy and CKD cats [20]. A single sample at 180' after-injection using corrected slope-intercept IOX clearance seemed to provide an accurate estimation of GFR in cats, although further investigations are still required for very low or very high values of GFR [18]. Nevertheless, there is a need of simplification of assay GFR protocols by validating detection methods of markers and reducing sampling times [21]. It is also important that each laboratory establishes its own reference range for a given GFR protocol in several animal species. Plasma concentration of IOX can be detected indirectly by measuring plasma levels of iodine or directly by the use of several methods including X-ray fluorescence [22, 23], inductively coupled plasma atomic emission spectroscopy [24], high-performance liquid chromatography (HPLC) [25–27], colorimetric assay [5, 13–28], and capillary electrophoresis [29]. However, HPLC is the most widely used technique for analysis of IOX in clinical practice due to its sensitivity and flexibility [30, 31]. In urine, plasma, and serum, IOX is present as two isomers, called endo- and exoiohexol both of which can be used for HPLC quantification and GFR measurement [25–31].

The aims of the present study were to develop a rapid and reliable HPLC analysis method for measuring IOX in feline plasma and to evaluate the accuracy of limited sampling models to establish an accurate, low-cost, and clinically suitable GFR test in cats.

2. Materials and Methods

2.1. Chemicals and Reagents.
IOX and the internal standard (IS) of iopentol were kindly supplied by Nycomed Amersham Sorin (Milan, Italy). Water was doubly distilled and purified using a Sartorius cellulose acetate filter (Göettingen, Germany). HPLC grade water, dichloromethane, and acetonitrile were supplied by LABSCAN (Hasselt, Belgium).

2.2. Chromatographic Conditions.
The HPLC system consisted of a Series 200 Perkin Elmer gradient Pump coupled to a Series 200 Perkin Elmer variable UV detector which was set at 254 nm. The reversed-phase column was a SunFire Waters C_{18} column (5 μm, 250 × 4.60 mm) connected to a Waters Guard-Pak C_{18} precolumn (4 μm) (Waters, Milford, MA, USA). The column was kept at room temperature. Turbochrom software was used for data processing. A 20 μL injection of sample was used each time. The mobile phase consisted in acetonitrile-water pH 2.7 (acidified by addition of H_3PO_4 85%). Both IOX and IS were eluted as two isomers. For analysis, the peak area of the major IOX and IS isomers was used because these constituted more than 80% of the combined peak areas and the ratio of both the isomer peaks remained constant at different IOX and IS concentrations under the current analytical condition. All calculations were performed using peak area ratios of the larger IOX peak to the IS peak (peak area ratio) by the use of Microsoft Excel (MS OFFICE, 2007).

2.3. Preparation of Stock Solutions.
Stock solutions of IOX and IS were prepared monthly as 1 mg/mL solutions in double-distilled water and stored at −20°C. IOX working solutions were made by further diluting the stock solutions and were prepared fresh daily. A total of seven concentrations of IOX including 2.5, 10, 25, 50, 125, 250, and 500 μg/mL in drug free feline plasma were used as calibrators. Three in-house quality control standards containing IOX at low (25 μg/mL), medium (125 μg/mL), and high (500 μg/mL) concentrations were also prepared in feline plasma and were used for assay validation. Aliquots of the IS stock solution were diluted in water to produce a working (50 μg/mL) IS solution. Aliquots of the calibrators, quality control samples, and reference standard solutions were stored at −20°C until use. A total of nine standard curves were prepared and all calibrators or quality control samples were injected in triplicate.

2.4. Validation.
The HPLC method was validated according to international rules [32]: specificity, sensitivity, linearity, limits of determination (LOD) and of quantification (LOQ), repeatability, and reproducibility were determined. For the linearity test calibration curves with IOX working as standard solutions at 0.5–100 μg/mL in water were prepared. Feline plasma samples spiked with IOX at 2.5, 10, 25, 50, 125, 250, and 500 μg/mL were analyzed using the HPLC method. Taking into account dilution step, these spiked samples corresponded to IOX standard concentrations of 0.5, 2, 5, 10, 25, 50, and 100 μg/mL. The experiment was repeated nine times. To evaluate specificity, blank samples of feline plasma containing no IOX or IS were analyzed to check for the presence of interfering peaks at the elution time of IOX and IS. The repeatability was tested by analyzing samples of feline plasma spiked with IOX (n = 63). Samples were spiked at the levels of 25 μg/mL (corresponding to 5 μg/mL), 125 μg/mL (corresponding to 25 μg/mL), and 500 μg/mL (corresponding to 50 μg/mL). All samples were measured in triplicate on the same day. For the within-laboratory reproducibility test, each spiked level was tested in triplicate over seven days. The results of these experiments were used also for the determination of the recovery. The analytical recovery of IOX was assessed by comparing the peak area ratio of spiked samples with the peak area ratio (analyte peak area/IOP peak area) of the reference standards prepared in water. The sensitivity of the method was expressed as the LOQ, which is the minimum concentration of IOX in plasma that can be quantitatively determined with a peak height to baseline ratio of at least 10 : 1, and the LOD, which has a peak height to baseline ratio of 3 : 1. To evaluate stability, aliquots of spiked samples were subjected to three cycles of freeze and thaw (freezing for 24 h at −20°C and thawing unassisted at room temperature). For short-term stability test, the aliquots of the spiked samples were thawed at room temperature and kept at this temperature for 6 h (the duration of analysis for a typical batch) before analysis. For long-term stability test, the aliquots of the spiked samples were thawed at room temperature and kept at this temperature for 12 and 24 h before analysis.

2.5. Animal Study. Fifty privately owned domestic short-hair cats, presented to the Department of Veterinary Science for minor surgery and/or neutering, were included in the study after the owner's informed consent and Ethical Committee approval (University of Pisa authorization number 8317). The cats were divided into two groups: nonazotaemic cats (PCr < 141 μmol/L) and azotaemic cats (PCr > 141 μmol/L) according to IRIS guidelines. The body weight of the cats ranged from 2 to 5.5 kg (mean 3.37 ± 0.71 kg) and their age from 1 to 3 years (mean 1.8 ± 0.7 years). All cats were assessed not to be affected by concurrent diseases on the basis of physical examination, complete blood count, plasma biochemical analysis, urinalysis, testing for FeLV and FIV, and abdominal ultrasound.

Each cat was fasted overnight (at least 12 h) before the experimental procedure, and no food was given during the trial. Water was given ad libitum. A commercially available IOX formulation was administered IV as a bolus (within 1 minute) at the dose of 64.7 mg/kg (0.1 mL/kg) through the right jugular catheter. The syringe and the needle used to infuse IOX were weighed before and after injection, in order to determine the exact administered dose. Samples were collected by the catheter positioned into the left jugular vein before marker's administration (time 0) and at 5, 30, 60, 120, 240, 360, and 480 minutes after the completion of the injection. Blood was collected into lithium heparin test tubes and centrifuged at 3500 rpm within 10 minutes from collection. Plasma was stored in aliquots at −20°C.

2.6. Preparation of Plasma Samples. Each plasma sample was submitted to a preparation method for the extraction of IOX. Fifty microliters of plasma was added to a 50 μL water solution of IS (50 μg/mL) and vigorously vortexed (60 seconds). The plasma sample was deproteinized by adding 100 μL of dichloromethane (CH_2Cl_2), extracted with double-distilled water (150 μL), vigorously vortexed (60 seconds), and centrifuged at 3500 rpm for 10 minutes. Twenty microliters of the supernatant was centrifuged at 3000 rpm for 10 minutes and then injected into the HPLC system.

2.7. Pharmacokinetic and Statistical Analysis. Pharmacokinetic analyses were performed by WinNonlin Version 5.1[a]. Plasma data were subjected to noncompartmental analysis with a statistical moment approach. The area under the plasma concentration *versus* time curve (AUC) was calculated by trapezoidal rule with extrapolation to infinity. Plasma clearance of IOX was determined by dividing dose administered by AUC, and indexed to body weight (BW) (mL/min/kg). The administered dose was established by assuming that the 85% of IOX was exoiohexol. The normalized seven-point clearance value was considered a reference for the evaluation of simplified methods. Correlation and agreement analysis between the GFR values obtained by the seven-point clearance method and the GFR values determined by the application of simplified sample combinations were performed using Pearson test, linear regression analysis, and Bland-Altman plots. In addition, the accuracy of the GFR estimates was determined as the percentage of results

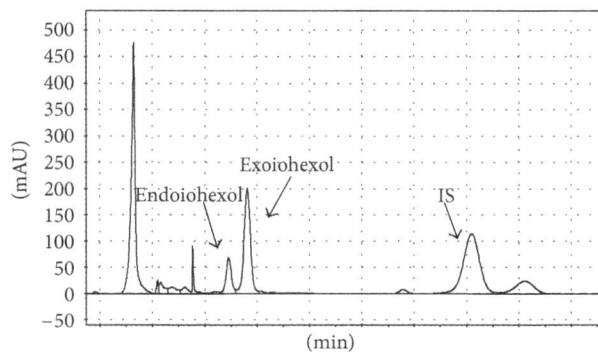

FIGURE 1: Chromatogram of the separation of IOX (10 μg/mL) and IS extracted from feline plasma; IS: internal standard.

not deviating more than 15%, 30%, and 50% from the GFR values obtained by the seven-point clearance method. The percentages between the formulas were compared using the Chi-square test.

For simplified methods GFR was calculated by using the same pharmacokinetic model of the reference method. Among the possible different models, four simplified sample combinations (Models A, B, C, and D) were chosen. Each model showed a different sample combination: Model A (5, 30, 60, and 240 minutes), Model B (5, 30, 60, and 120 minutes), Model C (5, 60, 120, and 240 minutes), and Model D (5, 30, and 60 minutes). Comparisons of nonazotaemic and azotaemic groups of cats were based on Student's *t*-test. A *P* value below 0.05 was considered significant.

3. Results

3.1. HPLC Method. Figure 1 illustrates chromatogram of IOX and IS in extracted feline plasma. IOX was eluted as two isomers endoiohexol and exoiohexol, at 6.4 and 6.8 min, respectively, whereas the IS was eluted as two isomers at 10.4 and 11.0 min. The specificity of the method was tested by analyzing feline plasma samples before the administration of IOX. No interfering peaks were observed at the elution times of IOX or IS isomers. IOX LOD and LOQ were found to be 0.01 and 0.1 μg/mL, respectively. Calibration graphs for IOX ($n = 9$) were constructed over the concentration range of 0.5–500 μg/mL and showed an average correlation coefficient (R^2) of 0.999. The accuracy of the estimated IOX concentration was more than 90% at three concentrations. The precision expressed as interday coefficient of variation (CV%) ranged from 3.8% to 6.5% and as the intraday CV% ranged from 1.5% to 4.0% (Table 1). The extraction method of IOX from plasma samples had an average recovery ranging from 96.0 ± 2.5% to 95.0 ± 2.1% for low-to-high spiked samples (Table 1). The recovery was reproducible over seven replications performed over 7 different days. IS had an average recovery ranging from 96.0 ± 2.5% to 95.0 ± 1.5%. The concentrations of IOX in freeze-thaw and short-term stability evaluation were not significantly different from the fresh calibrators. The accuracy of the spiked samples ranged from 98% to 100% and from 98% to 101% after the freeze-thaw stability and short-term

TABLE 1: Recovery and intra- and interday precision results for the assay; CV: coefficient of variation; intraday $n = 9$ in one day; interday $n = 9$ for 7 consecutive days.

Sample	Nominal IOX concentrations	Recovery (%)	Intraday precision (% CV)	Interday precision (% CV)
Low	25 μg/mL	96 ± 2.5	1.5	3.8
Medium	125 μg/mL	96 ± 1.8	2.5	3.2
High	500 μg/mL	95 ± 2.1	4.0	6.5

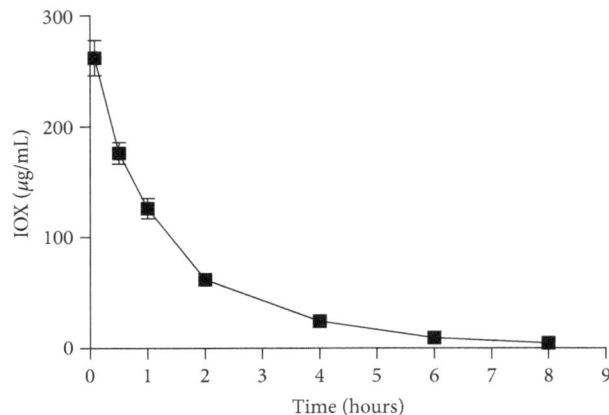

FIGURE 2: Plasma exoiohexol concentration *versus* time profile from 50 cats after a single administration of IOX (at a nominal dose of 64.7 mg/kg); data are expressed as mean ± standard error bars.

stability testing, respectively. The formal ruggedness test was conducted when the method was validated on a second HPLC system (Thermo Finnigan, Waltham, MA, USA) by another analyst (results not shown). Using the optimized parameters, the method was found to be equally robust.

3.2. Clearance of IOX. The GFR protocol used was well tolerated in all animals and no adverse effect was noticed or reported by the owner after the test. The plasma concentrations *versus* time profiles for IOX obtained from seven-point clearance method (5, 30, 60, 120, 240, 360, and 480 minutes) in all analyzed cats are reported in Figure 2. The extrapolated part of the AUC in all the analyzed models did not exceed 25% of the total AUC.

The nonazotaemic group consisted of 35 cats. PCr ranged from a minimum of 78 μmol/L to a maximum of 140 μmol/L (mean: 106 μmol/L). Reference GFR (7-point clearance method) ranged from a minimum of 1.21 mL/min/kg to a maximum of 8.62 mL/min/kg, with a mean value of 3.40 ± 0.29 mL/min/kg. Model A GFR ranged from a minimum of 1.52 mL/min/kg to a maximum of 6.80 mL/min/kg, with a mean value of 3.32 ± 0.47 mL/min/kg. Model B GFR ranged from a minimum of 1.64 mL/min/kg to a maximum of 6.62 mL/min/kg, with a mean value of 3.28 ± 0.38 mL/min/kg. Model C GFR ranged from a minimum of 1.40 mL/min/kg to a maximum of 6.87 mL/min/kg, with a mean value of 3.08 ± 0.41 mL/min/kg. Model D GFR ranged from a minimum of 1.51 mL/min/kg to a maximum of 8.30 mL/min/kg, with a mean value of 3.43 ± 0.39 mL/min/kg.

The azotaemic group consisted of 15 cats with PCr above the reference range (141 μmol/L). PCr ranged from a minimum of 143 μmol/L to a maximum of 209 μmol/L (mean: 160 μmol/L). Reference GFR (7-point clearance method) ranged from a minimum of 1.36 mL/min/kg to a maximum of 3.47 mL/min/kg, with a mean value of 2.38 ± 0.19 mL/min/kg. Model A GFR ranged from a minimum of 1.25 mL/min/kg to a maximum of 2.99 mL/min/kg, with a mean value of 2.11 ± 0.17 mL/min/kg. Model B GFR ranged from a minimum of 1.49 mL/min/kg to a maximum of 4.17 mL/min/kg, with a mean value of 2.57 ± 0.23 mL/min/kg. Model C GFR ranged from a minimum of 1.35 mL/min/kg to a maximum of 3.66 mL/min/kg, with a mean value of 2.28 ± 0.19 mL/min/kg. Model D GFR ranged from a minimum of 1.45 mL/min/kg to a maximum of 3.81 mL/min/kg, with a mean value of 2.26 ± 0.26 mL/min/kg.

t-test analysis showed a significant difference in GFR, PCr, and PU values between nonazotaemic and azotaemic cats at $P = 0.003$, $P < 0.0001$, and $P = 0.0006$, respectively (Table 2). t-test analysis showed no significant difference in bodyweight values between nonazotaemic and azotaemic cats ($P > 0.05$) (Table 2).

3.3. Correlation Analysis: Nonazotaemic Cats. Pearson correlation testing between GFR values obtained by reference method and Model A (5, 30, 60, and 240 mins) showed a positive linear correlation ($R^2 = 0.92$, $P = 0.95$; Figure 3(a)). Pearson correlation testing between GFR values obtained by reference method and Model B (5, 30, 60, and 120 mins) showed a positive linear correlation ($R^2 = 0.95$, $P = 0.97$; Figure 3(b)). Pearson correlation testing between GFR values obtained by reference method and Model C (5, 60, 120, and 240 mins) showed a positive linear correlation ($R^2 = 0.88$, $P = 0.94$; Figure 3(c)). Pearson correlation testing between GFR values obtained by reference method and Model D (5, 30, and 60 mins) showed a positive linear correlation ($R^2 = 0.83$, $P = 0.91$; Figure 3(d)). The results from Bland-Altman analysis are given in Figure 4. The accuracies of all models tested were not significantly different from those of the reference method (Table 3).

3.4. Correlation Analysis: Azotaemic Cats. Pearson correlation testing between GFR values obtained by reference method and Model A (5, 30, 60, and 240 mins) showed a positive linear correlation ($R^2 = 0.90$, $P = 0.95$; Figure 5(a)). Pearson correlation testing between GFR values obtained by reference method and Model B (5, 30, 60, and 120 mins) showed a positive linear correlation ($R^2 = 0.97$, $P = 0.98$; Figure 5(b)). Pearson correlation testing between GFR values

TABLE 2: The mean of bodyweight (BW), plasma urea (PU), plasma creatinine concentration (PCr), 7-point reference clearance of IOX (GFR 7 samples: 5, 30, 60, 120, 240, 360, and 480 minutes), and simplified models clearance of IOX in nonazotaemic and azotaemic cats. *Significantly different to nonazotaemic cats at $P < 0.05$.

Cats	BW (kg)	PU (mmol/L)	PCr (μmol/L)	GFR (mL/min/kg) 7 samples	GFR (mL/min/kg) Model A	GFR (mL/min/kg) Model B	GFR (mL/min/kg) Model C	GFR (mL/min/kg) Model D
Nonazotaemic ($n = 35$)	3.5 (2.0–5.0)	15.29 (6.92–24.13)	106 (78–140)	3.40 (1.21–8.62)	3.32 (1.52–6.80)	3.28 (1.64–6.62)	3.08 (1.40–6.87)	3.43 (1.51–8.30)
Azotaemic ($n = 15$)	3.36 (2.0–5.5)	19.78 (16.63–31.38)	160 (143–209)*	2.38 (1.36–3.47)*	2.11 (1.25–2.99)*	2.57 (1.49–4.17)*	2.28 (1.35–3.66)*	2.26 (1.45–3.81)*

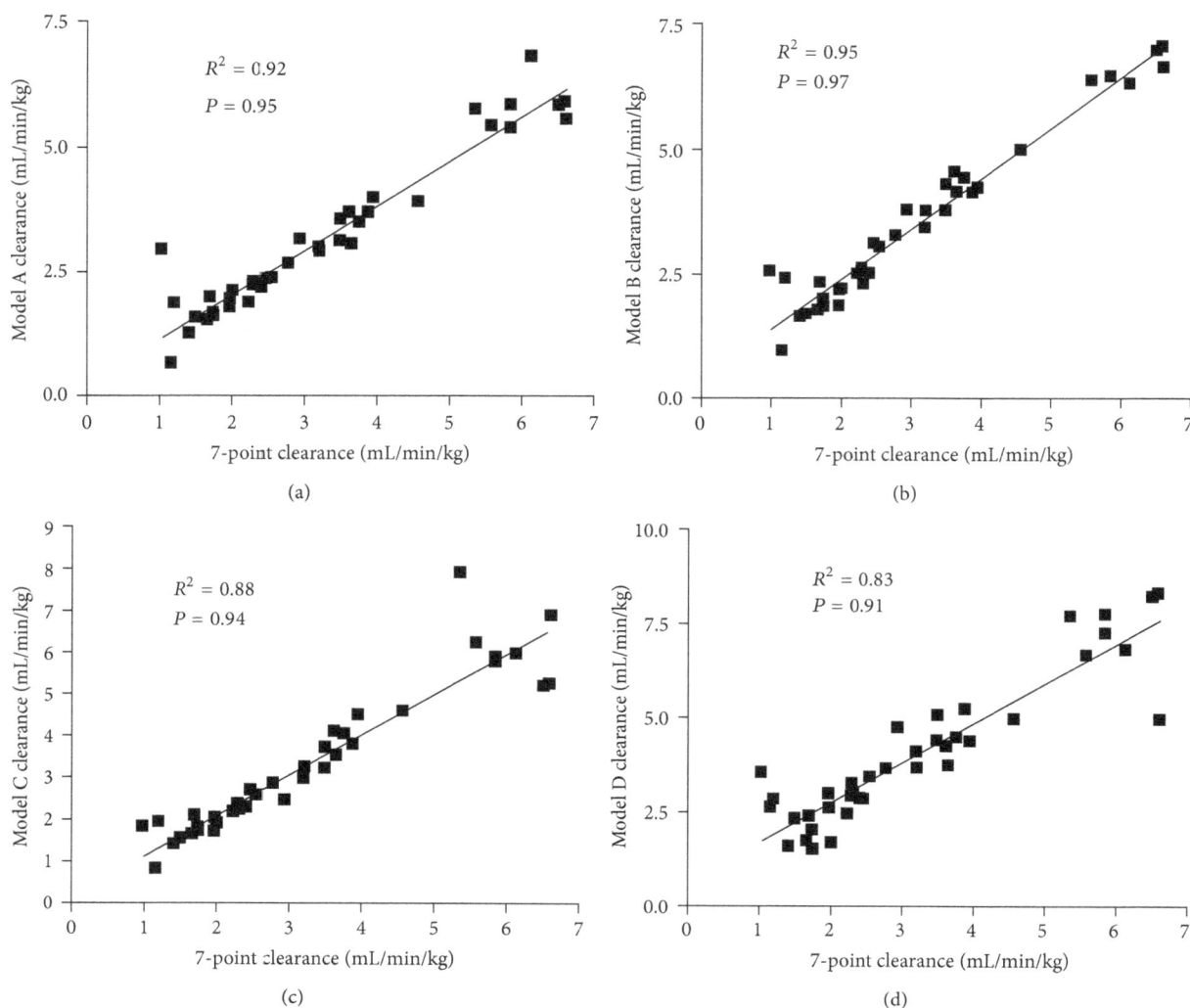

FIGURE 3: The correlation between the 7-point reference clearance and simplified clearance models (a), (b), (c), and (d) in nonazotaemic cats ($n = 35$).

TABLE 3: Results of the accuracies of four simplified clearance Models A, B, C, and D in nonazotaemic cats ($n = 35$) and azotaemic cats ($n = 15$) when compared to GFR determination with 7-point reference clearance. There are no significant differences between the different methods neither at the 15%, the 30% levels nor at the 50% level.

Model	Nonazotaemic Accuracy within			Azotaemic Accuracy within		
	15%	30%	50%	15%	30%	50%
A	87	92	95	92	100	100
B	66	92	95	77	100	100
C	79	92	95	100	100	100
D	47	64	87	53	80	93

obtained by reference method and Model C (5, 60, 120, and 240 mins) showed a positive linear correlation ($R^2 = 0.97$, $P = 0.98$; Figure 5(c)). Pearson correlation testing between

GFR values obtained by reference method and Model D (5, 30, and 60 mins) showed a positive linear correlation ($R^2 = 0.64$, $P = 0.80$; Figure 5(d)). The results from Bland-Altman analysis are given in Figure 6. The accuracies of all models tested were not significantly different from those of the reference method (Table 3).

Plasma clearance of IOX, determined with 3-point clearance Model D, in analyzed nonazotaemic cats ranged from 1.51 to 8.30 mL/min/kg (mean ± SEM, 4.07 ± 0.34 mL/min/kg) while in azotaemic cats it ranged from 1.45 to 3.81 mL/min/kg (mean ± SEM 2.26 ± 0.21 mL/min/kg). There were significant differences between the two groups in GFR ($P = 0.008$) (Table 2).

4. Discussion

The importance of early diagnosis in slowing down the progression of CKD has been widely demonstrated both in veterinary medicine and in human medicine [33–35].

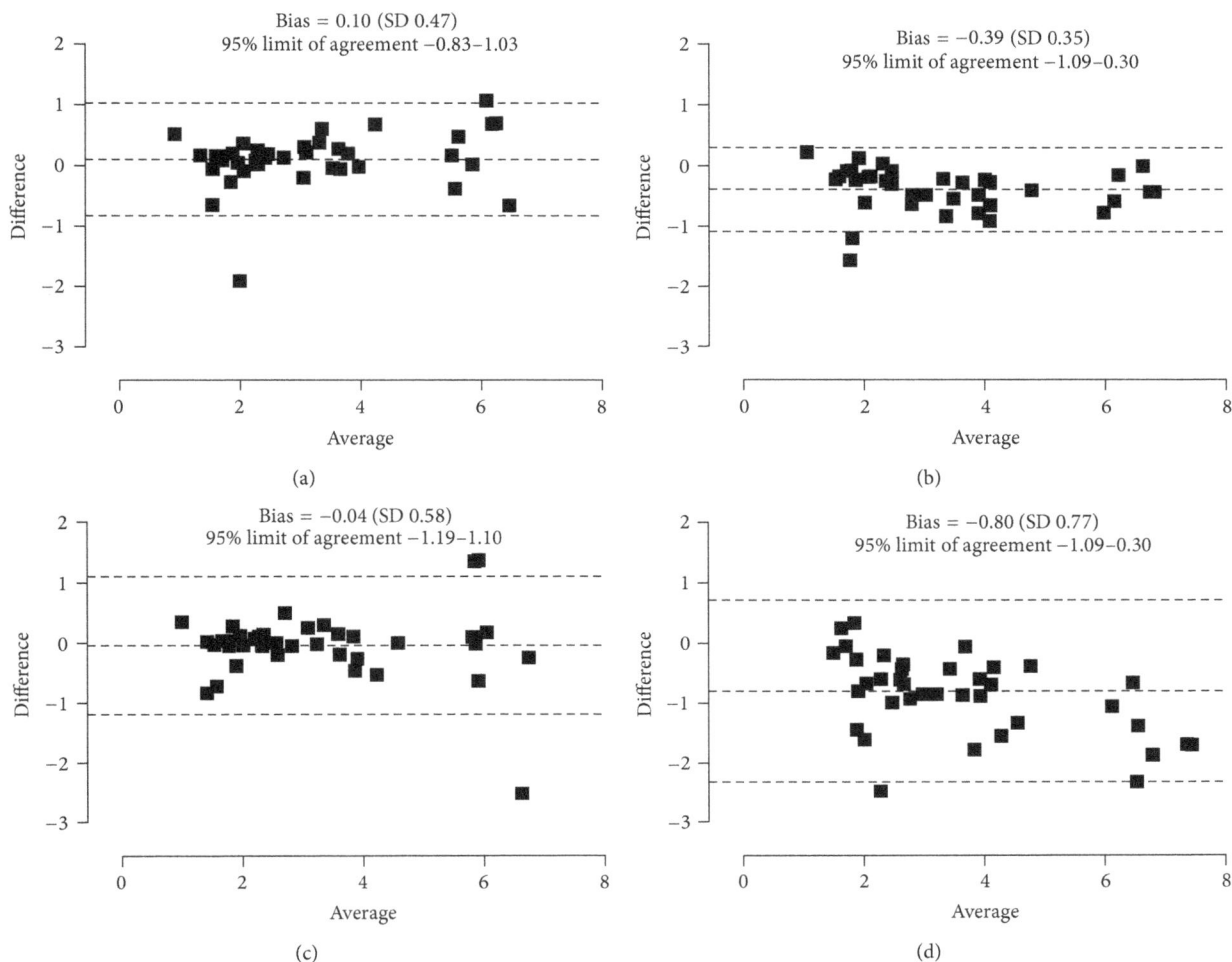

FIGURE 4: Bland-Altman plots of difference *versus* average of GFR between the 7-point reference clearance and simplified clearance models (a), (b), (c), and (d) in nonazotaemic cats ($n = 35$).

Unfortunately, although GFR is universally considered the gold standard test to evaluate overall renal function, its use in veterinary clinical practice is still uncommon, due to technical difficulties, high number of samples, and low availability of markers.

The present study showed a fast, accurate, and relatively simple method for GFR determination in feline patients by using IOX plasma clearance evaluation. Plasma clearance methods are easier to be performed compared to urinary clearance methods and represent an attractive way of GFR determination. IOX has been shown to be a good alternative to inulin and radioactive tracers in human [36], pig [37, 38], horse [39], donkey [40], dog and cat [13–41].

Currently available HPLC systems to determine plasma IOX concentration have been proven to give reliable data, but they still present some disadvantages to be routinely used for the early diagnosis of CKD in a clinical setting. The method investigated in the present study has combined an easy sample preparation and a rapid HPLC run with a simple mobile phase. Analysis has been performed with inexpensive, nonhazardous, and readily available chemicals.

The robustness of the method enables ease for operators to learn the technique and to generate reproducible results. The method indeed is very economical, with an approximate cost per sample of less than two Euros for supplies and materials. In fact, a single analytical column, under the assay condition, has lasted for the entire period of method validation and clinical study. Furthermore, the stability test has indicated that plasma samples can be frozen or sent by mail, and this would be attractive for general practitioners, who could send samples to a reference laboratory. This HPLC method requires a very small volume of plasma (50 μL). Such limited amounts of plasma may be a significant advantage in a feline clinical setting, especially when anaemic or dehydrated animals are involved. At the dosage used in this study, IOX can be safely utilized even in debilitated or severely azotaemic subjects. Furthermore, no one of the enrolled cats has shown immediate or subsequent side effects. In the authors' experience the use of two intravenous catheters (one utilized for IOX injection and the other one for taking blood samples) has increased the compliance of owners and patients.

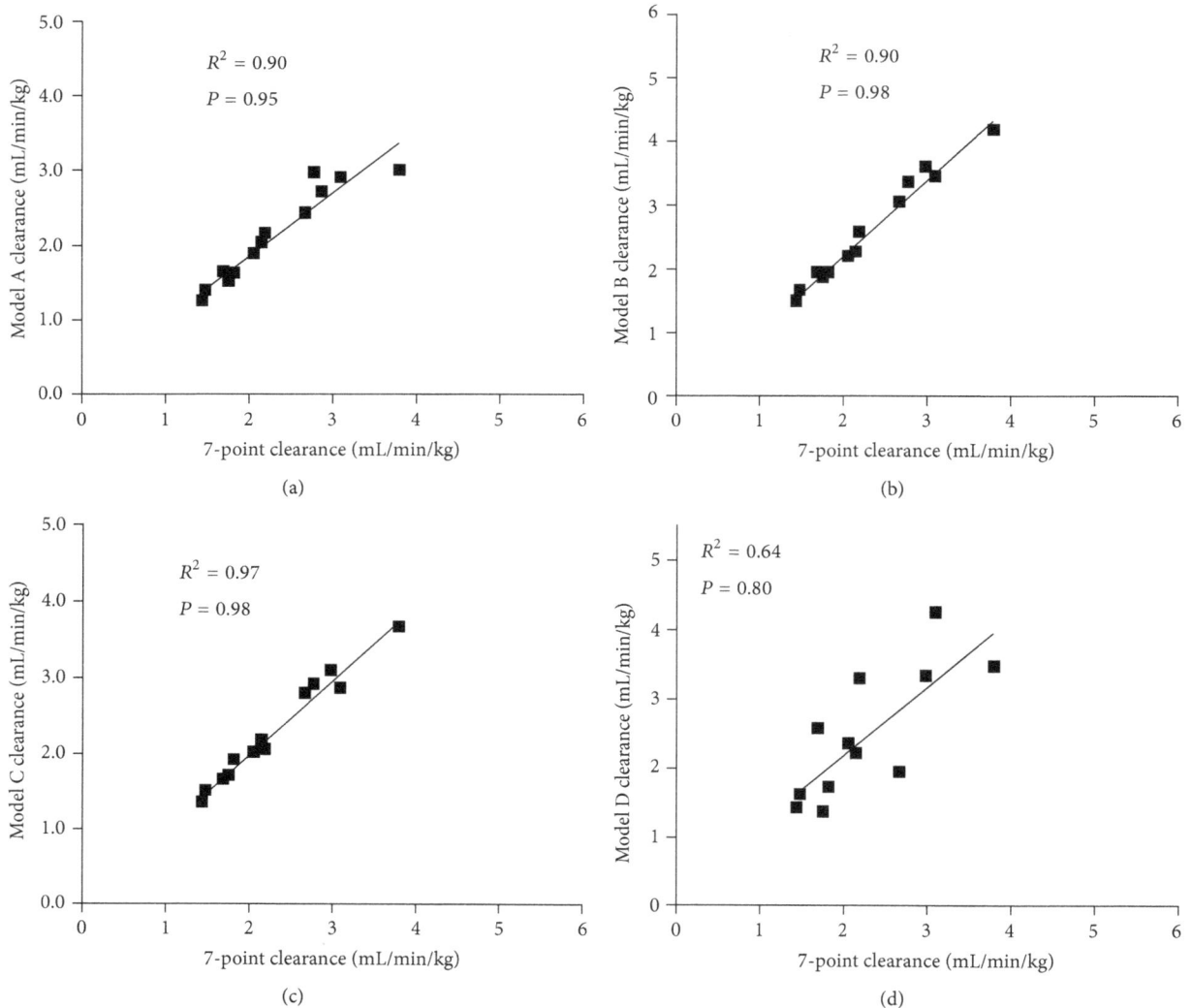

FIGURE 5: The correlation between the 7-point reference clearance and simplified clearance models (a), (b), (c), and (d) in azotaemic cats ($n = 15$).

The use of a seven-sample method to estimate plasma clearance of a tracer is an extremely accurate way of performing curve fitting with nonlinear regression analysis, but it is too time consuming and expensive and it could be excessively stressful for feline patients. Furthermore, the high number (seven) of blood samples required is too cumbersome to be used in a clinical setting. Limited sampling strategies for plasma clearance procedures have been investigated extensively in humans [42] and more recently in animals [43, 44] for establishing a quick, inexpensive, and clinically accurate value of GFR.

In the present study, plasma clearance values were determined by a noncompartmental approach. This approach is more convenient if the sampling period covers a sufficient period because it does not require specific mathematical modelling. The only parameter required, and which is easily calculated, is the AUC. The dose/AUC approach has shown to be both highly reproducible and the most precise and accurate strategy for GFR determination in healthy humans using sinistrin as marker [45]. It was demonstrated in the same study that a better estimation of GFR was obtained by extrapolating to infinity. The extrapolated part of the AUC should not exceed 20% of the total AUC. In the present study the extrapolated part of the AUC did not exceed 25% with all the simplified models analysed, and this in combination with fast, cheap, and accurate methods of analysis is therefore adequate for GFR estimation in cats in clinical settings. All simplified models, that have been taken into consideration in the present study, have shown a high accuracy in determining GFR, in both nonazotaemic and azotaemic patients, and have been a significant simplification of the reference method, in terms of time and number of samples. Anyway, among different models, Model D has shown the best solution because it has combined an enough accurate GFR determination with a very quick and easy-to-perform method. Model D was chosen as the best simplified

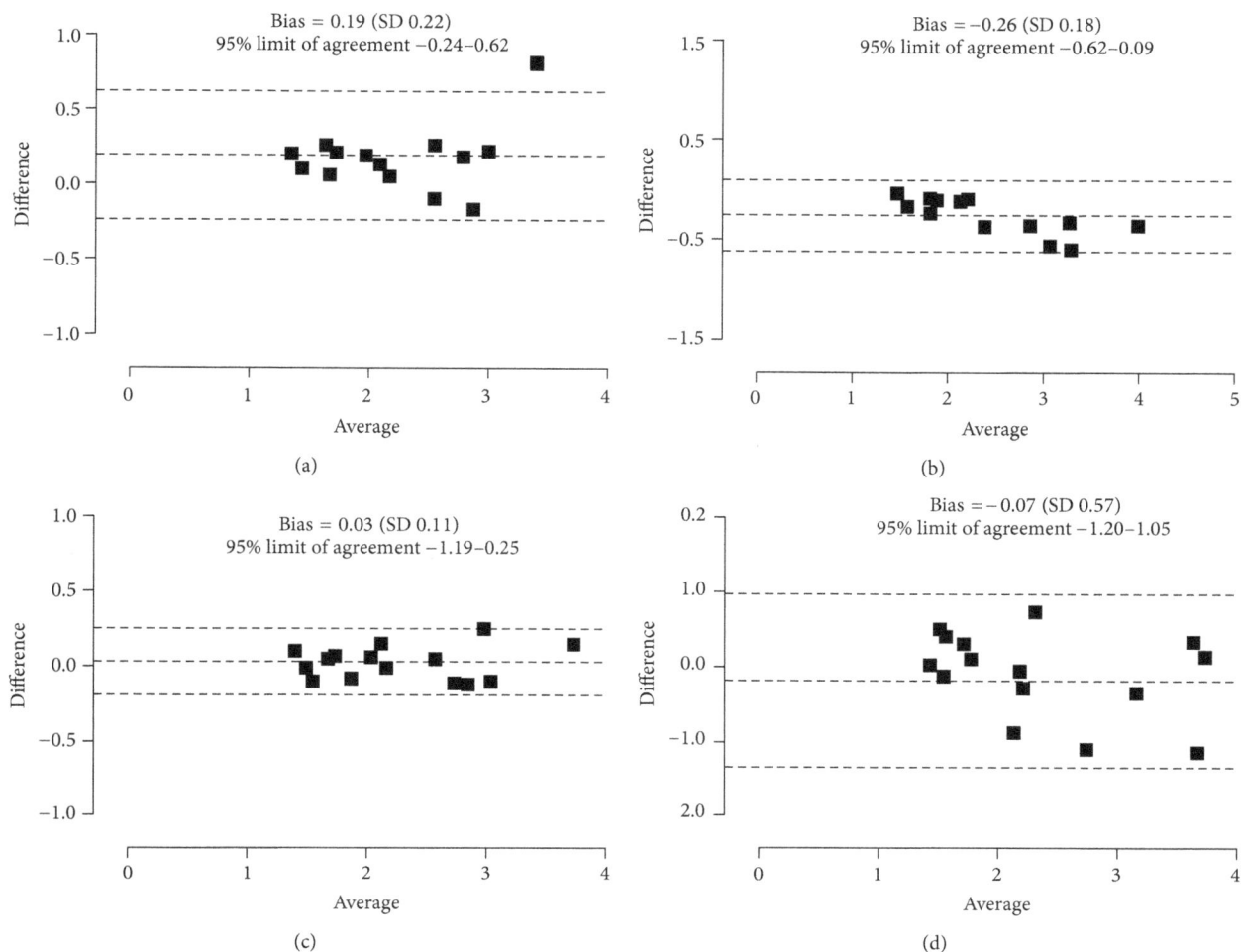

FIGURE 6: Bland-Altman plots of difference *versus* average of GFR between the 7-point reference clearance and simplified clearance models (a), (b), (c), and (d) in azotaemic cats ($n = 15$).

method also because it provided an enough accurate and precise GFR value using 3 blood samples only in one hour. This model is not the most precise one among all tested, but it represents a good compromise between precision and owner and patient compliance. An easy and rapid assay to determine GFR would be extremely useful for an early diagnosis of CKD in feline patients.

In conclusion, the present study has validated a safe, simple, and accurate three-sample HPLC method for the determination of GFR through the plasma clearance of IOX in feline patients. This method represents an attractive and cheap alternative to cumbersome plasma clearance methods, with a dramatic applicatory potential in different clinical settings. The accuracy of HPLC analysis, the possibility to mail plasma sample to a referring laboratory, and the high compliance of this method would lead general practitioners to an even more easy diagnosis of subclinical stages of CKD and to a better management of the disease.

Sources and Manufacturers

Pharsight, Mountain View, CA, USA.

References

[1] E. M. Lund, P. J. Armstrong, C. A. Kirk, L. M. Kolar, and J. S. Klausner, "Health status and population characteristics of dogs and cats examined at private veterinary practices in the United States," *Journal of the American Veterinary Medical Association*, vol. 214, no. 9, pp. 1336–1341, 1999.

[2] A. D. J. Watson, "Indicators of renal insufficiency in dogs and cats presented at a veterinary teaching hospital," *Australian Veterinary Practitioner*, vol. 31, no. 2, pp. 54–59, 2001.

[3] D. R. Finco, S. A. Brown, S. L. Vaden et al., "Relationship between plasma creatinine concentration and glomerular filtration rate in dogs," *American Journal of Veterinary Research*, vol. 33, pp. 2447–2450, 1995.

[4] A. Gleadhill, "Evaluation of screening tests for renal insufficiency in the dog," *Journal of Small Animal Practice*, vol. 35, pp. 391–396, 1994.

[5] Y. Miyagawa, N. Takemura, and H. Hirose, "Assessments of factors that affect glomerular filtration rate and indirect markers of renal function in dogs and cats," *Journal of Veterinary Medical Science*, vol. 72, no. 9, pp. 1129–1136, 2010.

[6] D. Polzin, C. Osborne, and S. Ross, "Chronic kidney disease," in *Textbook of Veterinary Internal Medicine*, S. J. Ettinger and E.

Feldman, Eds., pp. 1698–1703, Elsevier Saunders, Philadelphia, Pa, USA, 6th edition, 2004.

[7] K. S. Rogers, A. Komkov, S. A. Brown, G. E. Lees, D. Hightower, and E. A. Russo, "Comparison of four methods of estimating glomerular filtration rate in cats," *American Journal of Veterinary Research*, vol. 52, no. 6, pp. 961–964, 1991.

[8] L. A. Ross and D. R. Finco, "Relationship of selected clinical renal function tests to glomerular filtration rate and renal blood flow in cats," *American Journal of Veterinary Research*, vol. 42, no. 10, pp. 1704–1710, 1981.

[9] S. A. Brown, C. Haberman, and D. R. Finco, "Use of plasma clearance of inulin for estimating glomerular filtration rate in cats," *American Journal of Veterinary Research*, vol. 57, no. 12, pp. 1702–1705, 1996.

[10] M. J. Fettman, T. A. Allen, W. L. Wilke, M. J. Radin, and M. C. Eubank, "Single-injection method for evaluation of renal function with 14C-inulin and 3H-tetraethylammonium bromide in dogs and cats," *American Journal of Veterinary Research*, vol. 46, no. 2, pp. 482–485, 1985.

[11] M. Haller, K. Rohner, W. Müller et al., "Single-injection inulin clearance for routine measurement of glomerular filtration rate in cats," *Journal of Feline Medicine and Surgery*, vol. 5, no. 3, pp. 175–181, 2003.

[12] M. E. Kerl and C. R. Cook, "Glomerular filtration rate and renal scintigraphy," *Clinical Techniques in Small Animal Practice*, vol. 20, no. 1, pp. 31–38, 2005.

[13] K. Miyamoto, "Evaluation of plasma clearance of inulin in clinically normal and partially nephrectomized cats," *American Journal of Veterinary Research*, vol. 62, no. 8, pp. 1332–1335, 2001.

[14] K. Miyamoto, "Use of plasma clearance of iohexol for estimating glomerular filtration rate in cats," *American Journal of Veterinary Research*, vol. 62, no. 4, pp. 572–575, 2001.

[15] D. Uribe, D. R. Krawiec, A. R. Twardock, and H. B. Gelberg, "Quantitative renal scintigraphic determination of the glomerular filtration rate in cats with normal and abnormal kidney function, using 99mTc-diethylenetriaminepentaacetic acid," *American Journal of Veterinary Research*, vol. 53, no. 7, pp. 1101–1107, 1992.

[16] R. Heiene, B. S. Reynolds, N. H. Bexfield, S. Larsen, and R. J. Gerritsen, "Estimation of glomerular filtration rate via 2- and 4-sample plasma clearance of iohexol and creatinine in clinically normal cats," *American Journal of Veterinary Research*, vol. 70, no. 2, pp. 176–185, 2009.

[17] N. C. Finch, H. M. Syme, J. Elliott et al., "Glomerular filtration rate estimation by use of a correction formula for slope-intercept plasma iohexol clearance in cats," *American Journal of Veterinary Research*, vol. 72, no. 12, pp. 1652–1659, 2011.

[18] N. C. Finch, R. Heiene, J. Elliott et al., "A single method for estimating glomerular filtration rate in cats," *Journal of Veterinary Internal Medicine*, vol. 27, pp. 782–790, 2013.

[19] Y. Miyagawa, N. Takemura, and H. Hirose, "Evaluation of a single sampling method for estimation of plasma iohexol clearance in dogs and cats with various kidney functions," *Journal of Veterinary Medical Science*, vol. 72, no. 3, pp. 271–278, 2010.

[20] R. Katayama, J. Saito, M. Katayama et al., "Simplified procedure for estimation of glomerular filtration rate following intravenous administration of iodixanol in cats," *American Journal of Veterinary Research*, vol. 73, pp. 1344–1349, 2012.

[21] I. Goy-Thollot, S. Besse, F. Garnier, M. Marignan, and P. Y. Barthez, "Simplified methods for estimation of plasma clearance of iohexol in dogs and cats," *Journal of Veterinary Internal Medicine*, vol. 20, no. 1, pp. 52–56, 2006.

[22] F. Gaspari, N. Perico, M. Matalone et al., "Precision of plasma clearance of iohexol for estimation of GFR in patients with renal disease," *Journal of the American Society of Nephrology*, vol. 9, no. 2, pp. 310–313, 1998.

[23] I. Goy-Thollot, C. Chafotte, S. Besse, F. Garnier, and P. Y. Barthez, "Iohexol plasma clearance in healthy dogs and cats," *Veterinary Radiology and Ultrasound*, vol. 47, no. 2, pp. 168–173, 2006.

[24] W. E. Braselton, K. J. Stuart, and J. M. Kruger, "Measurement of serum iohexol by determination of iodine with inductively coupled plasma-atomic emission spectroscopy," *Clinical Chemistry*, vol. 43, no. 8, pp. 1429–1435, 1997.

[25] V. Meucci, A. Gasperini, G. Soldani, G. Guidi, and M. Giorgi, "A New HPLC method to determine glomerular filtration rate and effective renal plasma flow in conscious dogs by single intravenous administration of iohexol and p-aminohippuric acid," *Journal of Chromatographic Science*, vol. 42, no. 2, pp. 107–111, 2004.

[26] I. van Hoek, H. P. Lefebvre, H. S. Kooistra et al., "Plasma clearance of exogenous creatinine, exo-iohexol, and endo-iohexol in hyperthyroid cats before and after treatment with radioiodine," *Journal of Veterinary Internal Medicine*, vol. 22, no. 4, pp. 879–885, 2008.

[27] I. van Hoek, E. Vandermeulen, L. Duchateau et al., "Comparison and reproducibility of plasma clearance of exogenous creatinine, exo-iohexol, endo-iohexol, and 51Cr-EDTA in young adult and aged healthy cats," *Journal of Veterinary Internal Medicine*, vol. 21, no. 5, pp. 950–958, 2007.

[28] S.-E. Bäck, P. Masson, and P. Nilsson-Ehle, "A simple chemical method for the quantification of the contrast agent iohexol, applicable to glomerular filtration rate measurements," *Scandinavian Journal of Clinical and Laboratory Investigation*, vol. 48, no. 8, pp. 825–829, 1988.

[29] Z. K. Shihabi and M. S. Constantinescu, "Iohexol in serum determined by capillary electrophoresis," *Clinical Chemistry*, vol. 38, no. 10, pp. 2117–2120, 1992.

[30] B. Frennby and G. Sterner, "Contrast media as markers of GFR," *European Radiology*, vol. 12, no. 2, pp. 475–484, 2002.

[31] P. Nilsson-Ehle, "Iohexol clearance for the determination of glomerular filtration rate: 15 years experience in clinical practice," *Electronic Journal Journal of the International Federation of Clinical Chemistry*, vol. 13, no. 2, 2001, http://www.ifcc.org/ifcc-communications-publications-division-(cpd)/ifcc-publications/ejifcc-(journal)/e-journal-volumes/ejifcc-2002-vol-13/vol-13-no-2/iohexol-clearance-for-the-determination-of-glomerular-filtration-rate-15-years-experience-in-cl/.

[32] "ICH harmonised tripartite guideline, validation of analytical procedures: text and methodology Q2(R1), current step 4 version," in *Proceedings of the International Conference on Harmanisation of Technical Requirements for Registration of Pharmaceuticals for Human Use*, November 2005, http://www.ich.org/fileadmin/Public_Web_Site/ICH_Products/Guidelines/Quality/Q2_R1/Step4/Q2_R1_Guideline.pdf.

[33] R. Heiene and H. P. Lefebvre, "Assessment of renal function," in *Manual of Canine and Feline Nephrology and Urology*, J. Elliott and G. F. Grauer, Eds., pp. 117–125, BSAVA, Gloucester, UK, 2nd edition, 2007.

[34] J. Coresh, E. Selvin, L. A. Stevens et al., "Prevalence of chronic kidney disease in the United States," *Journal of the American Medical Association*, vol. 298, no. 17, pp. 2038–2047, 2007.

[35] Q.-L. Zhang and D. Rothenbacher, "Prevalence of chronic kidney disease in population-based studies: systematic review," *BMC Public Health*, vol. 8, article 117, 2008.

[36] L. A. Stevens and A. S. Levey, "Measured GFR as a confirmatory test for estimated GFR," *Journal of the American Society of Nephrology*, vol. 20, no. 11, pp. 2305–2313, 2009.

[37] B. Frennby, G. Sterner, T. Almén, C. M. Chai, B. A. Jönsson, and S. Månsson, "Clearance of iohexol, chromium-51-ethylenediaminetetraacetic acid, and creatinine for determining the glomerular filtration rate in pigs with normal renal function: comparison of different clearance techniques," *Academic Radiology*, vol. 3, no. 8, pp. 651–659, 1996.

[38] B. Frennby, G. Sterner, T. Almén, C.-M. Chai, B. A. Jönsson, and S. Månsson, "Clearance of iohexol, 51Cr-EDTA and endogenous creatinine for determination of glomerular filtration rate in pigs with reduced renal function: a comparison between different clearance techniques," *Scandinavian Journal of Clinical and Laboratory Investigation*, vol. 57, no. 3, pp. 241–252, 1997.

[39] K. E. Wilson, J. R. Wilcke, M. V. Crisman, D. L. Ward, H. C. McKenzie, and W. K. Scarratt, "Comparison of serum iohexol clearance and plasma creatinine clearance in clinically normal horses," *American Journal of Veterinary Research*, vol. 70, no. 12, pp. 1545–1550, 2009.

[40] I. Lippi, V. Meucci, M. Sgorbini, C. Michele, and G. Guidi, "Valutazione della velocità di filtrazione glomerulare nellasino sorcino crociato dellAmiata mediante clearance plasmatica dello ioexolo con metodica HPLC," in *Proceed of the Società Italiana Veterinari per Equini (SIVE '10)*, pp. 1–2, Montesilvano, Italy, 2010.

[41] N. H. Bexfield, R. Heiene, R. J. Gerritsen et al., "Glomerular filtration rate estimated by 3-sample plasma clearance of iohexol in 118 healthy dogs," *Journal of Veterinary Internal Medicine*, vol. 22, no. 1, pp. 66–73, 2008.

[42] G. J. Schwartz and S. L. Furth, "Glomerular filtration rate measurement and estimation in chronic kidney disease," *Pediatric Nephrology*, vol. 22, no. 11, pp. 1839–1848, 2007.

[43] A. D. J. Watson, H. P. Lefebvre, D. Concordet et al., "Plasma exogenous creatinine clearance test in dogs: comparison with other methods and proposed limited sampling strategy," *Journal of Veterinary Internal Medicine*, vol. 16, no. 1, pp. 22–33, 2002.

[44] I. Lippi, V. Meucci, G. Guidi et al., "Velocita di filtrazione glomerulare mediante clearance plasmatica dello ioexolo nel cane: confronto tra metodi semplificati," *Veterinaria*, vol. 22, pp. 53–60, 2008.

[45] T. Buclin, A. Pechère-Bertschi, R. Séchaud et al., "Sinistrin clearance for determination of glomerular filtration rate: a reappraisal of various approaches using a new analytical method," *Journal of Clinical Pharmacology*, vol. 37, no. 8, pp. 679–692, 1997.

10

Hemostatic Markers in Congestive Heart Failure Dogs with Mitral Valve Disease

Kreangsak Prihirunkit,[1] **Amornrate Sastravaha,**[2]
Chalermpol Lekcharoensuk,[2] **and Phongsak Chanloinapha**[3]

[1] *Department of Pathology, Faculty of Veterinary Medicine, Kasetsart University, Bangkok 10900, Thailand*
[2] *Department of Small Animal Sciences, Faculty of Veterinary Medicine, Kasetsart University, Bangkok 10900, Thailand*
[3] *Veterinary Teaching Hospital, Kasetsart University, Bangkok 10900, Thailand*

Correspondence should be addressed to Kreangsak Prihirunkit; fvetksp@ku.ac.th

Academic Editor: Alejandro Plascencia

Prothrombin time (PT), activated partial thromboplastin time (APTT), fibrinogen, D-dimer, antithrombin III (AT III), protein C (PC), factor VII (F.VII), and factor VIII (F.VIII), as well as hematocrit (HCT), platelets number (PLT), total plasma protein (TP), and albumin (ALB), were studied on fifty-eight congestive heart failure (CHF) dogs with mitral valve disease (MVD) and fifty control dogs. All of variables of MVD group, except APTT, were significantly different ($P < 0.5$) from control group. The variables were also compared among functional classes of CHF dogs and control dogs. It was determined that the higher the functional class of CHF dogs was, the greater the levels of fibrinogen and D-dimer were, whereas the lesser the activities of AT III and PC were presented. Additionally, TP had linear correlation with fibrinogen, D-dimer, HCT, and PLT ($r = 0.31$, 0.30, 0.43, and 0.38, resp., $P < 0.5$). These findings suggested that fibrinogen and D-dimer were the factors predisposing hypercoagulability through an increase in blood viscosity. The hemorheological abnormalities would shift an overall hemostatic balance toward a more thrombotic state in CHF dogs with MVD.

1. Introduction

Degenerative valve disease is one of the most common forms of canine heart disease and is also known as endocardiosis [1]. The most commonly affected valve in the dog is the mitral valve [2]. It is a well-compensated disease with a long evolution [3]. A genetic tendency to develop the disease has been proved in Cavalier King Charles Spaniel and Dachshunds [4]. Grossly, mitral valve disease (MVD) is a markedly thickened valve with the swollen free edge. As the disease progresses, the regurgitation of blood from the ventricle into the atrium causes volume overload and possibly leads to congestive heart failure (CHF) [5].

CHF has been associated with the profound clinical effects of hemostasis. The high plasma markers of thrombin activity, fibrinolytic activity, and platelet activation have been reported [6, 7]. Even though heart failure in human is associated with thromboembolic stroke risk, the prevalence of overt clinical thromboembolism in dogs with CHF is rarely reported [8].

Thromboembolic complications have been attributed to an imbalance between procoagulant and anticoagulant factors, including thrombocytosis, hemoconcentration, hyperviscosity, and immobilization [9]. Protein C (PC) and antithrombin III (AT III) are major natural anticoagulants. They play an important role in preventing excessive coagulation, whereas fibrinogen and D-dimer indicate the thromboembolic tendency [10].

The diagnosis of hypercoagulation is essential for identification of individuals at higher risk of thrombosis and for an early treatment of thrombotic disorders. Since the investigations relevant to the determination of coagulation in dogs with MVD remain scanty, the aims of the present study therefore are (1) to compare the levels of hemostatic markers between the MVD and the control dogs and (2) to investigate the alteration of coagulation parameters among groups of functional class of CHF dogs.

2. Materials and Methods

2.1. The Study Site. The study was carried out at the Veterinary Teaching Hospital, Kasetsart University, Thailand. In total, 108 dogs were categorized into MVD group ($n = 58$) and control group ($n = 50$). On the basis of physical examination, chest radiography, electrocardiography, and echocardiographic performance with cardiac alteration score, as previously described [5], 58 CHF dogs with MVD were selected from cardiology clinic. All patients were diagnosed and classified as the functional class of CHF by only one cardiologist. To classify CHF in dogs, New York Heart Association (NYHA) Classification was applied [11]. Patients were excluded if they had other thrombotic risk factors, such as infection, disseminated intravascular coagulation, diabetes, Cushing's disease, and neoplasm. Complete blood count (CBC) was performed to exclude ongoing inflammation. Dogs in control group were recruited from blood donors and were checked up by veterinarians as clinically healthy. None of the dogs received antithrombotic agents within 6 months prior to sample collection.

2.2. Collection and Preparation of Blood Samples. In each patient and each control dog, a CBC was conducted from the blood collected under aseptic conditions in tubes containing K_3EDTA as an anticoagulant. Clotted blood samples were used for clinical chemistry analysis, including total plasma protein (TP) and albumin (ALB). Blood samples for a coagulation profile: prothrombin time (PT), activated partial thromboplastin time (APTT), fibrinogen, D-dimer, antithrombin III (AT III), protein C (PC), factor VII (F.VII), and factor VIII (F.VIII), were collected using siliconized vacutainer tubes containing 3.18% trisodium citrate as an anticoagulant with a ratio of 9 : 1 (vol/vol). The samples were centrifuged at 4,500 rpm for 15 min to obtain platelet-poor plasma and were stored at −80°C until evaluation.

2.3. Sample Analysis. The CBCs were done by an automated hematology analyzer (Cell-Dyn 3500, Abbot Diagnostics, Illinois, USA); blood chemical tests were evaluated by an automated chemical analyzer (Liasys, AMS Diagnostics, Rome, Italy). According to the manufacturer's guidelines, the coagulation profiles were assayed, using Dade Behring (Marburg, Germany) diagnostic kits. The coagulation tests were carried out on an automated blood coagulation analyzer (Sysmex CA-1500, Kobe, Japan) with coagulometric, chromogenic, and immunoturbidimetric methods. PT and APTT were measured automatically as clotting tests using commercial reagents. The test results were reported in seconds. Fibrinogen concentration was determined by clotting assay. The enzyme thrombin converted the soluble plasma fibrinogen into its insoluble fibrin and was then inversely proportional to the fibrinogen concentration by a comparison with the fibrinogen calibration curve [12]. D-dimer

concentration was measured with an immunoturbidimetric method. The assay detected an antigen-antibody reaction according to the endpoint method. The result was reported as μg/mL fibrinogen equivalent units. Measurement of both F.VII and F.VIII was performed in PT and APTT assays with a mixture of the F.VII and F.VIII deficient substrate plasmas, respectively. The results were interpreted, using a standard calibration curve. AT III and PC activities were assessed by functional chromogenic assay. Two steps for AT III activity measurement were performed. First, the test plasma was incubated with an excessive amount of thrombin reagent in the presence of heparin. Second, the color was measured by the reaction between the chromogenic substrate and the residual thrombin after being neutralized by AT III in the sample. The color of the reaction was inversely proportional to the AT III level monitored kinetically at 405 nm. The percentage activity was read using the standard calibration curve [13]. For the measurement of PC, a specific snake venom activator was used to activate PC in the sample which was converted to activated PC. Then, the color of the reaction was proportional to the PC level monitored kinetically at 405 nm. The percentage activity was read by the standard calibration curve [14].

All of calibration curves prepared for the coagulation profile were modified using canine-pool plasma instead of commercial, lyophilized human plasma. Thirty canine plasma were mixed and used as normal pooled plasma. To generate the standard curves of AT III, PC, F.VII, and F.VIII, the canine-pool plasma was assigned as 100% activity. Subsequently, it was diluted through a dynamic linear range from 0% to 100% activity of each assay.

2.4. Statistical Analysis. Data were analyzed by the NCSS software [15]. The results of all variables: PT, APTT, fibrinogen, D-dimer, AT III, PC, F.VII, F.VIII, hematocrit (HCT), platelets number (PLT), TP, and ALB, were expressed as a mean ± SD. Differences of these variables between MVD and control groups and among functional classes of CHF dogs were determined by using a general linear model. Age, weight, and breed were not included in the model as covariates for multivariate analysis. If the model showed significance, Fisher's LSD multiple comparison was used to compare the means. Spearman's rank correlation coefficient (r) was used for the correlation analyses. The linear relationship was interpreted as follows: r between 0 and 0.3 (0 and −0.3) indicated a weak positive (negative), r between 0.3 and 0.7 (−0.3 and −0.7) indicated a moderate positive (negative), and r between 0.7 and 1.0 (−0.7 and −1.0) indicated a strong positive (negative) linear relationship, respectively. All tests were two-tailed, and a value with $P < 0.05$ was considered of statistical significance.

3. Results

Fifty-eight CHF dogs with MVD were included in final analyses. They were consisting of 38 males and 20 females of various breeds, including 1 Dachshund, 1 Spitz, 2 Miniature Pinschers, 2 Golden Retrievers, 3 Dalmatians, 14 Shih Tzus,

TABLE 1: Demographic data from 50 control dogs and 58 CHF dogs with MVD.

	Control ($n = 50$)	NYHA classification				Total CHF ($n = 58$)
		I ($n = 2$)	II ($n = 19$)	III ($n = 32$)	IV ($n = 5$)	
Age (year)	5.5 ± 1.4	13 ± 4.2	10.2 ± 3.4	10.8 ± 3.0	11.6 ± 2.1	10.8 ± 3.1
Weight (Kgs)	33.3 ± 8.4	17.1 ± 10.5	8.5 ± 6.4	7.3 ± 5.4	15.8 ± 10.5	8.8 ± 6.8
Sex (male/female)	33/17	1/1	14/5	18/14	5/0	38/20

TABLE 2: Comparison of selected coagulation, hematology, and blood chemistry parameters among various NYHA functional classes of CHF group and control group.

	Control ($n = 50$)	NYHA functional class				Total patients ($n = 58$)
		I ($n = 2$)	II ($n = 19$)	III ($n = 32$)	IV ($n = 5$)	
PT (sec.)	7.1 ± 0.5^{1a}	7.0 ± 0.1^{abc}	6.9 ± 0.3^{ab}	6.8 ± 0.3^{bc}	6.5 ± 0.3^{c}	6.9 ± 0.3^{2}
APTT (sec.)	12.2 ± 0.7^{1a}	12.3 ± 0.3^{a}	12.0 ± 0.4^{a}	12.0 ± 0.6^{a}	11.7 ± 0.4^{a}	12.0 ± 0.5^{1}
Fibrinogen (mg/dL)	175.2 ± 37.4^{1a}	223.5 ± 55.0^{ab}	268.8 ± 88.5^{b}	275.9 ± 99.5^{b}	351.8 ± 83.9^{c}	278.3 ± 94.9^{2}
D-dimer (μg/mL)	117.2 ± 36.9^{1a}	197.0 ± 45.3^{ab}	419.2 ± 173.2^{b}	742.8 ± 300.6^{c}	1349.8 ± 445.4^{d}	670.3 ± 380.7^{2}
ATIII (%)	112.6 ± 16.5^{1a}	88.7 ± 4.5^{abc}	87.2 ± 21.0^{b}	84.7 ± 27.1^{b}	59.2 ± 23.1^{c}	83.5 ± 25.2^{2}
PC (%)	110.2 ± 12.9^{1a}	99.8 ± 8.3^{ab}	101.2 ± 24.6^{ab}	93.3 ± 33.3^{b}	57.3 ± 21.7^{c}	93.0 ± 31.1^{2}
F.VII (%)	99.9 ± 15.8^{1a}	101.0 ± 8.5^{ab}	124.6 ± 36.5^{b}	125.8 ± 23.5^{b}	132.9 ± 15.9^{b}	125.2 ± 27.7^{2}
F.VIII (%)	98.1 ± 12.9^{1a}	112.4 ± 10.5^{ab}	124.7 ± 29.0^{b}	124.0 ± 26.0^{b}	139.3 ± 10.2^{b}	125.1 ± 25.8^{2}
HCT (%)	37.4 ± 3.0^{1a}	42.5 ± 2.3^{ab}	42.4 ± 6.7^{b}	41.8 ± 7.0^{b}	41.0 ± 8.2^{ab}	42.0 ± 6.7^{2}
PLT ($\times 10^{3}/\mu$L)	259.8 ± 45.5^{1a}	257.5 ± 109.6^{ab}	359.5 ± 122.8^{b}	355.5 ± 136.3^{b}	304.8 ± 104.7^{ab}	349.1 ± 128.0^{2}
TP (g/dL)	6.5 ± 0.5^{1a}	7.0 ± 0.3^{ab}	7.6 ± 1.0^{b}	7.5 ± 1.5^{b}	6.7 ± 1.1^{ab}	7.5 ± 1.3^{2}
ALB (g/dL)	3.1 ± 0.3^{1a}	3.4 ± 0.6^{ab}	3.5 ± 0.6^{b}	3.4 ± 0.5^{b}	2.9 ± 0.5^{a}	3.4 ± 0.6^{2}

[1,2] Different superscript numbers indicate statistical significance between MVD group and control group at $P < 0.05$. [a,b,c,d] Different superscript letters indicate statistical significance among various NYHA classes of CHF group and control group at $P < 0.05$.

14 mixed breeds, and 21 Poodles. On the criterion of NYHA, the CHF dogs were classified into Class I ($n = 2$), Class II ($n = 19$), Class III ($n = 32$), and Class IV ($n = 5$). Besides, 50 clinically healthy dogs (33 males and 17 females) were enrolled in the control group. They consisted of 3 Siberian Huskies, 4 German Shepherds, 4 Labrador Retrievers, 14 Golden Retrievers, and 25 mixed breed dogs. Descriptive data is demonstrated in Table 1.

The comparison of selected coagulation, hematology, and blood chemistry profiles: PT, APTT, fibrinogen, D-dimer, AT III, PC, F.VII, F.VIII, hematocrit (HCT), platelets number (PLT), TP, and ALB, between MVD and control groups showed that only APTT was not statistically different ($P > 0.05$) (Figure 1). Those variables were also compared among functional classes of CHF dogs and control dogs. They were summarized in Table 2. It was shown that the more the functional class of CHF dogs was, the more the concentration of fibrinogen and D-dimer increased, whereas the lesser the activity of AT III and PC decreased. However, these were noted significantly ($P < 0.05$) in Class IV CHF dogs. PT of CHF Class III and Class IV was statistically less than that of dogs in control group ($P < 0.05$), but APTT was not significantly different ($P > 0.05$) among functional classes of CHF group and control group. According to the percentage activities of F.VII and F.VIII, only Class I CHF dogs had no

significant difference ($P > 0.05$) compared to that of control dogs, while the levels of HCT, PLT, TP, and ALB of CHF dogs in Class II and Class III were of significant difference ($P < 0.05$) compared to that of dogs in control group.

The simple correlation among variables of the 58 dogs with CHF caused by MVD is shown in Table 3. Fibrinogen correlated positively with D-dimer, F.VII, F.VIII, and TP ($r = 0.54, 0.36, 0.37$, and 0.31, resp.; $P < 0.05$), but negatively correlated with AT III and PC ($r = -0.44$ and -0.33, resp.; $P < 0.05$). D-dimer negatively correlated with AT III and PC ($r = -0.57$ and -0.36, resp.; $P < 0.05$), whereas it was positively correlated with F.VII, F.VIII, HCT, PLT, and TP ($r = 0.44, 0.49, 0.33, 0.31$, and 0.30, resp.; $P < 0.05$). Additionally, a linear correlation was found between hematologic and protein variables.

4. Discussion

Disturbance in hemostasis was a common complication of CHF. In human, the incidence of hypercoagulability was a surrogate for clinical events which potentially caused thromboembolism and mortality in heart failure patients [16]. The thromboembolic complication was not found in the current study, judged by the lack of clinical signs;

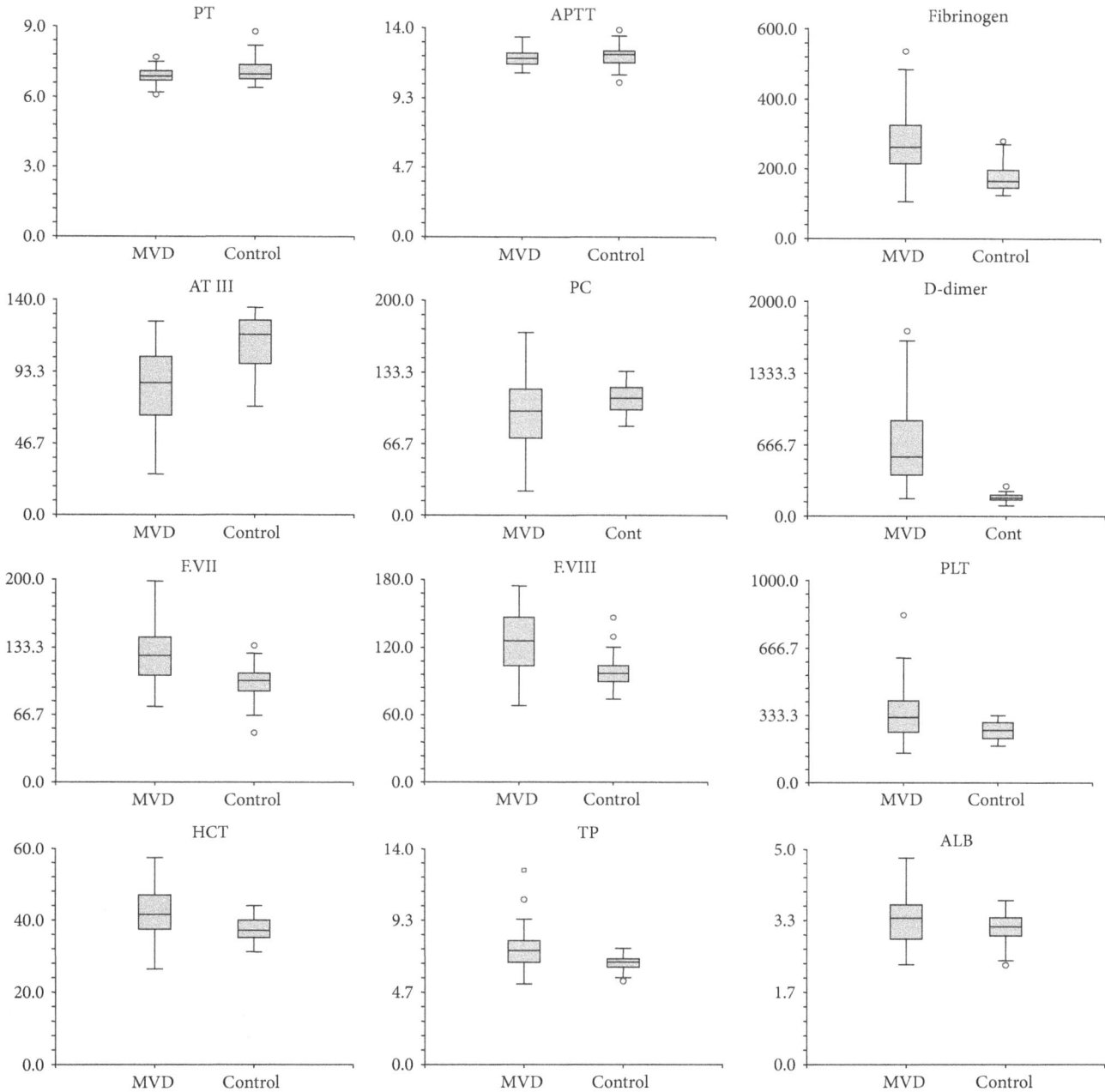

FIGURE 1: Comparison of all parameters; prothrombin time (PT), activated partial thromboplastin time (APTT), fibrinogen, antithrombin III (ATIII), protein C (PC), D-dimer, factor VII (F.VII), factor VIII (F.VIII), platelets number (PLT), hematocrit (HCT), total plasma protein (TP), and albumin (ALB), between dogs with mitral valve disease (MVD) and control (cont.) dogs observed in the study. Data are presented as boxes and whiskers. Each box includes the interquartile range, whereas the line within a box represents the median; the whiskers represent the range and extend to a maximum of 1.5 times the interquartile range. Outliers are depicted by circles.

however, the hypercoagulable parameters were observed. The hemostatic markers: fibrinogen, D-dimer, AT III, and PC, were significant difference between MVD and control groups. Prothrombotic parameters: fibrinogen and D-dimer, concentration increased, whereas natural anticoagulants: AT III and PC, decreased. We also found that the alteration of hemostatic variables related to the severity of heart failure. The higher the functional class of CHF group was, the greater

the levels of fibrinogen and D-dimer were, whereas the lesser the activities of AT III and PC presented. Moreover, correlations among these parameters were remarked. PT and APTT were screening tests and did not correlate with other variables. Likewise, F.VII and F.VIII were not statistically different among NYHA classes of CHF group, but they trended to have an increased percentage activity in higher functional class of CHF dogs. There were also significant

TABLE 3: Correlation between variables of 58 CHF dogs with MVD.

	PT	APTT	Fibrinogen	D-dimer	ATIII	PC	F.VII	F.VIII	HCT	PLT	TP	ALB
PT	1.00											
APTT	0.12	1.00										
Fibrinogen	−0.09	−0.01	1.00									
D-dimer	−0.25	−0.24	0.54[a]	1.00								
AT III	0.22	0.13	−0.44[a]	−0.57[a]	1.00							
PC	0.09	0.01	−0.33[a]	−0.36[a]	0.24	1.00						
F.VII	−0.28	−0.08	0.36[a]	0.44[a]	−0.22	−0.19	1.00					
F.VIII	−0.26	−0.19	0.37[a]	0.49[a]	−0.25	−0.05	0.38[a]	1.00				
HCT	−0.04	0.07	0.20	0.33[a]	−0.26	−0.13	0.24	0.24	1.00			
PLT	−0.11	0.07	0.23	0.31[a]	−0.18	−0.15	0.17	0.18	0.34[a]	1.00		
TP	0.03	−0.20	0.31[a]	0.30[a]	−0.26	−0.12	0.14	0.19	0.43[a]	0.38[a]	1.00	
ALB	0.08	−0.01	0.06	0.14	−0.21	0.04	0.07	0.00	0.44[a]	0.43[a]	0.56[a]	1.00

[a]Significant difference at $P < 0.05$ and r between 0.3 and 0.7 (−0.3 and −0.7) indicate a moderate positive (negative) linear relationship.

linear correlations with fibrinogen and D-dimer; therefore these two variables were supportive laboratory findings.

The altered hemostatic markers suggested that they were important in disease progression and thromboembolic complication. An increased fibrinogen concentration reflected quite well an increased coagulation potential. D-dimers were a specific degradation product of plasmin-cleaved cross-linked fibrin and, therefore, were considered a more specific indicator of hypercoagulable condition [17]. Even though the human D-dimer was applied in the current study, it was able to cross-react with canine D-dimer [18]. AT III and PC were major natural anticoagulants. A decreased level of AT III and PC enhanced thrombin generation which increased coagulation activity [19].

As a result of a further reduction in cardiac output and a worsening of abnormalities in regional blood flow, a hypercoagulable state in patients with CHF was associated with a reduction in plasma volumes [20]. The current study was undertaken to determine the hemorheology of the dogs with CHF. Blood viscosity was determined by an increased level of TP. It significantly increased and positively correlated with fibrinogen, D-dimer, HCT, and PLT. The result indicated that the hematological change has been along with an elevated marker of fibrin turnover: fibrinogen and D-dimer. Although it is important to realize that an increase in plasma fibrinogen concentration may occur as a result of transient fluid shift out of the intravascular space, leading to hemoconcentration, but D-dimer concentration was elevated only by the degradation of cross-linked fibrin [17]. A manifestation of hyperfibrinogenemia may be a factor predisposing hypercoagulability through increase in blood viscosity and formation of platelet aggregation [21]. Together with the viscosity, the increase in hematologic parameters would shift an overall hemostatic balance toward a more hypercoagulable state in the dogs with CHF [22].

Limitation of the current study was that the dogs with MVD and control dogs were not strictly matched regarding breed, age, and sex. Within the MVD group, dogs were small to medium breeds, while the control dogs were recruited from blood donors which were mainly medium to large breed dogs. Moreover, average age of MVD group was older than that of control dogs. Coincidentally, the studied population was male dominant. Based on physical examination and echocardiographic evaluation, a limited number of dogs with NYHA Class I and Class IV were made. Because of mild clinical signs with unlimited physical activity, CHF Class I dogs in this study were found incidentally. On the other hand, a complication was usually found in CHF Class IV dogs. Therefore, these dogs were excluded. Finally, it was the fact that an increased fibrin turnover may also enhance platelet aggregation. Anyhow, the platelet function test was not available in our settings.

5. Conclusion

To a lesser extent of the relationship between thromboembolism and MVD in veterinary study, the present study added up knowledge regarding the hemostatic markers in CHF dogs caused by MVD. The most important determinants of prothrombotic state were increased fibrinogen and D-dimer concentrations and decreased AT III and PC activities. Additionally, the abnormalities of hemorheological function would deteriorate hypercoagulability in CHF dogs with MVD.

Conflict of Interests

The authors declare that there is no conflict of interests regarding the publication of this paper.

Acknowledgment

The research was financially supported by Kasetsart University Research and Development Institute (KURDI), Thailand.

References

[1] J. E. Rush, N. D. Lee, L. M. Freeman, and B. Brewer, "C-reactive protein concentration in dogs with chronic valvular disease,"

Journal of Veterinary Internal Medicine, vol. 20, no. 3, pp. 635–639, 2006.

[2] H. D. Pedersen, B. O. Kristensen, K. A. Lorentzen, J. Koch, A. L. Jensen, and A. Flagstad, "Mitral valve prolapse in 3-year-old healthy Cavalier King Charles Spaniels: an echocardiographic study," *Canadian Journal of Veterinary Research*, vol. 59, no. 4, pp. 294–298, 1995.

[3] H. D. Pedersen and J. Häggström, "Mitral valve prolapse in the dog: a model of mitral valve prolapse in man," *Cardiovascular Research*, vol. 47, no. 2, pp. 234–243, 2000.

[4] L. H. Olsen, M. Fredholm, and H. D. Pedersen, "Epidemiology and inheritance of mitral valve prolapse in Dachshunds," *Journal of Veterinary Internal Medicine*, vol. 13, no. 5, pp. 448–456, 1999.

[5] P. Serfass, V. Chetboul, C. C. Sampedrano et al., "Retrospective study of 942 small-sized dogs: Prevalence of left apical systolic heart murmur and left-sided heart failure, critical effects of breed and sex," *Journal of Veterinary Cardiology*, vol. 8, no. 1, pp. 11–18, 2006.

[6] C. J. Davis, P. A. Gurbel, W. A. Gattis et al., "Hemostatic abnormalities in patients with congestive heart failure: diagnostic significance and clinical challenge," *International Journal of Cardiology*, vol. 75, no. 1, pp. 15–21, 2000.

[7] R. Marcucci, A. M. Gori, F. Giannotti et al., "Markers of hypercoagulability and inflammation predict mortality in patients with heart failure," *Journal of Thrombosis and Haemostasis*, vol. 4, no. 5, pp. 1017–1022, 2006.

[8] I. Tarnow, T. Falk, A. Tidholm et al., "Hemostatic biomarkers in dogs with chronic congestive heart failure," *Journal of Veterinary Internal Medicine*, vol. 21, no. 3, pp. 451–457, 2007.

[9] A. Citak, S. Emre, A. Şirin, I. Bilge, and A. Nayir, "Hemostatic problems and thromboembolic complications in nephrotic children," *Pediatric Nephrology*, vol. 14, no. 2, pp. 138–142, 2000.

[10] O. L. Nelson, "Use of the D-dimer assay for diagnosing thromboembolic disease in the dog," *Journal of the American Animal Hospital Association*, vol. 41, no. 3, pp. 145–149, 2005.

[11] The Criteria Committee of the New York Heart Association, *Nomenclature and Criteria for Diagnosis of Diseases of the Heart and Great Vessels*, Little Brown, Boston, Mass, USA, 9th edition, 1994.

[12] C. F. Arkin, D. M. Adcock, H. J. Day et al., *Procedure for the Determination of Fibrinogen in Plasma: Approved Guideline*, Document H30-A2, National Committee for Clinical Laboratory, Wayne, Pa, USA, 2nd edition, 2001.

[13] G. F. Handeland, U. Abildgaard, and A. O. Aasen, "Simplified assay for antithrombin III activity using chromogenic peptide substrate. Manual and automated method," *Scandinavian Journal of Haematology*, vol. 31, no. 5, pp. 427–436, 1983.

[14] A. Sturk, W. M. Morrien-Salomons, M. V. Huisman, J. J. J. Borm, H. R. Büller, and J. W. T. Cate, "Analytical and clinical evaluation of commercial protein C assays," *Clinica Chimica Acta*, vol. 165, no. 2-3, pp. 263–270, 1987.

[15] J. Hintze, *NCSS, PASS and GESS*, NCSS, Kaysville, Utah, USA, 2007.

[16] E. Sbarouni, A. Bradshaw, F. Andreotti, E. Tuddenham, C. M. Oakley, and J. G. F. Cleland, "Relationship between hemostatic abnormalities and neuroendocrine activity in heart failure," *The American Heart Journal*, vol. 127, no. 3, pp. 607–612, 1994.

[17] T. Stokol, "Plasma D-dimer for the diagnosis of thromboembolic disorders in dogs," *Veterinary Clinics of North America: Small Animal Practice*, vol. 33, no. 6, pp. 1419–1435, 2003.

[18] O. L. Nelson and C. Andreasen, "The utility of plasma D-dimer to identify thromboembolic disease in dogs," *Journal of Veterinary Internal Medicine*, vol. 17, no. 6, pp. 830–834, 2003.

[19] T. J. Rabelink, J. J. Zwaginga, H. A. Koomans, and J. J. Sixma, "Thrombosis and hemostasis in renal disease," *Kidney International*, vol. 46, no. 2, pp. 287–296, 1994.

[20] M. S. Feigenbaum, M. A. Welsch, M. Mitchell, K. Vincent, R. W. Braith, and C. J. Pepine, "Contracted plasma and blood volume in chronic heart failure," *Journal of the American College of Cardiology*, vol. 35, no. 1, pp. 51–55, 2000.

[21] E. M. Albella, "Hemostatic problems associated with renal disease," *Journal of Pediatric Hematology/Oncology*, vol. 1, pp. 43–51, 1994.

[22] G. Y. H. Lip and C. R. Gibbs, "Does heart failure confer a hypercoagulable state? Virchow's triad revisited," *Journal of the American College of Cardiology*, vol. 33, no. 5, pp. 1424–1426, 1999.

11

Whole Body Computed Tomography with Advanced Imaging Techniques: A Research Tool for Measuring Body Composition in Dogs

Dharma Purushothaman,[1] **Barbara A. Vanselow,**[2] **Shu-Biao Wu,**[1]
Sarah Butler,[3] **and Wendy Yvonne Brown**[1]

[1] *School of Environmental and Rural Science, Department of Animal Science, University of New England, Armidale, NSW 2351, Australia*
[2] *NSW Department of Primary Industries, Beef Industry Centre, University of New England, Armidale, NSW 2351, Australia*
[3] *North Hill Vet Clinic, Armidale, NSW 2350, Australia*

Correspondence should be addressed to Wendy Yvonne Brown; wbrown@une.edu.au

Academic Editor: Juan G. Chediack

The use of computed tomography (CT) to evaluate obesity in canines is limited. Traditional CT image analysis is cumbersome and uses prediction equations that require manual calculations. In order to overcome this, our study investigated the use of advanced image analysis software programs to determine body composition in dogs with an application to canine obesity research. Beagles and greyhounds were chosen for their differences in morphology and propensity to obesity. Whole body CT scans with regular intervals were performed on six beagles and six greyhounds that were subjected to a 28-day weight-gain protocol. The CT images obtained at days 0 and 28 were analyzed using software programs OsiriX, ImageJ, and AutoCAT. The CT scanning technique was able to differentiate bone, lean, and fat tissue in dogs and proved sensitive enough to detect increases in both lean and fat during weight gain over a short period. A significant difference in lean : fat ratio was observed between the two breeds on both days 0 and 28 ($P < 0.01$). Therefore, CT and advanced image analysis proved useful in the current study for the estimation of body composition in dogs and has the potential to be used in canine obesity research.

1. Introduction

Obesity is a common nutritional disorder in dogs with a reported incidence of between 22% and 40% globally [1, 2]. The most commonly used methods to evaluate body composition in canine obesity research are dual-energy X-ray absorptiometry (DXA) and deuterium oxide dilution [3]. When fat estimated by deuterium oxide dilution was validated against fat determined by ether extraction of the carcass using male and female dogs, a coefficient of determination, $r^2 = 0.95$, was obtained [4]. When DXA methodology was validated in dogs using chemical analysis of dissected carcasses, it was found to have an overall coefficient of determination, $r^2 = 0.96$, for fat mass; however, greater inaccuracies were observed in some individual

animals mainly due to skeletal muscle hydration [5]. This was further confirmed in a more recent study in pigs [6] that evaluated the DXA methodology using whole dissection and ashing and concluded that DXA provided inaccurate and misleading results without taking into consideration the hydration and lipid content variability within tissues. A recent study investigated a potentially new method for detecting body composition in dogs: bioimpedance spectroscopy [7]. The method was validated against DXA and found good agreement with the two methods (correlation coefficient $r = 0.93$ for fat) at a population level, but was limited in accuracy when used for individual animal measurements. Quantitative magnetic resonance (QMR) also has been shown to be a useful technique in dogs particularly because the dogs do not require sedation or anaesthesia [8].

Computed tomography (CT) works on the principle of acquiring information based on the X-ray radiation being transmitted in many directions through a specific volume of tissue. These transmitted radiations account for the linear attenuation coefficient which are transformed to CT values or Hounsfield units (HU), a quantitative scale for measuring radio-density ranging between −1024 for air, 0 for water, and +1000 for bone, with muscle having a positive HU value, while fat has a negative HU value. From human studies it has been suggested that computed tomography (CT) may be a more accurate method for measuring body composition than DXA [9]. Validation of CT in pigs using dissection and near-infrared spectroscopy showed a coefficient of determination $r^2 = 0.93$ [10]. The use of CT to evaluate body composition has been reported for other species: cats [11], minipigs [12], and particularly sheep [13–15], but only one study has utilized CT for measuring body composition in dogs [16]. This study demonstrated that the fat content measured at the third lumbar vertebra (L3) using the attenuation range of −135/−105 HU had the best correlation; correlation coefficient $r = 0.98$, with the body fat content estimated by deuterium oxide dilution method. However, CT slices analyzed were limited to only three levels: 12th thoracic vertebra (T12), the third lumbar vertebra (L3), and the fifth lumbar vertebra (L5), and were only investigated in beagles. The canine study [16] also demonstrated the potential for fat to be overestimated at −190/−30 HU. This further emphasized the need for an improved CT method in dogs. Traditional CT image analysis is cumbersome in a whole body scan because of the large number of CT images involved and the manual calculations required in the prediction equations. The application of advanced image analysis software programs simplifies and automates this process [13].

It has been noted that some breeds of dogs [2] are more prone to obesity than others. Therefore, the present study aimed to investigate the use of advanced imaging software techniques with CT to measure body composition in two breeds of dogs. Beagles and greyhounds were chosen because of their differences in morphology and propensity to obesity.

2. Materials and Methods

2.1. Experimental Animals and Design. Twelve dogs: six beagles and six greyhounds weighing 10.7 ± 0.9 kg (beagles) and 24.7 ± 2.0 kg (greyhounds), were recruited for the study. The veterinarian inspected all the dogs at the commencement of the experiment and only healthy dogs were used. Initial body condition, assessed using a 5-point body condition score, found that all dogs were within ideal range. The dogs were scanned using CT on day 0 and subjected to a weight gain protocol by incorporating saturated fat of coconut oil origin in the diets for 28 days, and whole body scans were repeated. The objective was to determine whether the CT scanning would be sensitive enough to detect fat deposition during weight gain over a short period.

For the duration of the 28-day study, dogs were housed at the University of New England (UNE) dog research facilities at Armidale, NSW, Australia. This study was approved by the University of New England Animal Ethics Committee (Authority no. AEC10/091), and written consent was obtained from the dog owners. All dogs participating in this study were privately owned and were returned to their owners at the end of the study.

2.2. Anaesthesia, CT Scanning, and Images. Following an overnight fast, dogs were sedated using medetomidine HCl (Domitor, Pfizer Australia Pty Ltd., West Ryde, NSW, Australia, 1 mg/mL) and butorphanol (Ilium Butorgesic, Troy Laboratories Pty Ltd., Smithfield, NSW, Australia, 10 mg/mL), each administered IV at 0.1 mL per 5 kg bodyweight (BW). Dogs were positioned in sternoabdominal recumbency on a fiberglass cradle lined with foam and gently strapped to prevent movement. A whole body scan with regular intervals was performed using a Picker UltraZ 2000 CT scanner, Philips (Philips Medical Imaging Australia, Sydney, NSW, Australia). The acquisition parameters of the CT scanner were as follows: 120 kV; 100 mA; 480 mm field of view; 5 mm thickness; 10 mm spacing and 1 s scanning time. After scanning, the sedation was reversed using atipamezole HCl (Antisedan, Pfizer Australia Pty Ltd., West Ryde, NSW, Australia, 5 mg/mL, IV) at 0.1 mL per 5 kg BW. Throughout the scanning process, the study veterinarian (SB) monitored the sedation of the dogs. The scanning procedure generated an average of 80 CT images for each beagle and 98 CT images for each greyhound in a single scan, and resulting images were analyzed using software programs—OsiriX, ImageJ, and AutoCAT.

2.3. OsiriX and ImageJ Programs. OsiriX, an open source software [17], was used to edit the digital images obtained from the CT scanner in DICOM format. The use of the OsiriX software program followed the published instructions [18]. Closed polygon region of interest (ROI) was drawn to remove extraneous objects such as the fiberglass cradle from each of the CT images. The area outside the ROI was set to −1024 (air). This new setting deleted the area outside the ROI and allowed ROI to be exported and saved in 16-bit black and white image in DICOM format. The saved images were then processed using ImageJ.

ImageJ is a public domain image analysis program [19] that can process images in DICOM format [20]. ImageJ was used to convert 16-bit CT images to 8-bit binary images. This modification was a prerequisite for the next image analysis program used: AutoCAT.

2.4. AutoCAT Program and Body Composition. AutoCAT is an automated image analysis program [10] developed using methods similar to the previously developed CATMAN program [15]. AutoCAT program partitions the CT images into fat, lean, and bone based on the HU range for each tissue and measures their area, mean pixel value, and variance. Tissue volumes are then calculated by integrating the area of the respective tissues [21], and tissue densities are calculated

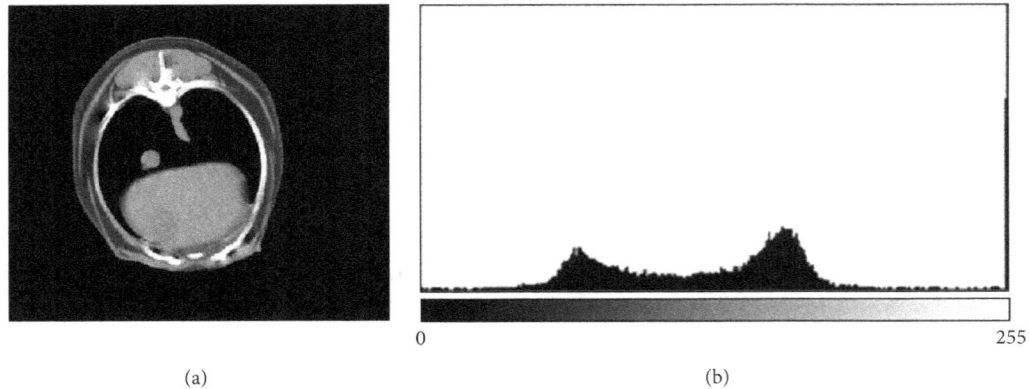

(a)   (b)

FIGURE 1: Representative CT image with a histogram to show the ranges in greyscale units 20–130 (fat), 131–220 (lean), and 221–255 (bone).

using a mathematical function relating HU values to tissue density:

$$\text{Tissue density} = 1.0062$$
$$+ (\text{mean tissue Hounsfield unit value}$$
$$\times 0.00601) \quad (\text{see } [22]).$$

(1)

AutoCAT then calculates tissue weight from the volume and density measurements. An additional function called CALC within the AutoCAT program calculated the total weight of lean, fat, and bone for each animal [10] using new ranges that were manually set to 20–130 (fat), 131–220 (lean), and 221–255 (bone) in greyscale units. These ranges were chosen for the canine species specifically in our study based on the histogram analysis in ImageJ program (see Figure 1). The equivalent values of the greyscale units in HU units were −214 to +7 for fat, 8 to 187 for lean, and 188 to 3072 for bone. These HU ranges were determined by the following formula:

$$HU = 2 * GU - 254 \quad (\text{see } [23]),$$

(2)

wherein GU is the greyscale value out of AutoCAT. The factor of 2 was used in the formula as 2 GU values were being combined into one HU value. The offset of 254 was an intercept adjustment to set water in the middle of a 256 GU range.

For clarification, total bodyweights obtained in this study from AutoCAT have been designated as CT-derived BW. The same researcher performed the various steps of CT image analysis to avoid biased analysis.

2.5. Bodyweight Measurement. Prior to CT scanning, the dogs were weighed on an electronic weigh scale, Provet Nuweigh Scales CHR-592 (Provet VMS Pty Ltd., Cameron Park, NSW, Australia) which was calibrated against a known weight before the initial use. The scales were set to "zero" before each weighing session, and dogs were weighed thrice to confirm the weight obtained. Throughout this study, the BW obtained from the electronic weigh scale has been designated as measured BW.

2.6. Statistical Analysis. Bland-Altman (BA) test of agreement was used to analyze the relationship between CT-derived BW and measured BW. To compare the differences in lean : fat ratios between the breeds, Mann-Whitney U test was used as the data was nonparametric in nature. MedCalc (MedCalc, Mariakerke, Belgium, Version 12.7.1.0) was used for statistical analysis, and $P < 0.05$ was considered statistically significant.

3. Results

3.1. Differences in Body Composition in Beagles and Greyhounds. For both beagles and greyhounds there was a nonsignificant increase in both lean and fat over the 28 days. Body composition data are presented in Table 1. A significant difference in the lean : fat ratio was seen between the two breeds on both days 0 and 28 ($P < 0.01$, Mann-Whitney U test).

3.2. CT-Derived BW versus Measured BW. Total BW were determined using the two methods CT-derived BW and measured BW described previously were compared. A Bland-Altman test of agreement (Table 2) shows that the two methods are interchangeable with respect to the BW as all the data points are within the mean $\pm$ 1.96 SD and that the BA ranges for the two measurements are not wide.

4. Discussion

The CT imaging and data analysis used in this study were able to differentiate bone, lean, and fat tissue in dogs. The CT scanning technique was sensitive enough to detect increases in both lean and fat during weight gain over a short period. In addition, the lean : fat ratio decreased in all dogs consistently with fat deposition. Importantly, the bone weights estimated by CT were identical on days 0 and 28 for each animal, supporting the reliability and repeatability of this technique.

The results obtained demonstrated a significant relationship between the CT-derived body weight and measured body weight, with the capacity to differentiate body composition such as lean : fat ratio in the two breeds of dogs.

TABLE 1: Body composition of individual dogs on day 0 and day 28.

Dog no.	Day	Bone (kg)	Lean (kg)	Fat (kg)	Lean/fat
Beagle 1	0	1.7	6.0	3.9	1.5
	28	1.7	6.7	4.8	1.4
Beagle 2	0	1.8	6.4	2.5	2.6
	28	1.8	7.4	3.4	2.2
Beagle 3	0	1.6	5.6	2.7	2.1
	28	1.6	6.2	3.3	1.9
Beagle 4	0	1.7	7.3	2.8	2.6
	28	1.7	7.9	3.1	2.5
Beagle 5	0	1.4	5.8	3.2	1.8
	28	1.4	6.1	3.9	1.6
Beagle 6	0	1.5	6.1	2.3	2.7
	28	1.5	6.6	2.9	2.3
Greyhound 1	0	3.5	19.7	3.5	5.6
	28	3.5	20.3	4.0	5.1
Greyhound 2	0	3.2	17.4	1.7	10.2
	28	3.2	18.3	2.6	7.0
Greyhound 3	0	3.4	20.2	2.6	7.8
	28	3.4	21.0	3.9	5.4
Greyhound 4	0	3.4	19.5	3.5	5.6
	28	3.4	20.3	4.0	5.1
Greyhound 5	0	3.0	17.1	2.6	6.6
	28	3.0	17.7	3.2	5.5
Greyhound 6	0	3.3	19.0	2.0	9.5
	28	3.3	20.0	3.5	5.7
Beagles (mean ± SD)	0	1.6 ± 0.1	6.2 ± 0.6	2.9 ± 0.6	2.2 ± 0.5
	28	1.6 ± 0.1	6.8 ± 0.7	3.6 ± 0.7	2.0 ± 0.4
Greyhounds (mean ± SD)	0	3.3 ± 0.2	18.8 ± 1.3	2.7 ± 0.7	7.5 ± 2.0
	28	3.3 ± 0.2	19.6 ± 1.3	3.5 ± 0.6	5.6 ± 0.7

The significant relationship between the two methods of bodyweight determination is similar to a study reported in sheep using the same research method wherein coefficient of determination, $r^2 = 0.96$, was observed when liveweight was correlated with CT estimates of liveweight [13]. In the present study, a consistent underestimation of CT-derived body weight was observed. This is partially similar to the findings of the sheep study wherein the author accounted for the underestimation to be due to the head and feet not being included in the CT analysis and the wool also not being accounted for as it does not absorb X-rays [13]. An underestimation was also reported in a pig study wherein the AutoCAT program was used to estimate the final weights of the fat, bone, and lean tissue [10]. In the pig study, CT-derived bone weight was significantly underestimated, lean tissue was significantly overestimated, when compared to weights measured by a combination of dissection and NIR, and fat was underestimated, though not significantly. The author accounted for the differences and inaccuracies in bone, and lean tissue weights due to the fundamental differences between the two methods that were compared, CT and combination of dissection and NIR. It is not clear why a consistent underestimation was observed in the present study in dogs. However, it is possible that the observed underestimation could have been due to the noncontinuous

nature of the CT slices. In addition, it is also not clear if the algorithm of the AutoCAT program previously tested in sheep and pigs requires a slight modification specifically for the canine species. Future work could involve a whole body scan with no gap between the slices, but this would increase the exposure time of the dogs to radiation and increase the number of CT slices for analyses.

The present study estimated body composition in dogs (total body fat, lean tissue, and bone), which was achieved using novel image analysis software program—AutoCAT together with software programs (OsiriX and ImageJ) to enhance the image analysis capabilities. When individual dogs were scanned on day 28, no change was seen in the estimated bone weight compared to day 0. This further emphasized the accuracy of the AutoCAT program. The use of AutoCAT program has been reported previously in sheep [14, 24, 25] and highlighted the diverse potential of the AutoCAT program for predicting body composition without the need of a validated prediction equation. This is the first study to report whole body CT scanning for measuring body composition in dogs. The challenge in developing an application of CT for body fat estimation is that the attenuation range set for fat can underestimate or overestimate the fat content. In the previously published CT study using beagles, the attenuation range for fat was proposed as −135/−105 [16]. In the present study wherein two different breeds were used, HU for fat was set as −214 to +7. This larger attenuation range for fat was chosen with the use of ImageJ software program to assist in detecting breed differences in fat composition. The CT techniques used in the present study demonstrated a significant breed difference in the lean : fat ratio.

Although there are advantages in applying CT to estimate body composition in dogs, the costs involved and the need to sedate the dogs limit the use of this methodology in a clinical setting. It is also recognized that the design of the present study could be strengthened with the inclusion of a comparison and validation with other existing methods, such as DXA and deuterium oxide dilution. Another aspect of body fat estimation, not explored in the present study, is the estimation of visceral/subcutaneous ratio (V/S). Auto-CAT software program has demonstrated the potential to estimate the total weight in kg of subcutaneous fat, as well as intramuscular fat in sheep [14]. Hence, future studies in canines using the present CT methodology should explore V/S ratio to determine visceral obesity, as it has been linked to metabolic diseases [26].

5. Conclusion

The findings of this study indicate that CT combined with advanced image analysis software is a promising candidate for an alternative noninvasive method for assessing body composition in dogs.

Conflict of Interests

The authors declare that there was no conflict of interests in the present study. None of the authors has any financial or

TABLE 2: Comparison of measured and CT-derived bodyweights (BW) using Bland-Altman (BA) test of agreement.

	Measured BW ± SD (kg)	CT-derived BW ± SD (kg)	Mean difference ± SD (kg)	BA limits (kg)	BA range (kg)	P
Beagles day 0	11.3 ± 1.0	10.7 ± 0.8	−0.63 ± 0.14	−0.90 to −0.37	−0.54	<0.0001
Beagles day 28	12.6 ± 1.1	12.0 ± 0.9	−0.58 ± 0.19	−0.96 to −0.20	−0.76	0.0035
Greyhounds day 0	25.8 ± 1.8	24.8 ± 2.0	−0.98 ± 0.24	−1.45 to −0.51	−0.94	0.0001
Greyhounds day 28	27.7 ± 1.9	26.4 ± 1.9	−1.30 ± 0.26	−1.81 to −0.79	−1.02	<0.0001

personal relationships that could inappropriately influence or bias the content of the paper.

Acknowledgments

The University of New England Postgraduate Research Grant funded this study. The authors thank the dog owners: Shirley Fraser for providing the beagles and Greg Nordstrom for the greyhounds. They thank Ms. Lynette McLean, Associate Lecturer, Animal Science, for the statistical advice and Mr. Andrew Blakely, Senior Technical Officer, Animal Science, for operating the CT scanner and providing technical comments during the preparation of the paper. An abridged version was presented as a poster presentation at the Nutrition Society of Australia's 36th Annual Scientific Meeting Program, 27th–30th November 2012, Wollongong, NSW, Australia.

References

[1] A. J. German, "The growing problem of obesity in dogs and cats," *Journal of Nutrition*, vol. 136, no. 7, pp. 1940S–1946S, 2006.

[2] A. T. Edney and P. M. Smith, "Study of obesity in dogs visiting veterinary practices in the United Kingdom," *The Veterinary Record*, vol. 118, no. 14, pp. 391–396, 1986.

[3] D. I. Mawby, J. W. Bartges, A. d'Avignon, D. P. Laflamme, T. D. Moyers, and T. Cottrell, "Comparison of various methods for estimating body fat in dogs," *Journal of the American Animal Hospital Association*, vol. 40, no. 2, pp. 109–114, 2004.

[4] W. J. Burkholder and C. D. Thatcher, "Validation of predictive equations for use of deuterium oxide dilution to determine body composition of dogs," *American Journal of Veterinary Research*, vol. 59, no. 8, pp. 927–937, 1998.

[5] J. R. Speakman, D. Booles, and R. Butterwick, "Validation of dual energy X-ray absorptiometry (DXA) by comparison with chemical analysis of dogs and cats," *International Journal of Obesity*, vol. 25, no. 3, pp. 439–447, 2001.

[6] J. P. Clarys, A. Scafoglieri, S. Provyn, O. Louis, J. A. Wallace, and J. De Mey, "A macro-quality evaluation of DXA variables using whole dissection, ashing, and computer tomography in pigs," *Obesity*, vol. 18, no. 8, pp. 1477–1485, 2010.

[7] L. C. Ward, L. Rae, D. Vankan, E. Flickinger, and J. Rand, "Prediction of body composition in dogs by bioimpedance spectroscopy," in *Proceedings of the Annual Scientific Meeting of the Nutrition Society of Australia*, p. 708, Wollongong, Australia, 2012.

[8] B. M. Zanghi, C. J. Cupp, Y. Pan et al., "Noninvasive measurements of body composition and body water via quantitative magnetic resonance, deuterium water, and dual-energy x-ray absorptiometry in awake and sedated dogs," *American Journal of Veterinary Research*, vol. 74, no. 5, pp. 733–743, 2013.

[9] J. T. Lane, L. R. Mack-Shipman, J. C. Anderson et al., "Comparison of CT and dual-energy DEXA using a modified trunk compartment in the measurement of abdominal fat," *Endocrine*, vol. 27, no. 3, pp. 295–299, 2005.

[10] N. B. Jopson, K. Kolstad, E. Sehested, and O. Vangen, "Computed tomography as an accurate and cost effective alternative to carcass dissection," *Proceeding of the Australian Association Animal Breeding and Genetics*, vol. 11, pp. 635–639, 1995.

[11] L. E. Buelund, D. H. Nielsen, F. J. Mcevoy, E. L. Svalastoga, and C. R. Bjornvad, "Measurement of body composition in cats using computed tomography and dual energy x-ray absorptiometry," *Veterinary Radiology and Ultrasound*, vol. 52, no. 2, pp. 179–184, 2011.

[12] J. Chang, J. Jung, H. Lee, D. Chang, J. Yoon, and M. Choi, "Computed tomographic evaluation of abdominal fat in minipigs," *Journal of Veterinary Science*, vol. 12, no. 1, pp. 91–94, 2011.

[13] F. E. M. Haynes, P. L. Greenwood, J. P. Siddell, M. B. McDonagh, and V. H. Oddy, "Computer tomography software program "Osirix" aids prediction of sheep body composition," *Proceedings of the Australian Society of Animal Production*, vol. 28, article 49, 2010.

[14] T. Kvame and O. Vangen, "Selection for lean weight based on ultrasound and CT in a meat line of sheep," *Livestock Science*, vol. 106, no. 2-3, pp. 232–242, 2007.

[15] B. Kinghorn and J. Thompson, "CATMAN—a program to measure CAT-Scans for predictions of body components in live animals," *Proceeding Australian Association Animal Breeding and Genetics*, vol. 10, pp. 560–564, 1992.

[16] K. Ishioka, M. Okumura, M. Sagawa, F. Nakadomo, K. Kimura, and M. Saito, "Computed tomographic assessment of body fat in beagles," *Veterinary Radiology and Ultrasound*, vol. 46, no. 1, pp. 49–53, 2005.

[17] A. Rosset, L. Spadola, and O. Ratib, "OsiriX: an open-source software for navigating in multidimensional DICOM images," *Journal of Digital Imaging*, vol. 17, no. 3, pp. 205–216, 2004.

[18] O. Ratib, A. Rosset, and J. Heuberger, *OsiriX: The Pocket Guide*, OsiriX Foundation, Geneva, Switzerland, 2nd edition, 2002.

[19] M. D. Abràmoff, P. J. Magalhães, and S. J. Ram, "Image processing with imageJ," *Biophotonics International*, vol. 11, no. 7, pp. 36–41, 2004.

[20] E. J. Escott and D. Rubinstein, "Free DICOM image viewing and processing software for your desktop computer: what's available and what it can do for you," *Radiographics*, vol. 23, no. 5, pp. 1341–1357, 2003.

[21] H. J. G. Gundersen, T. F. Bendtsen, L. Korbo et al., "Some new, simple and efficient stereological methods and their use in pathological research and diagnosis," *Acta Pathologica*,

Microbiologica, et Immunologica Scandinavica, vol. 96, no. 5, pp. 379–394, 1988.

[22] G. D. Fullerton, "Tissue imaging and characterisation," in *Medical Physics of CT and Ultrasound. Medical Physics Monograph*, G. D. Fullerton and J. A. Zagzebski, Eds., vol. 6, p. 125, American Institute of Physics, 1980.

[23] N. B. Jopson, *Physiological adaptations in two seasonal cervids [dissertation]*, Armidale, New South Wales, Australia, Animal Science, University of New England, 1993.

[24] T. Kvame and O. Vangen, "In-vivo composition of carcass regions in lambs of two genetic lines, and selection of CT positions for estimation of each region," *Small Ruminant Research*, vol. 66, no. 1–3, pp. 201–208, 2006.

[25] F. E. M. Haynes, P. L. Greenwood, M. B. McDonagh, and V. H. Oddy, "Myostatin allelic status interacts with level of nutrition to affect growth, composition, and myofiber characteristics of lambs," *Journal of Animal Science*, vol. 90, no. 2, pp. 456–465, 2012.

[26] R. N. Bergman, S. P. Kim, K. J. Catalano et al., "Why visceral fat is bad: mechanisms of the metabolic syndrome," *Obesity*, vol. 14, pp. 16S–19S, 2006.

12

Vaginoscopy in Ewes Utilizing a Laparoscopic Surgical Port Device

Jeremiah Easley, Desiree Shasa, and Eileen Hackett

Department of Clinical Sciences, Colorado State University Veterinary Teaching Hospital, 300 West Drake Road, Colorado State University, Fort Collins, CO 80523, USA

Correspondence should be addressed to Eileen Hackett; eileen.hackett@colostate.edu

Academic Editor: Antonio Ortega-Pacheco

Vaginoscopy allows for diagnostic evaluation and treatment of the vaginal vault. A laparoscopic surgical port device and rigid telescope were utilized for serial vaginoscopy in 8 healthy anesthetized ewes. Vaginoscopy examinations were performed in each ewe at days 1, 14, and 28. This technique was well-tolerated and facilitated carbon dioxide vaginal inflation, complete vaginal examination, identification of the cervix, and targeted biopsy collection. No complications were encountered during or following the vaginoscopy procedures. The laparoscopic port device was well-suited to the ewe vulvar size. This technique could be applied to clinical evaluation in ewes for the purposes of examination, biopsy, culture, foreign body removal, and minor surgical procedures.

1. Introductions

Vaginoscopy is a useful diagnostic procedure to evaluate the vaginal vault and corresponding structures, such as the cervix, vaginal fornix, and external urethral orifice. It can aid in the diagnosis of genital tract malignancies, foreign bodies, infection, and genital trauma or malformations in both humans and animals [1, 2]. Vaginoscopy is also an effective tool for reproductive management, identifying stages of estrus, predicting optimum stage for breeding, and facilitating transcervical insemination [1, 3]. Vaginal examination has traditionally been performed utilizing a vaginal speculum and light source; however traditional approaches can result in discomfort and are poorly suited for smaller patients or in cases of vaginal stenosis [2]. More recently, vaginoscopy has been performed with flexible and rigid endoscopes, combined with vaginal inflation with gas or fluid, in order to improve examination comfort and efficacy [2, 4].

Single incision laparoscopic surgery has gained popularity and can be facilitated through use of a laparoscopic surgical port device. Port devices have been described in a variety of applications in dogs, including exploratory laparoscopy, ovariectomy, ovariohysterectomy, cryptorchidectomy, gastropexy, splenectomy, and thoracoscopy [5–10]. Port devices can accommodate multiple cannulas and insufflation channels, offering entry points for a variety of instruments through a single port. Because of their flexibility, these devices could be applied to vaginoscopy, allowing simultaneous insufflation, telescopic examination, and insertion of instruments for aspiration, biopsy, or infusion.

The purpose of the present study was to evaluate vaginoscopy in ewes using a laparoscopic surgical port device. We hypothesized that the port device would allow simultaneous insufflation and telescope insertion, resulting in complete visualization of the vaginal walls, identification of the vestibulovaginal junction and cervix, and targeted biopsy procedures.

2. Materials and Methods

All research procedures were approved by the Colorado State University Institutional Animal Care and Use Committee (12-3692A) prior to study commencement. Eight mature healthy Rambouillet × Columbia cross bred ewes, approximately six years old and with a mean body weight of $82 \pm SD\ 15$ kg, were evaluated as part of a separate study [11]. Food was withheld for 24 hours and sheep were administered phenylbutazone (10 mg/kg per os) and procaine penicillin (30,000 IU/kg subcutaneous) 30–60 min prior to the procedure. Water was not withheld before the procedure. The ear was aseptically prepared and venous and arterial catheters were inserted. Sheep were induced with intravenous ketamine (3.3 mg/kg) and diazepam (0.1 mg/kg) and intubated. Sheep were then moved onto a surgery table in dorsal recumbency and the limbs were secured to the table prior to tilting into a 5-degree Trendelenburg position. Anesthesia was maintained with isoflurane in oxygen and mechanical ventilation, with the % isoflurane administered varying to obtain the appropriate anesthetic depth between 1.5 and 3, and oxygen flow rate of 1.5 L/min. Direct arterial blood pressure was continuously monitored, in addition to electrocardiography, pulse oximetry, and end-tidal capnography. Hypotension was considered in ewes in which the mean arterial blood pressure fell below 65 mmHg and was treated with a single dose of ephedrine between 0.05 and 0.1 mg/kg. All ewes were administered isotonic lactated ringers crystalloid fluids at 3–5 mL/kg body wt per hour IV during anesthesia. Wool surrounding the vulvar region was clipped and the perineum and vulva were aseptically prepared prior to draping the site with sterile towels in preparation for vaginoscopy.

A laparoscopic surgical port device (SILS Port, Medtronic, Minneapolis, MN) was lubricated and inserted into the vagina with curved hemostats until securely in place within the vaginal cavity in all ewes, regardless of variation in body weight. Three cannulas, two 5 mm and one 12 mm, were inserted via the port device. Insufflation tubing was connected from the insufflator (Electronic Endoflator 264305 20, Karl Storz Veterinary Endoscopy-America, Goleta, CA) to the port device for carbon dioxide gas delivery, which was maintained at a pressure of approximately 6 mmHg. A 10 mm diameter, 30°, 33 cm rigid laparoscopic telescope (Hopkins II Telescope 26003BA, Karl Storz Veterinary Endoscopy-America, Goleta, CA) connected to a viewing tower with a camera (Image 1 HD H3 2 camera and 222010 20 processor, Karl Storz Veterinary Endoscopy-America, Goleta, CA) and light source (495NE light cable and Xenon 300 201331 20 light source, Karl Storz Veterinary Endoscopy-America, Goleta, CA) was inserted via the 12 mm cannula within the port device (Figure 1). Upon entering the vagina, visible structures were identified and the examination was video recorded. A 5 mm × 2 mm laparoscopic biopsy punch forcep was inserted through a 5 mm portal within the laparoscopic surgical port device and vaginal mucosal biopsies were obtained from the right and left dorsolateral and right and left ventrolateral vaginal walls. Total procedure duration, including anesthetic induction, positioning, perineal preparation, and vaginoscopy, was recorded.

Following vaginoscopy, sheep were relocated to a recovery area, where heart rate, respiratory rate, position, and swallowing were monitored until anesthetic recovery and extubation. The sheep were reintroduced to feed and maintained in barn confinement for 28 days, with daily monitoring of health.

3. Results and Discussion

The laparoscopic surgical port device was easily inserted into the ewe vagina and insufflation was maintained via the

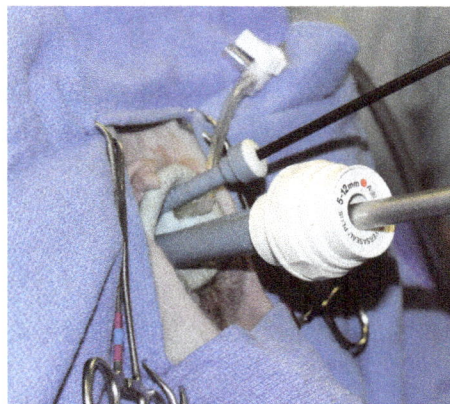

FIGURE 1: Vaginoscopy is conducted in an anesthetized ewe in dorsal recumbency. The laparoscopic surgical port device is inserted in the vulva, allowing insufflation with carbon dioxide gas and insertion of a 10 mm diameter rigid telescope for complete examination. A 5 mm biopsy instrument has also been inserted through one of the 5 mm portals.

dedicated insufflation port, despite variation in ewe body weight. A cannula within the port device allowed rigid telescope insertion. The vestibule-vaginal junction, vaginal wall and fornices, and cervix were visible in each sheep evaluated via vaginoscopy facilitated by the port device (Figure 2). Minor manipulation of the laparoscopic telescope visual field and insertion distance was necessary to examine each structure. Insufflation resulted in vaginal expansion and panoramic surface visibility. The right and left anterolateral and right and left posterolateral vaginal walls were easily visualized and biopsies were successfully and accurately performed with minor manipulation of insufflation pressure to reduce tension along the vaginal wall. Three vaginoscopy examinations and biopsy procedures were performed in each ewe for a total of 24 procedures. Hypotension occurred immediately following induction in 7 of 24 anesthetic episodes and corrected within 5 minutes following treatment. Mean procedure duration was 23 minutes ± 4 minutes SD. No secondary vaginal trauma was visible from vaginal examination or port device insertion. Gas vaginal insufflation was released upon removal of the port device. All ewes salivated during general anesthesia and regurgitation was observed in 10% of anesthetic episodes. All sheep recovered well following the procedure, with return to consciousness, extubation, and ability to maintain sternal recumbency within 15 minutes and standing within 30 minutes. No adverse events occurring during the 28-day monitoring period.

Vaginoscopy using the laparoscopic surgical port device was performed in all ewes without procedural or postvaginoscopy complications. Vaginal cavity examination was excellent, compared with previous experience using various specula adapted from other species, due to both vaginal inflation and laparoscopic telescope magnification and illumination. The 30° laparoscopic telescope could be rotated to expand the field of view without losing orientation within the vaginal cavity, similar to previous reports where telescopes

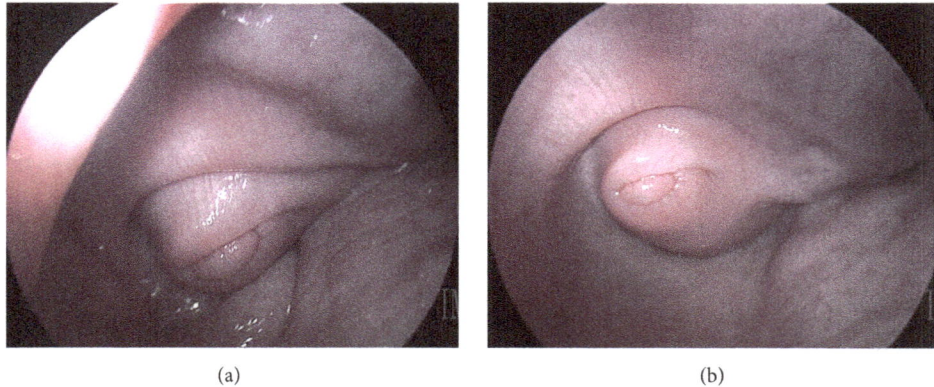

(a)   (b)

FIGURE 2: (a) Vaginoscopy image following partial insufflation and expansion of the vaginal vault. (b) Vaginoscopy image following complete insufflation and expansion of the vaginal vault with improved visibility of the cranial vagina and cervix tubercle.

with optical angles allowed improved visibility [1]. Vaginal inflation prior to telescope insertion decreases the likelihood of inadvertent trauma to the vaginal wall upon insertion. The rigid telescope could easily be removed, cleaned of mucus, and reinserted without requiring removal of the port device and loss of inflation. The laparoscopic port device was well sized for the ewe vagina and prevented escape of gas insufflation, allowing examination of the vaginal walls, fornices, and cervix, as well as accurate biopsy collection. Inflation of the vaginal cavity did not require addition of balloon dilation or manual compression, which is often necessary with other methods [12]. Image capture for medical recording was also easily performed using this described vaginoscopy method, with image recording preferred to written description for the purposes documentation and evaluating response to treatment.

Vaginoscopy allows inspection of the vaginal cavity, often prompted by abnormal clinical signs of bleeding or persistent vulvovaginitis, and is an excellent diagnostic complement to transabdominal ultrasound examination [1, 12]. Vaginal discharge is a common sign observed in small ruminants with uterine neoplasia and vaginoscopy could be considered to differentiate between or determine the severity of vaginal, cervical, and uterine neoplasms [13, 14]. One benefit of the technique described in the present report is the ease of insertion of examination probes or biopsy forceps through the additional instrument portals in the port device, which could be used to obtain samples for microscopic tissue evaluation and identification of neoplasms. Use of the port device also allows collection of samples for culture, application of topical treatments, and performance of surgery within the vaginal cavity [15]. The laparoscopic surgical port device could be considered for vaginoscopy of animals of similar size, but further validation in other species would be required.

Excellent viewing when utilizing a laparoscopic port device paired with rigid endoscopic equipment for vaginoscopy in ewes could outweigh the associated equipment costs, especially when examinations are performed in hospitals equipped for laparoscopic procedures. In the present report, ewes underwent vaginoscopy under general anesthesia in dorsal recumbency. Ruminants will often regurgitate while under general anesthesia, especially when in Trendelenburg position; therefore fasting prior to the procedure and tracheal intubation with a cuffed tube during anesthesia is necessary to prevent aspiration. Trendelburg positioning in ruminants poses an additional risk of regurgitation under general anesthesia and this informed our use of prophylactic antibiotics. Trendelenburg positioning has been associated with decreased dynamic lung compliance due to increased pressure on the diaphragm and reduction of lung volume, which can contribute to decreased cardiac venous return, cardiac output, and tissue oxygen delivery [16]. Future study is recommended to evaluate the contribution of Trendelenburg position on physiologic parameters in anesthetized sheep. Sedation or other restraint protocols could be considered for ewe vaginoscopy, though further investigation would be needed to evaluate these protocols relative to patient cooperation, ease of examination, and safety [1]. Application of this technique to ewes with vaginal or cervical pathology will be necessary to further investigate its utility in these cases.

4. Conclusions

A commercially available laparoscopic surgical port device was successfully utilized for vaginoscopic examination and biopsy collection in ewes. By manipulation of the endoscope and insufflation pressures, it was possible to visualize the cervix and vaginal wall. Thus, application of this technique would be appropriate for complete vaginal examination to detect anatomical alterations, investigate diseases associated with vaginal discharge, and obtain targeted biopsies within the vagina.

Conflicts of Interest

The authors declare that there are no conflicts of interest regarding the publication of this article.

Acknowledgments

The authors acknowledge the support of Mrs. Kimberly Lebsock in the preparation of this manuscript.

References

[1] X. Lévy, "Videovaginoscopy of the canine vagina," *Reproduction in Domestic Animals*, vol. 51, supplement 1, pp. 31–36, 2016.

[2] A. Di Spiezio Sardo, B. Zizolfi, G. Calagna, P. Florio, C. Nappi, and C. Di Carlo, "Vaginohysteroscopy for the diagnosis and treatment of vaginal lesions," *International Journal of Gynecology and Obstetrics*, vol. 133, no. 2, pp. 146–151, 2016.

[3] N. Tison, E. Bouchard, L. DesCôteaux, and R. C. Lefebvre, "Effectiveness of intrauterine treatment with cephapirin in dairy cows with purulent vaginal discharge," *Theriogenology*, vol. 89, pp. 305–317, 2017.

[4] J. P. Lulich, "Endoscopic vaginoscopy in the dog," *Theriogenology*, vol. 66, no. 3, pp. 588–591, 2006.

[5] F. M. Sánchez-Margallo, A. Tapia-Araya, and I. Díaz-Güemes, "Preliminary application of a single-port access technique for laparoscopic ovariohysterectomy in dogs," *Veterinary Record Open*, vol. 2, no. 2, Article ID e000153, 2015.

[6] A. Khalaj, J. Bakhtiari, and A. Niasari-Naslaji, "Comparison between single and three portal laparoscopic splenectomy in dogs," *BMC Veterinary Research*, vol. 8, article 161, 2012.

[7] M. Manassero, D. Leperlier, R. Vallefuoco, and V. Viateau, "Laparoscopic ovariectomy in dogs using a single-port multiple-access device," *Veterinary Record*, vol. 171, no. 3, p. 69, 2012.

[8] E. Gonzalez-Gasch and E. Monnet, "Comparison of Single Port Access Versus Multiple Port Access Systems in Elective Laparoscopy: 98 Dogs (2005–2014)," *Veterinary Surgery*, vol. 44, no. 7, pp. 895–899, 2015.

[9] M. L. Wallace, J. B. Case, A. Singh, G. W. Ellison, and E. Monnet, "Single Incision, Laparoscopic-Assisted Ovariohysterectomy for Mucometra and Pyometra in Dogs," *Veterinary Surgery*, vol. 44, no. 1, pp. 66–70, 2015.

[10] J. J. Runge, P. G. Curcillo, S. A. King et al., "Initial application of reduced port surgery using the single port access technique for laparoscopic canine ovariectomy," *Veterinary Surgery*, vol. 41, no. 7, pp. 803–806, 2012.

[11] J. A. Moss, I. Butkyavichene, S. A. Churchman et al., "Combination pod-intravaginal ring delivers antiretroviral agents for HIV prophylaxis: Pharmacokinetic evaluation in an ovine model," *Antimicrobial Agents and Chemotherapy*, vol. 60, no. 6, pp. 3759–3766, 2016.

[12] A. Golan, "Continous flow vaginoscopy in children," *Journal of Lower Genital Tract Disease*, vol. 5, no. 2, pp. 85-86, 2001.

[13] C. V. Löhr, "One hundred two tumors in 100 goats (1987–2011)," *Veterinary Pathology*, vol. 50, no. 4, pp. 668–675, 2013.

[14] M. Heller, "Uterine Neoplasia in Small Ruminants: Retrospective Study," *Journal of Veterinary Internal Medicine*, vol. 26, no. 3, pp. 761-761, 1991.

[15] V. Billone, C. Amorim-Costa, S. Campos et al., "Laparoscopy-like operative vaginoscopy: A new approach to manage mesh erosions," *Journal of Minimally Invasive Gynecology*, vol. 22, no. 1, p. 10, 2015.

[16] Y. Moens, "Mechanical Ventilation and Respiratory Mechanics During Equine Anesthesia," *Veterinary Clinics of North America—Equine Practice*, vol. 29, no. 1, pp. 51–67, 2013.

13

Frequency and Clinical Epidemiology of Canine Monocytic Ehrlichiosis in Dogs Infested with Ticks from Sinaloa, Mexico

Carolina Guadalupe Sosa-Gutierrez,[1,2] Maria Teresa Quintero Martinez,[2] Soila Maribel Gaxiola Camacho,[3] Silvia Cota Guajardo,[3] Maria D. Esteve-Gassent,[4] and María-Guadalupe Gordillo-Pérez[1]

[1] *Unidad de Investigacion Medica en Enfermedades Infecciosas y Parasitarias, Hospital de Pediatria, Centro Medico Nacional Siglo XXI, Instituto Mexicano del Seguro Social, 07300 Mexico City, Mexico*
[2] *Departamento de Parasitologia, Facultad de Medicina Veterinaria y Zootecnia, Universidad Nacional Autonoma de México, Mexico City, Mexico*
[3] *Departamento de Parasitologia, Facultad de Medicina Veterinaria y Zootecnia, Universidad Autonoma de Sinaloa, SIN, Mexico*
[4] *Department of Veterinary Pathobiology, College of Veterinary Medicine and Biomedical Sciences, Texas A&M University, TX, USA*

Correspondence should be addressed to Carolina Guadalupe Sosa-Gutierrez; mcarososagtz@yahoo.com.mx

Academic Editor: Masanori Tohno

Ehrlichia canis is a rickettsial intracellular obligate bacterial pathogen and agent of canine monocytic ehrlichiosis. The prevalence of this disease in veterinary medicine can vary depending on the diagnostic method used and the geographic location. One hundred and fifty-two canine blood samples from six veterinary clinics and two shelters from Sinaloa State (Mexico) were analyzed in this study. All animals were suspected of having Canine Monocytic Ehrlichiosis (CME). The diagnostic methods used were the ELISA (Snap4Dx, IDEXX) together with blood smear and platelet count. From all dogs blood samples analyzed, 74.3% were positive to *E. canis* by ELISA and 40.1% were positive by blood smear. The sensitivity and specificity observed in the ELISA test were 78.8% and 86.7%. In addition, thrombocytopenia was presented in 87.6% of positive dogs. The predominant clinical manifestations observed were fever, anorexia, depression, lethargy, and petechiae. Consequently, this is the first report in which the morulae were visualized in the blood samples, and *E. canis*-specific antibodies were detected in dogs from Sinaloa, Northwest of Mexico.

1. Introduction

Ehrlichia canis is the causative agent of canine monocytic ehrlichiosis (CME). Moreover, CME is an emerging disease in veterinary medicine, and *E. canis* has been considered in the last decade as a potential zoonotic pathogen [1, 2]. It is a worldwide disease transmitted by a tick bite. The competent vector for its transmission is the Ixodidae ticks *Rhipicephalus sanguineus* and *Dermacentor variabilis* [3]. In dogs, the CME is a multiphase disorder that progresses in three stages: acute, subclinical, and chronic. Each phase is characterized by several clinical and hematologic abnormalities. Thrombocytopenia is a common finding in *E. canis* infected dogs and

many clinicians tend to use it as an indication for antibiotic treatment, and it is observed in 84% of the cases and its severity varies in the different disease phases [4]. During the subclinical stage a moderate thrombocytopenia is observed, while the chronic phase is characterized by severe leukopenia and anemia. In this stage dogs show other complications such as hypocellular marrow, suppressed splenic sequestration, decreased life of platelets, and an increase of circulating migration-factor platelet inhibitor [3, 4]. The relationship between the magnitude of thrombocytopenia and prevalence of *E. canis* has been established in countries such as Brazil in 2004 where 84.1% of infected dogs showed thrombocytopenia [3]. Taken together, more data is necessary to determine the environmental factors and infected vector prevalence in Mexico due to high incidence of CME in this region of the country. The purpose of this study was to evaluate the frequency and clinical manifestations of dogs from Sinaloa, Mexico, with clinical suspicion of CME by ELISA (SNAP4Dx) and blood smears and with a history of tick infestation.

2. Material and Methods

2.1. Location. The study was conducted in Culiacan, Sinaloa, Mexico, located north 27° 02′, south 22° 29′ north latitude east 105° 23′, to 109° 28′ west longitude.

2.2. Samples and Serological Analysis. Samples were collected between March 2006 and July 2007, and 152 blood samples from dogs were collected in six veterinary clinics and two shelters from Sinaloa State, Mexico. Blood samples were chosen by dogs (males and females) with tick infestation and clinical signs suggesting CME (fever, anorexia, lethargy, depression, petechiae, bruising of the skin or prone to bleeding in mucous membranes, and epistaxis). Three ml of blood sample in EDTA tubes was obtained from each dog by the radial vein. All samples were processed using two techniques to detect *E. canis* specific IgG antibodies, the IDDEX ELISA kit and the Snap test. Samples were processed according to the manufacturer's recommendations. In addition, blood smears were done immediately after the blood was drawn to detect forms of *E. canis* morulae in monocytes, using Wright's stain. Finally platelet count was performed by an Automatic Hematology Analyzer (IDEXX QBC VetAutoread). All counts less than 200,000 platelets/μL were considered as thrombocytopenia [4].

2.3. Statistical Analysis. The platelet counts from each sample were compared with the seropositive and seronegative results. Qualitative variables such as sex (female, male), age (<1 year, 1–3 years, 3–5 years, >5 years), presence of thrombocytopenia (yes, no), fever (yes, no), anorexia (yes, no), lethargy (yes, no), depression (yes, no), petechiae (yes, no), skin ecchymosis (yes, no), epistaxis (yes, no), bleeding tendency (yes, no), and anorexia (yes, no) were evaluated and used on the chi square or Fisher exact tests using EpiInfo 3.5, which provides regression analysis estimating linear 95% confidence interval (95% CI).

3. Results

Among the canine individuals with suspected CME 74.5% (113/152) have *E. canis*-specific antibodies. In addition, 40.1% (61/152) were found positive when examined by smear to detect *E. canis* morulae in monocytes (Figure 1). Overall the clinical manifestations observed (Table 1) were fever (91.2%), anorexia (86.7%), depression (85.0%), lethargy (72.6%), and petechiae (72.6%). The male-female ratio was 1 : 1, and the most affected age was 1-2 years old (53%), followed by under 1 year (28%) and 3–5 years (19%). We compare the results obtained from the blood smear technique and Snap 4DX; of the 152 samples analyzed; 60 (38.2%) and 21 (13.7%) were

TABLE 1: Clinical manifestations presented by dogs positive for antibodies to *E. canis*.

Clinical manifestation	Positive N = 113	Frequency (%)	Odds ratio (CI)	P value
Fever	103	91.2	3.6 (1.3–10.2)	<0.01
Anorexia	98	86.7	4.08 (1.6–10.3)	<0.01
Lethargy	82	72.6	NS	NS
Depression	96	85.0	3.93 (1.6–9.7)	<0.01
Petechiae	82	72.6	2.5 (1.1–5.7)	<0.01
Ecchymosis	22	19.5	NS	NS
Epistaxis	80	70.8	NS	NS
Thrombocytopenia	106	93.8	5.2 (1.7–12.9)	<0.01

NS: Not Significant. Evaluated by chi square test and calculating odds ratio (OR) and 95% confidence intervals (CI).

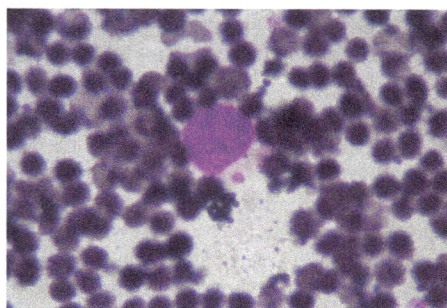

FIGURE 1: Observed using light microscopy; this is an image created from a peripheral blood smear of a dog infected with Canine Monocytic Ehrlichiosis. This image shows the morulae within the cytoplasm of a monocyte. Wright's stain.

positive and negative for both methods diagnostically, with a sensibility of 78.8% (95% CI 69.8–85.6) and specificity 86.7% (95% CI 74.3–99.1), and were assessed by chi square test by calculating odds ratios (OR) and 95% confidence intervals (CI) with a 2.12 (95% CI 1.01–4.45) $P < 0.05$. The 87.6% (106) of the dogs with thrombocytopenia were positive to the presence of antibodies of *E. canis* and were evaluated by chi square test by calculating odds ratios (OD) and 95% confidence intervals (CI) with a 24.2 (95% CI 8.9–65.9) $P < 0.01$; this parameter is a risk factor for disease and showed high rates of exposure, consistent with previous reports [5].

4. Discussion

The results obtained in this study were similar to those observed in 2002, in which the authors compared five serodiagnostic methods for *E. canis* and found 79.2% positive samples using the same ELISA techniques as the one utilized in our study [6]. In Mexico (2000) a national study reported a 33% of seroprevalence for *E. canis* using the same diagnostic method as those presented in here [7]. Contrary to what was found in this study, our results showed the highest ehrlichiosis case. In Yucatan, Mexico, a 44.1% seroprevalence for CME has been reported using the same diagnostic method. Yucatan is in a climate zone similar to that of Sinaloa. Taken together, our study shows a frequency for CME similar if not higher than that observed in other regions of the country, as well as in other countries of Center and South America, which suggests the increasing importance of this disease in the canine population. *E. canis* has been described as a potential zoonotic pathogen for humans [5], and therefore our findings and current studies suggest its importance as human pathogen in Latin American countries.

A positive result for *E. canis* by ELISA indicates that the dog was or is exposed to this bacterial pathogen and does not necessarily imply that there is a latent infection. On the other hand, when using the ELISA test, cross-reactivity with other *Ehrlichia* species may occur since it is not specific for *E. canis*. Antibodies against this pathogen decrease approximately 6 to 9 months after infection. This together with the presence of subclinical infection in canids causes difficulties in the diagnosis of the disease by the clinicians. Consequently, there is a need of tools to support the diagnosis of the disease with hematological tests to evaluate thrombocytopenia, since this sign implies bacterial growth and its effect on antibody-producing organs.

Previous *E. canis* experimental studies [3, 4] reported thrombocytopenia in 89% of the infected dogs. In addition, thrombocytopenia was described in every stage of infection, and it persisted during subclinical stages of the disease. The morulae are easily identified by light microscopy during the acute phase of infection (4-5 days after exposure) but difficult to detect when the disease progressed undetected. Some studies reported that only 4% of the blood samples studied showed morulae in blood smears [8–10]. In this case 40.1% were found positive, which indicates that the search for the morulae in peripheral blood was done in the acute phase [11]. Moreover, dogs in endemic areas may have high IgG titers specific to *E. canis* without clinical signs and this can cause false positive serological tests [3], reinforcing the necessity for more specific test to be used in veterinary medicine.

5. Conclusions

In this study we have introduced the presence of the Canine Monocytic Ehrlichiosis in Sinaloa, Mexico. Dogs infested with ticks showed high frequency for *E. canis* in dogs which suggests the classification of this region of Mexico as an endemic area for the disease. Based on our findings and previous studies done in Mexico and other Latin American countries, we suggest that, in the absence of molecular methodologies for the diagnostics of CME, a serology test to detect *E. canis*-specific antibodies plus the presence of clinical manifestations and thrombocytopenia is a basic tool for its diagnosis in endemic areas.

References

[1] Y. Rikihisa, "The tribe Ehrlichieae and ehrlichial diseases," *Clinical Microbiology Reviews*, vol. 4, no. 3, pp. 286–308, 1991.

[2] A. Unver, M. Perez, N. Orellana, H. Huang, and Y. Rikihisa, "Molecular and antigenic comparison of *Ehrlichia canis* isolates from dogs, ticks, and a human in Venezuela," *Journal of Clinical Microbiology*, vol. 39, no. 8, pp. 2788–2793, 2001.

[3] C. Bulla, R. Kiomi Takahira, J. Pessoa Araújo Jr., L. A. Trinca, R. Souza Lopes, and C. E. Wiedmeyer, "The relationship between the degree of thrombocytopenia and infection with *Ehrlichia canis* in an endemic area," *Veterinary Research*, vol. 35, no. 1, pp. 141–146, 2004.

[4] T. Waner and S. Harrus, "Ehrlichiosis monocytic canine," in *Recent Advances in Canine Infectious Diseases*, L. Carmichael, Ed., 2004.

[5] R. I. Rodriguez-Vivas, R. E. F. Albornoz, and G. M. E. Bolio, "*Ehrlichia canis* in dogs in Yucatan, Mexico: Seroprevalence, prevalence of infection and associated factors," *Veterinary Parasitology*, vol. 127, no. 1, pp. 75–79, 2005.

[6] M. Bélanger, H. L. Sorenson, M. K. France et al., "Comparison of serological detection methods for diagnosis of *Ehrlichia canis* infections in dogs," *Journal of Clinical Microbiology*, vol. 40, no. 9, pp. 3506–3508, 2002.

[7] O. L. Nuñez, "Estudio de la seroprevalencia de *Ehrlichia canis* en México," *Revista AMMVEPE*, vol. 14, no. 3, pp. 83–85, 2003.

[8] E. Elias, "Diagnosis of Ehrlichiosis from the presence of inclusion bodies of morulae of *E. canis*," *Journal of Small Animal Practice*, vol. 33, pp. 540–543, 1991.

[9] J. A. Benavides and G. F. Ramírez, "Casos Clínicos: Ehrlichiosis canina," *Revista Colombiana de Ciencias Pecuarias*, vol. 16, no. 3, pp. 268–294, 2003.

[10] W. C. Buhles Jr., D. L. Huxsoll, and M. Ristic, "Tropical canine pancytopenia: clinical, hematologic, and serologic response of dogs to *Ehrlichia canis* infection, tetracycline therapy, and challenge inoculation," *Journal of Infectious Diseases*, vol. 130, no. 4, pp. 357–367, 1974.

[11] L. Bockino, P. M. Krimer, S. L. Kenneth, and J. B. Perry, "An Overview of Canine Ehrlichiosis," 2013, http://www.vet.uga.edu/vpp/clerk/Bockino.

14

Seroprevalence of Canine Parvovirus in Dogs in Lusaka District, Zambia

Ngonda Saasa,[1] King Shimumbo Nalubamba,[2] Ethel M'kandawire,[1] and Joyce Siwila[2]

[1]*Department of Disease Control, University of Zambia, School of Veterinary Medicine, P.O. Box 32379, 10101 Lusaka, Zambia*
[2]*Department of Clinical Studies, University of Zambia, School of Veterinary Medicine, P.O. Box 32379, 10101 Lusaka, Zambia*

Correspondence should be addressed to Ngonda Saasa; nsaasa@yahoo.co.uk

Academic Editor: Paola Paradies

Canine parvovirus (CPV) enteritis is a highly contagious enteric disease of young dogs. Limited studies have been done in Zambia to investigate the prevalence of CPV in dogs. Blood was collected from dogs from three veterinary clinics (clinic samples, $n = 174$) and one township of Lusaka (field samples, $n = 56$). Each dog's age, sex, breed, and vaccination status were recorded. A haemagglutination assay using pig erythrocytes and modified live parvovirus vaccine as the antigen was used. Antibodies to CPV were detected in 100% of dogs (unvaccinated or vaccinated). The titres ranged from 160 to 10240 with a median of 1280. Vaccinated dogs had significantly higher antibody titres compared to unvaccinated ($p < 0.001$). There was a significant difference in titres of clinic samples compared to field samples ($p < 0.0001$) but not within breed ($p = 0.098$) or sex ($p = 0.572$). Multiple regression analysis showed that only age and vaccination status were significant predictors of antibody titres. The presence of antibody in all dogs suggests that the CPV infection is ubiquitous and the disease is endemic, hence the need for research to determine the protection conferred by vaccination and natural exposure to the virus under local conditions.

1. Introduction

Canine parvovirus (CPV) is a major cause of morbidity and mortality in dogs worldwide. Infection with CPV results in a highly contagious enteric disease affecting mainly young naïve dogs or may result from vaccination failure due to maternal antibody interference [1]. Three antigenic variants, CPV-2a, CPV-2b, and CPV-2c, that differ by single amino acid residues of the VP2 capsid protein have so far been identified [1–3]. The clinical signs of CPV infection range from mild to severe foul-smelling haemorrhagic enteritis, fever, vomiting, and often death in severe cases [4]. Transmission of the parvovirus is most commonly through the faecal-oral route via contaminated food and water and the environment [5]. After being ingested, a viraemia develops with subsequent spread throughout the small intestines. The stability of the virus when shed in the environment promotes the spread through indirect transmission. Apart from domestic dogs, the virus has also been detected in several other species such as wild dogs and lions [6].

In Zambia, limited studies have been conducted to determine the prevalence of CPV in dogs. Only a single study found exposure of wild carnivores to CPV although no domestic dogs were examined [6]. There is also no study that has been conducted to evaluate the effectiveness of the vaccination or whether the dogs are protected or not. The majority of cases reported as being attributed to CPV by veterinary surgeons are based purely on clinical presentation since confirmatory diagnostic tests such as SNAP® tests and PCR are rarely done. Vaccination against CPV is routinely done using Vanguard Plus-CPV-2 strain NL-35-D vaccine (Pfizer) containing a monovalent modified live parvovirus which is given at 6 weeks of age. In addition, a multivalent preparation Vanguard Plus-5L containing canine distemper (CD) virus, canine adenovirus type 1 (CAV-1), canine adenovirus type 2 (CAV-2), canine parainfluenza (CPI) virus, canine parvovirus (CPV), and *Leptospira* antigens is also used.

The majority of dogs in high density communities are either free-roaming or semistray. These dogs receive minimal prophylactic or therapeutic veterinary care. The disease status of these free-roaming dogs is usually not known, nor is the history of previous exposure to common infections. Although the CPV cases in dogs (based on clinical presentation) have been reported in several veterinary clinics in Zambia, no seroprevalence study has yet been conducted to establish the extent of CPV exposure among dogs in Zambia. Therefore, the aim of this study was to provide information on the prevalence of antibodies to CPV in the dog population of Lusaka district in Zambia.

2. Materials and Methods

2.1. Study Area, Design, and Sampling. The samples used in this study were collected during a cross-sectional study conducted in Lusaka, to investigate filarial infections in dogs as previously described [7]. The samples were collected over a period of 5 months. Whole blood was collected in plain tubes for serum preparation from dogs aged six months and above that were presented for medical consultation at the School of Veterinary Medicine, University of Zambia ($n = 111$), or other nearby veterinary clinics ($n = 63$). Field samples ($n = 56$) from one of the townships of Lusaka were collected during an antirabies vaccination campaign. Consent to collect blood from the dogs was obtained from the owners after explaining the purpose of the study. Subject data was captured on a preprinted form.

Age was determined from owner's information and corroborated from dental examination when in doubt. The ages of all the dogs were then categorized as 1 (0–3 years), 2 (4–7 years), 3 (8–11 years), 4 (≥12 years), and 5 (adults of unknown age) because of the difficulty in determining the exact age of most of the subjects. There were equal numbers of unvaccinated ($n = 115$) and vaccinated ($n = 115$) dogs. The vaccinated dogs had received either a monovalent parvovirus vaccine or a multivalent vaccine. Vaccination status was obtained by a vaccination history and/or vaccination certificate. Other parameters collected included breed, sex, and source of subject (either clinic or field samples). The main outcome variable in the analysis was the presence of antibodies to canine parvovirus. The haemagglutination inhibition assay was used to determine the presence of antibodies specific to CPV.

2.2. Haemagglutination (HA) and Inhibition (HI) Assay. The HA test was carried out by preparing serial twofold dilutions of the modified live parvovirus vaccine (Vanguard Plus-CPV®) in 50 μL of normal saline and 50 μL of 1.0% fresh pig erythrocytes. The titre was expressed as the reciprocal of the highest dilution of haemagglutination. Newcastle disease Lasota vaccine virus strain was used as negative control antigen for the pig erythrocytes. The HI test was performed in 96-well microplates using 8 HA units of the parvovirus modified live vaccine virus. Twenty-five microlitres of the vaccine antigen was added to 25 μL of twofold serial dilution of test serum and incubated for 1 hr at room temperature. Thereafter, 50 μL of 1% pig erythrocytes suspension was added to all the wells, and the mixture was incubated in a refrigerator at 4°C. The reading of results was carried out after 1 hr and repeated after 24 hrs. The HI titre was expressed as the reciprocal of the highest dilution of serum showing

TABLE 1: Summary of the dogs sampled, vaccination status, age distribution ($n = 230$), and associated p values.

Variable	Number	Unvaccinated (%)	Vaccinated (%)	p value
Source				
Clinics	174	59	115	<0.0001
Field	56	56	0	
Sex				
Male	130	63	67	0.572
Female	100	52	48	
Breed				
Pure	50	11	39	0.098
Mixed	180	104	76	
Site				
A (clinic)	9	8 (89)	1 (11)	
B (clinic)	111	33 (30)	78 (70)	0.001*
C (clinic)	54	18 (33)	36 (67)	
D (field)	56	56 (100)	0 (0)	
Age group (years)				
1 (0–3)	163	85	78	
2 (4–7)	43	22	21	
3 (8–11)	6	4	2	0.006*
4 (≥12)	2	2	0	
5 (unknown)	16	2	14	

*ANOVA.

complete inhibition of haemagglutination of pig erythrocytes [8].

2.3. Data Analysis. Data was entered into a Microsoft Excel® spreadsheet and examined for correctness and completeness. Descriptive statistical analysis and graphing was performed in R statistical software (R Core Team, 2014, Vienna, Austria). The analysis was performed after log transforming the antibody titre results. Statistical analysis was undertaken using a t-test for independent samples to determine the differences in the parvovirus antibody titres of unvaccinated and vaccinated dogs. Determination of predictors of antibody titres was performed using multiple linear regression models. The predictor variables analysed included source of subjects, sex, breed, and age (Table 1). Results were considered significant at $p < 0.05$.

3. Results

A total of 230 serum samples were collected comprising 130 male and 100 female dogs from four sources: 3 clinics (A; $n = 9$, B; $n = 111$, C; $n = 54$) and a field vaccination campaign ($n = 56$) (Table 1). The majority of the dogs (180/230; 78.3%) were of the mixed breed type while 50/230 (21.7%) were pure breeds (Boerboel, German shepherd, Jack Russell, Labrador retriever, Maltese poodles, Bull mastiff, Pomeranian, and Rottweiler).

TABLE 2: Pairwise comparison of antibodies titres of dogs in various clinics/sites, ($n = 230$).

Site	A	B	C
D (field)	$p < 0.0001$	$p < 0.0001$	$p < 0.0001$
A (clinic)	—	$p = 1.000$	$p = 0.259$
B (clinic)		—	$p = 0.013$

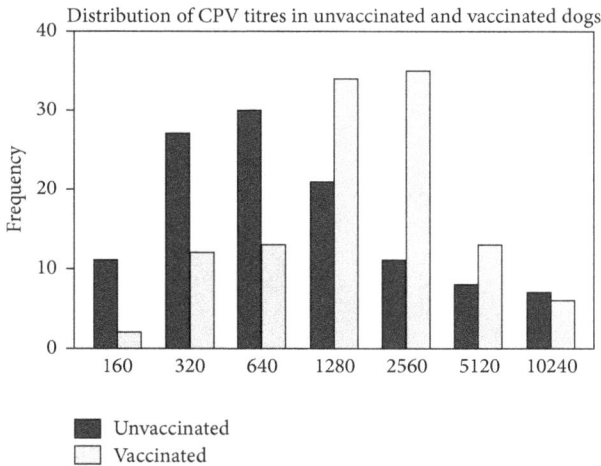

FIGURE 1: Distribution of CPV titres in dogs.

Seroprevalence in both unvaccinated and vaccinated dogs was 100%. The distribution of antibody titres ranged from 160 to 10240 (log = 2.2–4.0) with a median of 1280 (log = 3.1) (Figure 1). The mean titre for samples collected from dogs from veterinary clinics (clinic samples) was 2560 (log = 3.4) and that from the field sampling (vaccination campaign) was 640 (log = 2.8). The t-test showed a significant difference in antibody titres between unvaccinated and vaccinated dogs ($p < 0.001$) (Table 1). The analysis also showed that there was a significant difference in titres of dogs that were brought to the clinics compared to those that were sampled from the field vaccination ($p < 0.000$) (Table 2). No significant differences in antibody titres were seen between breed ($p = 0.098$) (Table 1) and sex ($p = 0.572$). A difference in titres among the age groups was also present but only between age groups 1 and 5 ($p = 0.006$) (Table 2).

A multiple regression model was performed to estimate the influence of the predictors (sex, breed, age, and source of the subjects) of the antibody titres. A significant model was developed for age and source of subjects (F-statistic: 13.29, adjusted $R^2 = 0.097$, df = 227, and $p = 0.000$).

4. Discussion

Canine parvovirus is a cause of morbidity and mortality in dogs, hence the need to investigate the prevalence of the antibodies to CPV. Although a few researchers have reported on CPV infection in Zambia [6], a number of putative cases are reported in veterinary clinics (Dr. Elizabeth Oparaocha, Showgrounds Vet clinic, personal communication). A number of these suspected cases are based on clinical presentation

of haemorrhagic enteritis with absence of prior vaccination against CPV especially in young dogs less than six months of age [9]. At least one case of CPV infection per week is seen by clinicians in small animal practices (Dr. Andrew M. Phiri, UNZAVET Clinics, personal communication). In a study conducted in wild and domestic canids, CPV neutralizing antibodies were detected in lions and hyenas, but this was not done in dogs due to sample limitation [6].

The present study found that CPV is prevalent in Lusaka. All dogs, whether vaccinated or not, had anti-CPV antibodies indicating that they had been exposed to the virus. This finding is similar to previous studies in Zimbabwe and South Korea that found a high proportion of seroconversion in dogs [10, 11]. The antibody titres in dogs previously vaccinated were, however, significantly higher than those not known to have been previously vaccinated. In nonendemic areas or where compliance with vaccination is very high, natural exposure to CPV is low, thereby making the puppy series of vaccinations necessary.

The estimation of the contribution of the various predictors towards the antibody status of the dogs showed that age and vaccination status of the dog were the only significant predictors. The low coefficient of determination ($R^2 = 0.10$) of the model suggested that age and vaccination status could only account for a small variation in antibody titres and that there are many other factors besides vaccination and age that influence the observed titres of parvovirus in the dogs.

Whether a higher CPV antibody titre would lead to more superior protection against the disease or less severe clinical signs or both, resulting in better care outcomes, cannot be determined without carrying out challenge protection and neutralization tests. Although revaccination confers higher serum antibody titres and possibly protection against related strains of parvovirus, antibody titre levels may still need to be established before revaccination [12, 13]. The CPV antibody prevalence of 100%, although higher antibody titres were observed in vaccinated dogs, is evidence of the ubiquitous nature of CPV in Lusaka.

It was evident from this study that dogs that had received prior vaccination had significantly higher titres than dogs that did not have a history of vaccination (field samples). The differences in the antibody titres of dogs that were presented to the various clinics would suggest that these dogs received better or appropriate vaccination. The fact that these dogs were presented to the clinic by owners is an indication that such dogs had at one time most likely received a vaccine against parvovirus. In contrast, nearly all dogs that were sampled from the field antirabies vaccination campaign were not immunized against rabies or canine parvovirus. In endemic areas, dogs are generally exposed to the CPV in the environment and natural acquisition of protection may take place in which unvaccinated dogs eventually seroconvert [10, 14].

In conclusion, we found that CPV is endemic and exposure is common in unvaccinated dogs aged more than six months in the greater Lusaka region. Vaccination of dogs accounts for a small proportion (10%) to the relatively high CPV antibody titres observed in vaccinated dogs. Follow-up work to include serosurvey of dogs less than 6 months and comparing the F_1 of vaccinated and unvaccinated dogs is recommended. A longitudinal study of antibody levels in puppies of vaccinated and unvaccinated dams until first vaccination at six weeks of age will be part of future studies.

Competing Interests

The authors declare that they have no conflict of interests.

References

[1] J. Meers, M. Kyaw-Tanner, Z. Bensink, and R. Zwijnenberg, "Genetic analysis of canine parvovirus from dogs in Australia," *Australian Veterinary Journal*, vol. 85, no. 10, pp. 392–396, 2007.

[2] C. R. Parrish, C. F. Aquadro, M. L. Strassheim, J. F. Evermann, J.-Y. Sgro, and H. O. Mohammed, "Rapid antigenic-type replacement and DNA sequence evolution of canine parvovirus," *Journal of Virology*, vol. 65, no. 12, pp. 6544–6552, 1991.

[3] S.-Y. Jeoung, S.-J. Ahn, and D. Kim, "Genetic analysis of VP2 gene of canine parvovirus isolates in Korea," *Journal of Veterinary Medical Science*, vol. 70, no. 7, pp. 719–722, 2008.

[4] H.-S. Moon, S.-A. Lee, S.-G. Lee et al., "Comparison of the pathogenicity in three different Korean canine parvovirus 2 (CPV-2) isolates," *Veterinary Microbiology*, vol. 131, no. 1-2, pp. 47–56, 2008.

[5] N. Decaro, G. Crescenzo, C. Desario et al., "Long-term viremia and fecal shedding in pups after modified-live canine parvovirus vaccination," *Vaccine*, vol. 32, no. 30, pp. 3850–3853, 2014.

[6] A. R. Berentsen, M. R. Dunbar, M. S. Becker et al., "Rabies, canine distemper, and canine parvovirus exposure in large carnivore communities from two zambian ecosystems," *Vector-Borne and Zoonotic Diseases*, vol. 13, no. 9, pp. 643–649, 2013.

[7] J. Siwila, E. T. Mwase, P. Nejsum, and P. E. Simonsen, "Filarial infections in domestic dogs in Lusaka, Zambia," *Veterinary Parasitology*, vol. 210, no. 3-4, pp. 250–254, 2015.

[8] M. Senda, N. Hirayama, O. Itoh, and H. Yamamoto, "Canine parvovirus: strain difference in haemagglutination activity and antigenicity," *Journal of General Virology*, vol. 69, no. 2, pp. 349–354, 1988.

[9] M. Ling, J. M. Norris, M. Kelman, and M. P. Ward, "Risk factors for death from canine parvoviral-related disease in Australia," *Veterinary Microbiology*, vol. 158, no. 3-4, pp. 280–290, 2012.

[10] A. McRee, R. P. Wilkes, J. Dawson et al., "Serological detection of infection with canine distemper virus, canine parvovirus and canine adenovirus in communal dogs from Zimbabwe," *Journal of the South African Veterinary Association*, vol. 85, no. 1, pp. 1–2, 2014.

[11] D.-K. Yang, S.-S. Yoon, J.-W. Byun, K.-W. Lee, Y.-I. Oh, and J.-Y. Song, "Serological survey for canine parvovirus type 2a (CPV-2a) in the stray dogs in South Korea," *Journal of Bacteriology and Virology*, vol. 40, no. 2, pp. 77–81, 2010.

[12] H.-P. Ottiger, M. Neimeier-Förster, K. D. C. Stärk, K. Duchow, and L. Bruckner, "Serological responses of adult dogs to revaccination against distemper, parvovirus and rabies," *Veterinary Record*, vol. 159, no. 1, pp. 7–12, 2006.

[13] S. Wilson, J. Illambas, E. Siedek et al., "Vaccination of dogs with canine parvovirus type 2b (CPV-2b) induces neutralising antibody responses to CPV-2a and CPV-2c," *Vaccine*, vol. 32, no. 42, pp. 5420–5424, 2014.

[14] M. Riedl, U. Truyen, S. Reese, and K. Hartmann, "Prevalence of antibodies to canine parvovirus and reaction to vaccination in client-owned, Healthy dogs," *Veterinary Record*, vol. 177, no. 23, article 597, 2015.

15

Epidemiological Overview of African Swine Fever in Uganda (2001–2012)

David Kalenzi Atuhaire,[1,2] Sylvester Ochwo,[1] Mathias Afayoa,[1]
Frank Norbert Mwiine,[1] Ikwap Kokas,[1] Eugene Arinaitwe,[3] Rose Anna Ademun-Okurut,[3]
Julius Boniface Okuni,[1] Ann Nanteza,[1] Christosom Ayebazibwe,[3] Loyce Okedi,[2]
William Olaho-Mukani,[4] and Lonzy Ojok[1]

[1] College of Veterinary Medicine, Animal Resources and Biosecurity, Makerere University, P.O. Box 7062, Kampala, Uganda
[2] National Agricultural Research Organization, National Livestock Resources Research Institute, P.O. Box 96, Tororo, Uganda
[3] Ministry of Agriculture, Animal Industry and Fisheries, National Animal Disease Diagnostics and Epidemiology Centre,
  P.O. Box 513, Entebbe, Uganda
[4] African Union-Inter African Bureau for Animal Resources, P.O. Box 30786, Nairobi, Kenya

Correspondence should be addressed to Frank Norbert Mwiine; mwiine@vetmed.mak.ac.ug

Academic Editor: Masanori Tohno

African swine fever (ASF) is a contagious viral disease, which can cause up to 100% mortality among domestic pigs. In Uganda there is paucity of information on the epidemiology of the disease, hence a study was carried out to elucidate the patterns of ASF outbreaks. Spatial and temporal analyses were performed with data collected monthly by the district veterinary officers (DVOs) and sent to the central administration at MAAIF from 2001 to 2012. Additionally, risk factors and the associated characteristics related to the disease were assessed based on semistructured questionnaires sent to the DVOs. A total of 388 ASF outbreaks were reported in 59 districts. Of these outbreaks, 201 (51.8%) were reported in districts adjacent to the national parks while 80 (20.6%) were adjacent to international borders. The number of reported ASF outbreaks changed over time and by geographical regions; however, no outbreak was reported in the North-Eastern region. ASF was ranked as second most important disease of pigs, and it occurred mostly during the dry season ($P = 0.01$). Pig movements due to trade (OR 15.5, CI 4.9–49.1) and restocking (OR 6.6, CI 2.5–17.3) were the major risk factors. ASF control strategies should focus on limiting pig movements in Uganda.

1. Introduction

African swine fever (ASF) is a highly fatal disease of domestic pigs and can cause mortality of up to 100% of affected pigs [1]. The disease is caused by double-stranded DNA virus with an icosahedral symmetry that belongs to genus *Asfivirus* and family *Asfarviridae* [2]. Since its first description in Kenya in the early 1920s [3], the disease has been reported in several countries around the world, remaining endemic in Sardinia, and in 2007 outbreaks was reported in Georgia, Russia, and neighbouring countries [4]. The epidemiology of ASF is complex, transmission is direct and vector-borne, and the disease has well-recognized sylvatic and domestic

cycles. In sub-Saharan Africa, ASFV is maintained by long-term, inapparent infection of wildlife hosts such as bush pigs (*Potamochoerus porcus*) and warthogs (*Phacochoerus africanus*) which are infected via tick bites of the argasid tick vector (*Ornithodoros* complex) [5].

ASF is highly contagious and is transmitted by direct contact between infected pigs and susceptible ones or by contact with or ingestion of infectious secretions/excretions. The virus is highly resistant in tissues and the environment, contributing to its transmission over long distances through swill feeding and fomites (e.g., contaminated material, vehicles, or visitors to pig premises) [6]. In subacute cases pigs lose condition and die of pneumonia. Chronically, survivors are characterized by emaciation, stunted growth, hemorrhagic necrosis of the skin overlying bony protuberances, followed by abscessation, and deep ulceration. Acute disease caused by the virus is characterized by high fever, hemorrhages in the reticuloendothelial system, and high morbidity and mortality rates with consequent economic losses [7]. Unlike domestic swine, ASFV infections of wild swine are asymptomatic with low viraemia titers [8]. The wild swine and soft ticks of the genus *Ornithodoros* act as a virus reservoir [5]. This large natural reservoir of virus poses a constant threat to domestic pig populations worldwide.

Pig farming is one of the fastest growing livestock activities in the rural areas of Uganda and has become very attractive through the country as a means of increasing food, but income and employment have on several occasions been hampered by ASF [9]. According to reports, Uganda has the largest and fastest growing pig production in Eastern Africa with the pig population standing at 3.2 million [10]. But ASF is an economically important and frequently lethal disease of domestic pigs which has hampered the development of the pig industry. The aim of the study was to elucidate the patterns of ASF outbreaks in Uganda based on the spatial and temporal retrospective data retrieved from monthly reports from district veterinary officers (DVOs) to the central administration at the Ministry of Agriculture, Animal Industry and Fisheries (MAAIF) for the years spanning 2001–2012 to give an insight in the epidemiology of the disease in Uganda.

2. Materials and Methods

Retrospective data on ASF outbreaks in Uganda during 2001–2012 were retrieved from MAAIF, Uganda. The information was based on the monthly ASF disease surveillance reports from the DVOs. For the period considered under this study, Uganda had a differing number of districts (80–120). The lowest administrative units reporting ASF outbreaks in Uganda are districts, and, in this work, these were used as epidemiological units of ASF outbreaks and classified as adjacent to the national park(s) and international border(s). The national parks considered in this study included: Queen Elizabeth National Park (QENP), Lake Mburo National Park (LMNP), Murchison Falls National Park (MFNP), Kidepo Valley National Park (KVNP), Rwenzori Mountains National Park (RMNP), Kibale National Park (KINP), Mount Elgon National Park (MENP), Bwindi Impenetrable National Park (BINP), Mgahinga Gorilla National Park (MGNP), and Semuliki National Park (SNP).

Rainfall values and the seasons for the different months, districts, and years (2001–2008) were obtained from the Meteorological Department, Ministry of Energy, Water and Mineral Resources, Uganda. For convenience of data handling and presentation, seven geographical regions, which in most cases vary by rainfall [11], agroecology, and farming production systems, were considered. The months of the year were categorized as having below average rainfall (dry season), above average rainfall (wet season), and average rainfall (neither wet nor dry season) based on long term mean monthly rainfall over the period 2001–2008. A nonparametric test (Kruskal-Wallis rank test) was used to assess the effect of

season on ASF (Stata 12.0). ArcGIS (version 10) was used to plot the district distribution of ASF outbreaks (2001–2012).

Semistructured questionnaires on the occurrence of ASF outbreaks and the perception of risk factors and characteristics of these outbreaks were administered to the DVOs in their respective districts. General subject introductions and clarifications were made immediately after the distribution of the questionnaires. Questions included whether there are cases of pig deaths or sickness, percentage of the pig population affected, rating of ASF as an important disease, seasons when incidence is most frequent, and actions taken to control ASF. Questions were answered by ticking prewritten choices, whilst additional information was supplied in the extra spaces provided. Opinions and data were collected, entered into Excel 2010, summarized, coded, and analyzed. Perceived risk factors were scored on a Likert scale [12] and categorized as less or not important (below 25%), important (26–100%), or not applicable so as to estimate the corresponding odds ratios (ORs) as described previously [13]. Both descriptive statistics (contingency tables) and inferential statistics such as confidence interval for odds ratio were computed so as to quantify the major reason for pig movement in the area.

3. Results

3.1. Temporal Patterns for the Occurrence of ASF. The regional monthly reports of ASF outbreaks from districts during the years 2001–2012 are summarized in Table 1. The total number of districts which reported ASF was 59 with a total of 388 outbreaks. The number of reported ASF outbreaks was highest (68) in 2011 and lowest (6) in 2009. More outbreaks were reported during the months of February (43), March (42), June (40), and January (38) than during the remaining months of the year. The months of October (19), May (20), and September (26) had the lowest number of outbreaks reported. In the districts and regions where rainfall data were available (Table 2), it was apparent that the occurrence of ASF was significantly associated with dry season ($P = 0.01$), when mean monthly rainfall (mm) was below average and the times when animal movement are more frequent.

3.2. Spatial Patterns for the Occurrence of ASF

3.2.1. Regional Occurrence of ASF Outbreaks. Regional occurrence of ASF outbreaks is summarized in Table 3. The Central region reported the highest number of ASF outbreaks (181) followed by the Eastern (100), Northern (60), Western (23), Southwestern (12), and West Nile (12). However, there was no ASF outbreak reported in the Northeastern region throughout the period covered by the study. It should be noted that outbreaks were sporadic in the Southwest and West Nile regions throughout the study period.

3.2.2. Occurrence of ASF Outbreaks Adjacent to National Parks. A total of 201 outbreaks were reported in districts adjacent to the national parks representing 51.8% of the total outbreaks reported during the period (2001–2012) as summarized in Table 4.

TABLE 1: Reported ASF outbreaks by year, month and region in Uganda (2001–2012).

Year	Region	J	F	M	A	M	J	J	A	S	O	N	D	Total	
2001	C	—	1	3	—	—	5	4	4	4	2	5	5	33	
	E	—	1	2	—	—	—	—	1	1	2	1	1	9	
	N	—	1	—	—	—	1	—	1	1	—	—	—	4	(49)
	W	—	—	—	—	—	—	—	—	1	—	1	1	3	
	SW	—	—	—	—	—	—	—	—	—	—	—	—	0	
	WN	—	—	—	—	—	—	—	—	—	—	—	—	0	
2002	C	1	1	3	3	3	5	4	4	4	2	4	5	39	
	E	1	1	2	2	1	—	—	1	1	2	2	1	14	
	N	—	1	—	—	—	1	—	1	1	—	—	—	4	(59)
	W	—	—	—	—	—	—	—	1	—	—	—	1	2	
	SW	—	—	—	—	—	—	—	—	—	—	—	—	0	
	WN	—	—	—	—	—	—	—	—	—	—	—	—	0	
2003	C	4	3	2	2	1	3	1	—	4	—	3	2	25	
	E	3	3	3	2	1	—	2	2	2	1	4	2	25	
	N	—	1	—	1	1	1	—	—	—	—	—	1	5	(64)
	W	—	—	1	1	1	2	2	—	—	—	—	—	7	
	SW	—	—	1	1	—	—	—	—	—	—	—	—	2	
	WN	—	—	—	—	—	—	—	—	—	—	—	—	0	
2004	C	1	2	1	2	3	4	2	2	2	1	1	4	25	
	E	4	3	4	2	2	3	1	3	—	—	—	—	22	
	N	—	1	1	—	—	—	—	—	—	1	2	—	5	(57)
	W	—	—	—	—	—	—	1	—	—	—	1	—	2	
	SW	—	—	—	—	—	—	1	—	1	1	—	—	3	
	WN	—	—	—	—	—	—	—	—	—	—	—	—	0	
2005	C	3	2	—	—	—	—	—	—	—	—	—	—	5	
	E	1	—	2	3	—	—	—	—	—	—	—	—	6	
	N	—	1	2	1	—	—	—	1	—	—	—	—	5	(17)
	W	—	—	—	—	—	—	—	—	—	—	—	—	0	
	SW	1	—	—	—	—	—	—	—	—	—	—	—	1	
	WN	—	—	—	—	—	—	—	—	—	—	—	—	0	
2006	C	—	—	—	—	—	—	—	—	—	—	—	—	0	
	E	1	1	2	1	1	—	—	—	—	—	—	1	7	
	N	—	—	—	—	—	—	—	—	—	—	1	1	2	(14)
	W	—	—	—	—	—	—	—	—	—	—	—	—	0	
	SW	—	—	—	—	—	—	—	—	—	—	—	—	0	
	WN	1	1	—	—	—	—	—	1	—	1	1	—	5	
2007	C	—	—	—	—	—	1	2	—	—	—	—	1	4	
	E	—	—	—	1	—	—	—	1	1	—	—	—	3	
	N	—	2	—	—	—	—	—	—	—	—	—	—	2	(9)
	W	—	—	—	—	—	—	—	—	—	—	—	—	0	
	SW	—	—	—	—	—	—	—	—	—	—	—	—	0	
	WN	—	—	—	—	—	—	—	—	—	—	—	—	0	
2008	C	—	2	1	1	2	—	1	—	—	1	1	1	10	
	E	—	1	1	—	—	—	—	—	—	—	1	1	4	
	N	—	—	—	—	—	—	—	—	—	—	—	—	0	(20)
	W	—	—	2	1	—	—	—	—	—	—	—	—	3	
	SW	—	—	—	—	—	—	—	—	—	1	1	1	3	
	WN	—	—	—	—	—	—	—	—	—	—	—	—	0	

TABLE 1: Continued.

Year	Region	J	F	M	A	M	J	J	A	S	O	N	D	Total	
2009	C	—	—	—	—	—	—	—	—	—	1	—	—	1	
	E	1	—	1	1	1	—	—	—	—	—	—	—	4	
	N	—	—	—	—	—	—	—	—	—	—	—	—	0	(6)
	W	—	—	—	—	—	—	—	—	—	—	—	—	0	
	SW	1	—	—	—	—	—	—	—	—	—	—	—	1	
	WN	—	—	—	—	—	—	—	—	—	—	—	—	1	
2010	C	—	—	—	—	—	—	1	—	—	—	1	—	2	
	E	—	—	—	1	—	—	1	1	—	—	1	—	4	
	N	—	—	—	—	—	1	—	—	1	—	—	—	2	(9)
	W	—	—	—	—	—	—	—	—	—	—	—	—	0	
	SW	—	—	—	—	—	1	—	—	—	—	—	—	1	
	WN	—	—	—	—	—	—	—	—	—	—	—	—	0	
2011	C	4	2	1	3	2	7	2	2	1	2	1	2	29	
	E	1	—	—	—	1	—	—	1	—	—	—	1	4	
	N	4	8	2	3	—	1	1	1	—	—	1	1	22	(68)
	W	—	1	1	—	—	1	—	—	—	—	—	—	3	
	SW	—	—	—	—	—	—	—	1	—	—	—	—	1	
	WN	3	—	—	—	—	—	—	1	1	1	1	2	9	
2012	C	—	2	1	—	—	1	—	—	—	—	—	—	4	
	E	—	—	—	—	—	—	—	—	—	—	—	—	0	
	N	3	1	2	—	—	1	1	1	1	—	—	—	10	(16)
	W	—	—	—	—	—	1	—	—	—	—	—	—	1	
	SW	—	—	—	—	—	—	—	—	—	—	—	—	0	
	WN	—	—	1	—	—	—	—	—	—	—	—	—	1	
	Total	38	43	42	32	20	40	27	32	26	19	34	35		(388)

C: central; E: eastern; N: northern; W: western; SW: southwestern; WN: west nile
Dashes (—) represent periods when there were no newly reported ASF outbreaks.

TABLE 2: Assessment of patterns of occurrence of ASF outbreaks and the distribution of rainfall in selected districts in Uganda (2001–2008).

Region	District	Mean annual rainfall (mm)	ASF outbreaks by rainfall (mm)			Total number of outbreaks
			Above average[a]	Average[b]	Below average[c]	
N	Apac	1489	4	0	9	13
N	Kitgum	1343	1	0	3	4
W	Masindi	1317	2	3	9	14
C	Wakiso	1216	7	1	6	14
C	Nakasongola	1046	0	1	4	5
C	Rakai	987	2	5	7	14
E	Kamuli	1387	3	5	8	16
SW	Kasese	884	0	1	4	5
WN	Moyo	1459	0	0	1	1
Total			19	16	51	86

Monthly rainfall (mm) was evaluated as average (normal season), below average (dry season), or above average (wet season) based on long-term mean. Mean annual rainfall values (mm) represent the distribution across selected weather stations and regions.
[a]Wet season.
[b]Neither dry nor wet season.
[c]Dry season.

TABLE 3: Regional reported ASF outbreaks 2001–2012.

Region	Number of outbreaks (%)
Central	181 (**46.6**)
Eastern	100 (**25.8**)
Northern	60 (**15.5**)
Southwestern	12 (**3.1**)
Western	23 (**5.9**)
West Nile	12 (**3.1**)
Total	388

3.2.3. Occurrence of ASF Outbreaks Adjacent to the International Borders. Uganda is landlocked and shares borders with Southern Sudan (435 km) on the northern side, Democratic Republic of Congo (DRC, 765 km) on the western side, Tanzania (396 km) and Rwanda (169 km) on the southern side, and Kenya (933 km) on the eastern side (Figure 1). The total number of districts adjacent to the international borders reporting ASF outbreaks was 18. Eighty (20.6%) ASF outbreaks occurred in 18 districts along the international borders compared to 308 outbreaks that occurred in districts that did not share an international border. The number of ASF outbreaks varied between the different international borders, the highest being adjacent with DRC (31 outbreaks in eight districts) and Tanzania borders (26 outbreaks in 2 districts) while only 3 districts bordering Kenya reported 13 outbreaks. The lowest number of ASF outbreaks was reported among the districts bordering Rwanda (one outbreak in one district) and Southern Sudan (9 outbreaks in 4 districts).

3.2.4. Responses of DVOs to the Semistructured Questionnaire about ASF Occurrence in Uganda. Opinions among the DVOs about the characteristics of occurrence and control of ASF in Uganda are summarized in Table 5. In all the 29 districts visited, all the DVOs reported that farmers valued pigs in their areas and that pig farming ranked third in relation to all the other livestock.

ASF was ranked as the second most important disease of pigs after helminthiasis. When faced with problems of pig health, all DVOs reported that they diagnose by use of clinical signs, and only 15 combined the use of clinical signs and laboratory testing. It was however established that the majority of laboratory testing is done at the National Disease Diagnostics and Epidemiological Center in Entebbe with few sending samples to the College of Veterinary Medicine, Makerere University. Twenty-five (86.2%) and 22 (75.9%) of the DVOs reported that the source of ASF outbreaks was as a result of pig movements due to trade (odds ratio OR 15.5, confidence interval CI 4.9–49.1) and pig restocking (odds ratio OR 6.6, confidence interval CI 2.5–17.3), respectively. However, the majority of the DVOs blamed a neighbouring district as a source of their own outbreaks. Only 2 DVOs attributed the outbreaks to wild pigs. Only 1 DVO (Kasese) reported a source of a former outbreak as from a neighbouring country (DRC).

4. Discussion

This study aimed at elucidating the patterns of African swine fever outbreaks in Uganda based on the spatial and temporal retrospective data retrieved from monthly reports from DVOs. The study also aimed at describing the perceptions of DVOs on the characteristics of ASF outbreaks in their areas by use of a questionnaire. ASF outbreaks occurred during the entire period of study (2001–2012). Our research findings have proved that ASF is endemic in Uganda since throughout the study period ASF was reported. These findings agree with a previous study in Uganda [14] (unpublished data). A report by the OIE has also indicated that ASF is an endemic disease in Uganda [15].

The distribution of ASF outbreaks showed no specific patterns; however, there was a significant difference in the regions on reported ASF outbreaks with the central region being the most affected (181 outbreaks), and yet it has the highest pig population [10]. Consumption of pork has increased in Uganda with the central region leading in demand. This could be the reason leading to a surge in movement of pigs by traders from most parts of the country to the central region, hence the highest number of outbreaks. The Eastern region reported 100 outbreaks followed by Northern (60) and Western (23) with Southwestern and West Nile reporting only 12 outbreaks each. However, there was no ASF outbreak reported in the North-Eastern region. This difference could be partly because of the proximity to the central administration at MAAIF, methods used in reporting, misdiagnosis, the different husbandry practices, and vigilance in disease control, animal movements, distribution of pig markets, and other virus transmission dynamics. In the North-Eastern region the majority of the population being majorly pastoralists could be the reason that no ASF was reported in that region. More so, the North-Eastern region has the lowest number of pigs and the lowest region household average in Uganda [10].

In the present study, there was a tendency to a seasonal pattern with higher frequency of ASF outbreaks reported during the months with lower or without rainfall. Rainfall distribution in Uganda has been shown to follow 14 distinct climate zones, which often span beyond the administrative partitions [11]. An exact analysis of time-specific rainfall data from a smaller number of districts confirmed that outbreaks were more common during the dry season compared to the parts of the year with average and above average rainfall (normal and wet season).

The spatial and temporal patterns of ASF outbreaks indicate that the virus can survive during periods without reports of ASF outbreaks. This could be partly because of underreporting or most importantly due to the transmission dynamics of the virus. The spreading of the infection through introduction of infected pigs, either during the incubation period or by persistently infected pigs, has been described as one of the most important transmission routes [16]. In addition, the fact that the virus is spread through both the sylvatic and the domestic cycles could be a reason for the observed patterns of outbreaks. The sylvatic cycle involves wild species of swine spreading the virus by soft ticks of the

TABLE 4: Occurrence of ASF outbreaks within the districts adjacent to the national parks (2001–2012).

National parks	Year of ASF occurrence												Total
	2001	2002	2003	2004	2005	2006	2007	2008	2009	2010	2011	2012	
BINP	—	—	—	2	1	—	—	—	—	—	—	—	3
KINP	—	—	2	5	—	—	—	—	—	—	3	—	10
KVNP	1	1	—	—	2	2	1	—	—	—	4	2	13
LMNP	4	4	3	—	—	—	—	1	—	—	4	1	17
MENP	5	7	16	10	4	2	3	4	1	3	3	—	58
MFNP	6	5	13	6	5	6	2	6	1	4	29	8	91
QENP	—	—	2	1	—	—	—	3	1	1	1	—	9

BINP: Bwindi impenetrable national park, KINP: Kibale national park, KVNP: Kidepo valley national park, LMNP: Lake Mburo national park, MENP: Mount Elgon national park, MFNP: Murchison Falls national park, QENP: Queen Elizabeth national park.

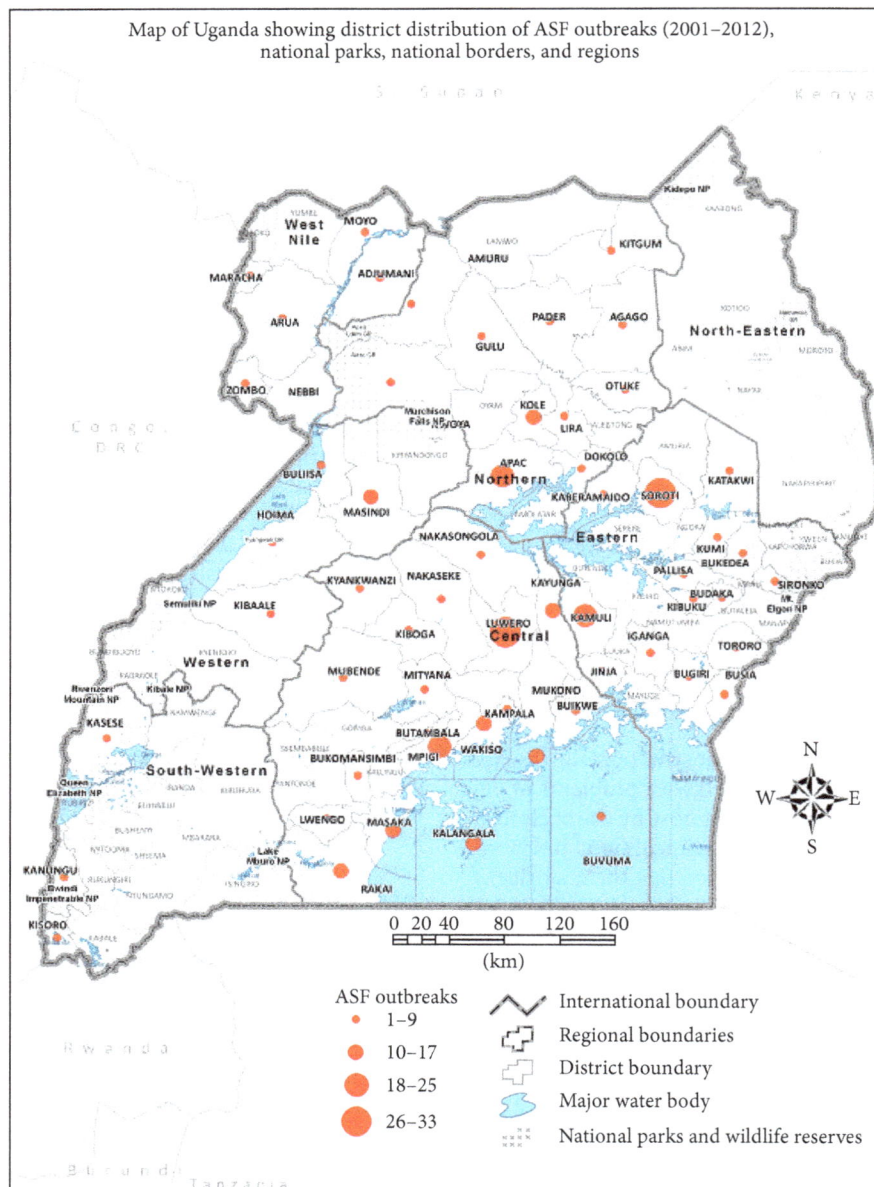

FIGURE 1: Map of Uganda showing distribution of ASF outbreaks (2001-2012), national parks, national borders, and regions.

TABLE 5: Perceived characteristics of ASF occurrence and control in Uganda.

Perceived variables	Parameters	Response (numbers/proportion)		
		Yes	No	NA
Cases of pig deaths or sickness		29 (1.00)	0 (0.00)	0 (0.00)
Percentage of the pig population affected	<5%	7 (0.24)	22 (0.76)	0 (0.00)
	5–15%	8 (0.28)	21 (0.72)	0 (0.00)
	20–25%	6 (0.21)	23 (0.79)	0 (0.00)
	Over 50%	8 (0.28)	21 (0.72)	0 (0.00)
Rating of ASF as an important disease in relation to other diseases	ASF (rank = 3.76)	24 (0.83)	5 (0.17)	0 (0.00)
	Helminthiasis/worms (rank = 2.21)	29 (1.00)	0 (0.00)	0 (0.00)
	Malnutrition (rank = 8.76)	11 (0.38)	18 (0.62)	0 (0.00)
	Piglet anaemia (rank = 11.72)	4 (0.14)	25 (0.86)	0 (0.00)
	Cysticercosis (rank = 12.62)	1 (0.03)	28 (0.97)	0 (0.00)
	Mange/Ectoparasites (rank = 6.41)	18 (0.64)	11 (0.36)	0 (0.00)
	Swine Dysentery (rank = 12.28)	4 (0.14)	25 (0.86)	0 (0.00)
	Swine erysipelas (rank = 12.31)	1 (0.03)	28 (0.97)	0 (0.00)
	Abortions (rank = 12.28)	2 (0.07)	27 (0.93)	0 (0.00)
	Pneumonia (rank = 12.31)	1 (0.03)	28 (0.97)	0 (0.00)
	Trypanosomosis (rank = 11.79)	4 (0.14)	25 (0.86)	0 (0.00)
	Lameness (rank = 12.69)	1 (0.03)	28 (0.97)	0 (0.00)
	Ticks (rank = 12.66)	1 (0.03)	28 (0.97)	0 (0.00)
Most recent incident of ASF outbreak	6 months ago	10 (0.35)	19 (0.65)	0 (0.00)
	Still ongoing	9 (0.31)	20 (0.69)	0 (0.00)
	1 year ago	5 (0.17)	24 (0.83)	0 (0.00)
	More than 1 year ago	5 (0.17)	24 (0.83)	0 (0.00)
	Shivering	1 (0.03)	28 (0.97)	0 (0.00)
Seasons when incidence is most frequent	Dry seasons	14 (0.48)	8 (0.28)	7 (0.24)
	Wet seasons	3 (0.10)	19 (0.66)	7 (0.24)
	Every after 5 years	1 (0.03)	21 (0.72)	7 (0.24)
	Every after 2 years	1 (0.03)	21 (0.72)	7 (0.24)
	Throughout the year	4 (0.14)	18 (0.62)	7 (0.24)
Months when ASF is frequent	January–March	3 (0.10)	26 (0.90)	0 (0.00)
	April–June	0 (0.00)	29 (1.00)	0 (0.00)
	July–September	2 (0.07)	27 (0.93)	0 (0.00)
	October–December	2 (0.07)	27 (0.93)	0 (0.00)
	January–June	1 (0.03)	28 (0.97)	0 (0.00)
	Throughout the year	8 (0.28)	21 (0.72)	0 (0.00)
	January–March, July–September	3 (0.10)	26 (0.90)	0 (0.00)
	January–March, October–December	2 (0.07)	27 (0.93)	0 (0.00)
	July–December	4 (0.14)	25 (0.84)	0 (0.00)
Actions taken to control ASF	Quarantine	23 (0.79)	5 (0.21)	1 (0.03)
	Slaughter	7 (0.24)	21 (0.76)	1 (0.03)
	Burial of the dead	6 (0.21)	22 (0.79)	1 (0.03)
	Avoid immediate restocking	1 (0.03)	27 (0.97)	1 (0.03)
	Community sensitization	8 (0.28)	20 (0.72)	1 (0.03)
	Disinfection	1 (0.03)	27 (0.97)	1 (0.03)

genus *Ornithodoros* [17]. In Africa the major host for the ASF virus is the warthog, but all wild species of swine in Africa can be silent carriers. The *Ornithodoros* ticks can survive for a long time and can harbour the virus for several years with only a gradual decrease of infectivity [17]. In commercial farms it is unlikely for the domestic pigs to come in contact with wild pigs and their ticks, but this is considered more common in traditional free-ranging systems [16]. A previous study carried out in Mubende district located in central Uganda suggested that free ranging and tethering could have an influence on the occurrence of ASF outbreaks [18]. In Uganda ASFV has been detected in the wild suids and in *Ornithodoros* ticks in Rakai district, and in the same study eight PCR-positive pigs were found with no known clinical disease [19]. In the intermediate cycle ASFV has been found in ticks collected in pig stys that have been empty of pigs for four years [20].

The domestic cycle involves domestic pigs spreading the virus to other domestic pigs through direct or indirect contact [17]. In the infected domestic pig the virus is shed in enormous amounts in all bodily secretions and excretions, tissues, and blood 24 to 48 hours before clinical symptoms are shown. Transmission through direct contact can occur up to 30 days after infection, whereas blood is infective for eight weeks [17] and in putrefied blood as long as 15 weeks [21]. Meat from infected pigs or contaminated pork products is another important source of infection due to the virus's long persistence in tissues [22]. The virus has been found in lymphoid tissues in domestic pigs for up to three–four months after infection [17]. The role of subclinical carriers has been widely described in several studies. Recovered pigs might remain persistently infected for 6 months and during this time act as a source of transmission to susceptible pigs [22]. In addition, symptomatic carrier animals play an important role in the persistence and dissemination of the disease in endemic areas [21]. In a recent study conducted in Gulu district in Northern Uganda, it was found out that in most rural areas, local slaughter places are small and poorly equipped and waste is directly accessible to other animals such as dogs or roaming pigs and that many pig owners sell their pigs as soon as they suspect ASF among them [23]. This could be one of the major modes of transmission and sources of outbreaks in other rural areas of Uganda.

In this study, a total of 201 outbreaks were reported in districts adjacent to the national parks representing 51.8% of the total outbreaks reported during the study period (2001–2012) with some national parks being more involved than others. This emphasizes the role of the wild suids in the epidemiology of ASF in Uganda. However, the results of this study cannot conclude on the dynamics of transfer of ASFV between domestic pigs and wild suids in Uganda. Eighty ASF outbreaks were reported in 18 districts along the international borders compared to 308 outbreaks reported in districts that did not share an international border. The number of ASF outbreaks varied between the different international borders, the highest being adjacent with DRC (31 outbreaks in eight districts) and Tanzania borders (26 outbreaks in 2 districts). Though the occurrence of ASF does not entirely depend on proximity to international borders, it is important to consider control of cross-border movements in the animal disease control programme in Uganda. The authors think that the porous nature along the two borders and the geography of the Eastern part of the DRC could be the cause of uncontrolled animal movements, hence the observed high number of ASF outbreaks. Notably, 26 outbreaks were reported in only 2 of the districts bordering Tanzania. A recent study has reported a genetic similarity in ASF disease outbreaks in Uganda and Kenya in 2003, 2006, and 2007 [24] emphasizing the role of cross-border animal movements in the epidemiology of ASF.

The perceptions of the DVOs on risk factors were highly suggestive that trade and restocking were the most important risk factors for the occurrence of ASF outbreaks. This important finding could not be obtained through analysis of spatial and temporal data. A combination of findings from the spatial and temporal studies and DVO-based analysis of risk factors and characteristics of ASF outbreaks in Uganda indicates that the risk is highest during the dry season. This could be as a result of lack of or limited feed resources by the farmers that lead to the sale of pigs or even due to the dynamics of pig movement in search of feeds. Twenty-seven of the 29 DVOs that responded reported that the ASF outbreaks in their districts originated from a neighbouring district indicating the role of animal movement in disease spread. Furthermore, this could probably be due to pig farmers' and traders' failure to adhere to quarantine measures when instituted during ASF outbreaks. One DVO (Kasese) reported the source of a previous outbreak to be across the border (DRC). This could be due to the porous nature of the border and lack of vigilance to enforce animal movement control. This could justify the high number of outbreaks along the DRC border compared to other international borders during the study.

The authors affirm that with regard to the validity of the data presented in this paper, the DVOs are well trained and experienced in animal disease surveillance and control measures, and it is highly likely that the information obtained through extracts from the regular reports to the central administration at MAAIF and through the questionnaire is too reliable. This study has found out that pig movement in the form of trade and restocking is an important factor in the transmission of ASF in Uganda. We strongly recommend that ASF control strategies should encompass a holistic value chain analysis. The government of Uganda through MAAIF should revise and enforce the restocking policy guidelines. More detailed and systematic studies should be undertaken to investigate further other specific risk factors and patterns of occurrence of ASF in Uganda.

Conflict of Interests

The authors declare that they have no conflict of interests.

Acknowledgments

This study was funded by the Millennium Science Initiative under the Uganda National Council of Science and Technology through a grant to LO, WO and JOB (Appropriate Animal diagnostic technologies project). Special thanks go to the staff of the Ministry of Agriculture, Animal Industry and Fisheries for the valuable information on the subject. The authors also thank the District Veterinary Officers who cooperated during data collection, Mr. Kennedy Jumanyol for giving valuable advice during data analysis, and Mr. Bernard Mwesigwa of FAO, Uganda, for his input in GIS mapping.

References

[1] M.-L. Penrith, G. R. Thomson, A. D. S. Bastos et al., "An investigation into natural resistance to African swine fever in domestic pigs from an endemic area in southern Africa," *OIE Revue Scientifique et Technique*, vol. 23, no. 3, pp. 965–977, 2004.

[2] L. K. Dixon, J. M. Escribano, C. Martins, D. L. Rock, M. L. Salas, and P. J. Wilkinson, "Asfarviridae," in *Virus Taxonomy*, C. M. Fauquet, M. A. Mayo, J. Maniloff, U. Desselberger, and L. A. Ball, Eds., Report of the ICTV, London, UK, 8th edition, 2005.

[3] R. E. Montgomery, "On a form of swine fever occurring in British East Africa (Kenya Colony)," *Journal of Comparative Pathology*, vol. 34, pp. 159–191, 1921.

[4] R. J. Rowlands, V. Michaud, L. Heath et al., "African swine fever virus isolate, Georgia, 2007," *Emerging Infectious Diseases*, vol. 14, no. 12, pp. 1870–1874, 2008.

[5] W. Plowright, J. Parker, and M. A. Peirce, "African swine fever virus in ticks (*Ornithodoros moubata*, murray) collected from animal burrows in Tanzania," *Nature*, vol. 221, no. 5185, pp. 1071–1073, 1969.

[6] P. J. Wilkinson, "African swine fever virus," in *Virus Infections of Porcines*, M. B. Pensaert, Ed., pp. 17–35, Elsevier Science Publishers, Amsterdam, The Netherlands, 1989.

[7] B. A. Lubisi, A. D. S. Bastos, R. M. Dwarka, and W. Vosloo, "Molecular epidemiology of African swine fever in East Africa," *Archives of Virology*, vol. 150, no. 12, pp. 2439–2452, 2005.

[8] E. C. Anderson, G. H. Hutchings, N. Mukarati, and P. J. Wilkinson, "African swine fever virus infection of the bushpig (*Potamochoerus porcus*) and its significance in the epidemiology of the disease," *Veterinary Microbiology*, vol. 62, no. 1, pp. 1–15, 1998.

[9] D. Muhanguzi, V. Lutwama, and F. N. Mwiine, "Factors that influence pig production in Central Uganda—case study of Nangabo Sub-County, Wakiso District," *Veterinary World*, vol. 5, no. 6, pp. 346–351, 2012.

[10] UBOS/MAAIF, *Uganda Census of Agriculture 2008/2009*, 2009.

[11] C. P. K. Basalirwa, "Delineation of Uganda into climatological rainfall zones using the method of principal component analysis," *International Journal of Climatology*, vol. 15, no. 10, pp. 1161–1177, 1995.

[12] R. Likert, "A technique for the measurement of attitudes," *Archives of Psychology*, vol. 22, no. 140, pp. 1–55, 1932.

[13] J. M. Bland and D. G. Altman, "Statistics notes. The odds ratio," *British Medical Journal*, vol. 320, no. 7247, article 1468, 2000.

[14] C. Rutebarika and A. O. Ademun, *Overview of African Swine Fever (ASF) Impact and Surveillance in Uganda. During African Swine Fever Diagnostics, Surveillance, Epidemiology and Control: Identification of Researchable Issues Targeted To the Endemic Areas Within Sub-Saharan Africa*, 2011.

[15] Office International des Epizooties (OIE), *Manual of Diagnostic Tests and Vaccines For Terrestrial Animals*, 2010.

[16] P. J. Wilkinson, "The persistence of African swine fever in Africa and the Mediterranean," *Preventive Veterinary Medicine*, vol. 2, no. 1–4, pp. 71–82, 1984.

[17] M.-L. Penrith and W. Vosloo, "Review of African swine fever: transmission, spread and control," *Journal of the South African Veterinary Association*, vol. 80, no. 2, pp. 58–62, 2009.

[18] A. Muwonge, H. M. Munang'andu, C. Kankya et al., "African swine fever among slaughter pigs in Mubende district, Uganda," *Tropical Animal Health and Production*, vol. 44, no. 7, pp. 1593–1598, 2012.

[19] L. Björnheden, "A study of domestic pigs, wild suids and ticks as reservoirs for African swine fever virus in Uganda," *Institutionen För Biomedicin Och Veterinär Folkhälsovetenskap*, 2011.

[20] J. Ravaomanana, F. Jori, L. Vial et al., "Assessment of interactions between African swine fever virus, bushpigs (Potamochoerus larvatus), Ornithodoros ticks and domestic pigs in northwestern Madagascar," *Transboundary and Emerging Diseases*, vol. 58, no. 3, pp. 247–254, 2011.

[21] J. M. Sánchez-Vizcaíno, L. Mur, and B. Martínez-López, "African swine fever: an epidemiological update," *Transboundary and Emerging Diseases*, vol. 59, no. 1, pp. 27–35, 2012.

[22] S. Costard, B. Wieland, W. de Glanville et al., "African swine fever: how can global spread be prevented?" *Philosophical Transactions of the Royal Society B*, vol. 364, no. 1530, pp. 2683–2696, 2009.

[23] E. Tejlar, *Outbreaks of African Swine Fever in Domestic Pigs in Gulu District, Uganda*, 2012.

[24] C. Gallardo, A. R. Ademun, R. Nieto et al., "Genotyping of African swine fever virus (ASFV) isolates associated with disease outbreaks in Uganda in 2007," *African Journal of Biotechnology*, vol. 10, no. 17, pp. 3488–3497, 2011.

16

Seroprevalence of Leptospiral Antibodies in Canine Population in and around Namakkal

N. R. Senthil, K. M. Palanivel, and R. Rishikesavan

Department of Veterinary Epidemiology and Preventive Medicine, Veterinary College and Research Institute and Tamilnadu Veterinary and Animal Sciences University, Tamilnadu, Namakkal 637 002, India

Correspondence should be addressed to K. M. Palanivel; drkmpalanivel@gmail.com

Academic Editor: Daniel A. Feeney

Leptospirosis is a reemerging and a complex zoonotic bacterial disease, caused by pathogenic serovars of *Leptospira interrogans*. A total of 124 sera samples of dogs belonging to different categories like vaccinated, unvaccinated-semiowned, and stray dogs were subjected to sampling. Microscopic agglutination test (MAT) was conducted by using *Leptospira* culture. Out of 42 vaccinated dogs, 24 (57%) were positive to one or more serovars. Of the 24, 22 (52.3%), 11 (26.19%), 4 (9.5%), 1 (3%), and 2 (4.7%) were positive to *icterohaemorrhagiae, canicola, pomona, grippotyphosa*, and *autumnalis*, respectively. Of the 48 unvaccinated semiowned dogs, 10 (28.8%) showed positive agglutination to one or more serovars. Of the 10 samples, 7 (14.5%), 2 (4.1%), 3 (6.2%), 3 (6.2%), and 5 (10.2%) were positive to *icterohaemorrhagiae, canicola, pomona, grippotyphosa*, and *autumnalis*, respectively. Among the 34 stray dogs, 12 showed positive agglutination to one or more leptospiral antibodies. Of the 12 samples, 6 (17.6%) showed positive agglutination to *icterohaemorrhagiae*, 2 (5.8%) to *canicola*, 5 (14.7%) to *pomona*, 7 (20.5%) to *grippotyphosa*, and 5 (4.7%) to *autumnalis*. This study emphasized the changing trends in the epidemiology of leptospirosis with higher prevalence of serovar *L. grippotyphosa* in street dogs.

1. Introduction

The five leptospiral serovars known to be endemic in and around Namakkal, Tamilnadu, are *L. interrogans* serovars *icterohaemorrhagiae, canicola, pomona, grippotyphosa*, and *autumnalis*. Exposure to leptospira organisms is common in dogs reported by [1–3]. Currently available leptospiral vaccines for dogs in India contain inactivated *Leptospira interrogans* serovars *icterohaemorrhagiae* and *canicola* [4] which are antigenically similar to serovar *copenhageni* being from the same serovars *icterohaemorrhagiae* [5] and will stimulate active immunity to both serovars. A serosurveillance study was conducted to provide further information on the changing epidemiological trend of canine leptospirosis infections in Tamilnadu. The aim in the present study was to investigate the prevalence of serum antibodies against five endemic leptospiral serovars in dogs identifying the patterns of risk and generating further hypotheses for investigation of canine leptospirosis infections in Tamilnadu, India.

2. Materials and Methods

2.1. Data Collection and Handling. The study population was a convenience sample of 124 canine serum samples submitted to the diagnostic laboratory of the Department of Veterinary Epidemiology and Preventive Medicine (DVEPMD), Veterinary College and Research Institute, Namakkal, Tamilnadu. Blood was collected in a plain vacutainer tubes and submitted to Leptospirosis laboratory (DVEPMD) for diagnostic purposes unrelated to this study. The samples were received from 8 different regions: 284 samples were from half of the Namakkal district and 174 from the same regions (Table 1) from resident dogs (vaccinated pet), resident semiowned dogs, and stray dogs (unvaccinated) in and around Namakkal. Information provided with the data included breed, sex, age, and the region the animal resided when the blood was collected and simultaneously the blood was collected from stray dogs with the help of animal attendants from the same regions randomly.

TABLE 1: Estimate of dog population at risk and number of sera samples per 10,000 dogs at risk population for each region of Namakkal district from a survey of MAT titres to leptospires, total: 18, 39,791.

Place	No. of sampled	Estimated population at risk	No. of sampled per 10,000 population
Vaccinated			
Erumaipatti	39	4200	92.8
Mohanur	31	3600	86.1
Namagiripet	35	2800	125.0
Namakkal town	56	6000	93.3
Puduchatram	27	2400	112.5
Rasipuram	45	5000	90.0
Sendamangalam	25	2000	125.0
Vennandur	26	1700	152.9
Total	**284**	**27,700**	**102.5**
Unvaccinated			
Erumaipatti	21	1100	190.9
Mohanur	19	1400	135.7
Namagiripet	21	1500	140.0
Namakkal town	32	2200	145.4
Puduchatram	19	1000	190.0
Rasipuram	26	1800	144.4
Sendamangalam	18	1200	150.0
Vennandur	20	800	250.0
Total	**176**	**11,000**	**160.0**

Population at risk data obtained from Veterinary Dispensaries and Regional Animal Disease Intelligence Unit Survey (2001).

TABLE 2: Number and percentage of each variable with MAT titre of >90 for any one of leptospira serovars.

Variable	Level	Number (% of study population)	Positive MAT (% of level)
Age	1-2 years	80 (17.4)	21 (26.3)
	2-3 years	90 (19.6)	26 (28.9)
	3-4 years	86 (18.7)	32 (37.2)
	4-5 years	94 (20.4)	18 (19.1)
	5 and above	110 (23.9)	7 (6.4)
Sex	Male	263 (57.2)	55 (20.9)
	Female	197 (42.8)	42 (21.0)
Breed size	Small breeds	112 (24.3)	19 (17.0)
	Larger breeds	143 (31.0)	21 (14.7)
	Mongrel	185 (40.2)	48 (26.0)
Vaccination status	Vaccinated	284 (61.7)	126 (44.4)
	Unvaccinated	176 (38.3)	143 (81.3)

for investigation and the association between prevalence of positive leptospiral titres for any serovars and protective titre of each individual were analysed.

3. Results and Discussion

The study population that included 460 dogs confirmed that leptospira interogans serovar icterohaemorrhagiae was the most common leptospiral serovars and that this population of dog had positive titre of 1 : 40. In addition, the prevalence of titres to leptospira interogans serovar icterohaemorrhagiae in dogs sampled 7.7 percent was similar to the prevalence of 9.5 percent reported by [2]. However 18.8 percent of positive cases of L. icterohaemorrhagiae were maintained in vaccinated dog population in this region. This could be the reason for higher prevalence of L. icterohaemorrhagiae in vaccinated dog population in these areas. However, if the dogs were exposed to natural infection before vaccination, naturally the antibody titres were increased and respond to given vaccine in this study. Prevalence of positive titres to L. icterohaemorrhagiae of 12 percent in region wise (Tamilnadu) was reported by [1]. There was a little change in the prevalence of pomona (1.4%), canicola (3.9%), grippotyphosa (0.4%), and autumnalis (0.7%) in vaccinated dogs when compared with unvaccinated dogs population: pomona (10.2%), canicola (9.1%), grippotyphosa (11.4%), and autumnalis (10.8%), respectively (Table 3). This finding is consistent with a report of [7]. The overall prevalence of any one leptospiral antibodies to L. icterohaemorrhagiae was 26 percent followed by 17 percent in small breeds and 14.7 percent in larger breeds. Similar findings were reported by [8, 9]. The reasons for higher prevalence of leptospira antibodies in Mongrel breeds than other breeds, thus the hypotheses that increased contact with rats and therefore having increased positive titre of leptospirosis by this survey group of the sample size in this breed group (n = 185) was low and may not have been sufficient to detect differences in prevalence of positive

2.2. Microscopic Agglutination Test (MAT).

2.2. Microscopic Agglutination Test (MAT). Sera were tested against five serovars most likely to cause disease in dogs in Namakkal regions which are L. interrogans: serovars icterohaemorrhagiae, pomona, canicola, autumnalis, and grippotyphosa. The MAT was performed as per the method of [6]. A homologous, high titred antiserum was included in each testing session. Serum dilutions were prepared in 8-well "U" bottomed disposable microtitre plates (Tarson). A serial twofold dilution of each serum was made in phosphate buffered saline (pH 7.2) starting with an initial dilution of 1 : 10. An equal volume (i.e., 50 μL) of culture was added to each well, mixed by gentle rocking, and incubated at 37°C for 2 hrs after sealing with polyethylene sheet. The MAT titre was the reciprocal of the highest dilution of the serum in which >50% of the antigen was agglutinated. A minimum titre of 1 : 40 and above was taken as the positive agglutination reaction in endemic areas.

2.3. Data Analysis. The variable age was divided into 5 categories (1-2 yrs; 2-3; 3-4; 4-5, and above). The breeds were classified into 3 broad categories. Small breeds (Pomeranian, Poodles, Pug, Dachshund, and Spitz), larger breeds (Labrador, Great Dane, Golden retriever, German shepherd, and English mastiff), and Terrier breeds (retriever, non-descript (Mongrel), Rajapalayam, Combi, etc.) were taken

TABLE 3: Count and prevalence of microscopic agglutination test titres >96 to individual serovars icterohaemorrhagiae, grippotyphosa, canicola, pomona, autumnalis, and any one of serovars in dogs.

Serovars	Vaccinated		Unvaccinated		Region wise	
	Count	Prevalence	Count	Prevalence	Count	Prevalence
icterohaemorrhagiae	22	7.7	33	18.8	55	12.0
grippotyphosa	1	0.4	20	11.4	21	4.6
canicola	11	3.9	16	9.1	27	5.9
pomona	4	1.4	18	10.2	22	4.8
autumnalis	2	0.7	19	10.8	21	4.6
Any one of serovars	53	18.7	92	52.3	145	31.5

leptospiral titres by breed in the total population of 80,239 in this region.

There is an anecdotal perception among veterinarians that urban dogs are at lesser role of exposure to leptospires than other dogs. In the present study small breeds live in urban environment did not have a lesser incidence of titres to *L. interrogans* serovar *icterohaemorrhagiae* than other breeds. This finding might be due to vaccination; however vaccine induced titres rarely result in >300 and these titres only persist for 3–12 weeks after vaccination, falling below MAT titres of 1 : 100. This finding is consistent with reported data of [2, 10] that reported that dogs most likely infect natural exposure in naive or vaccinated dogs.

Vaccine induced titres against serovars *icterohaemorrhagiae* and *canicola* make interpretation of multiple positive titres and *pomona, grippotyphosa,* and *autumnalis* titres more difficult. The elevated MAT titres to leptospires reflect natural exposure and not by vaccination as reported by [11]. In this study, nonvaccinated dogs will have increased antibody response when compared to vaccinated dogs. The higher antibody prevalence of serovars *grippotyphosa, autumnalis, pomona,* and *canicola* in this study may reflect a population of vaccinated dogs responding to natural challenge, rather than increase in titres after natural infection unrelated to vaccine administration [12, 13].

There was statistically significant difference in prevalence of positive leptospiral titres between the vaccinated and non vaccinated dogs. The reason for increased leptospiral antibody titers might be the changing epidemiology of canine leptospirosis. The changes include increased incidence or recognition of clinical disease caused by serovars not currently included in commercially available canine vaccines and may also be due to contact with wild and livestock reservoir hosts.

Dogs aged 5 years or older had a significant reduced prevalence of positive titres to leptospiral serovars when compared to dogs less than 5 years of age. There was a positive association that could be made with both sexes (male or female) and the presence of a leptospiral MAT titre of ≥96 (Table 2). This finding is in contrast to other reports which showed significantly higher titre in male dogs which were thought to be more likely to roam and therefore be exposed to infection [14].

The titre value of 1 : 100 or greater was considered as positive for leptospirosis [2]. For this study we recorded titres of 1 : 40 and above considered as positive. This cut-off will increase specificity of the positive results thus making conclusions regarding factors associated with the prevalence of positive leptospiral titres more compelling. There is no variability in titres reported by different laboratories testing identical samples [15].

The prevalence of higher leptospiral antibodies in canine population indicated that testing for multiple serovars is known to be circulating in the local canine population especially in the diagnosis of acute disease. Similarly, [16, 17] also found that multiple serovars are circulating in vaccinated and non vaccinated canine population throughout the world.

Generally, vaccination against leptospirosis has been recommended for dogs, because of the prevalence of serovars *icterohaemorrhagiae* and *canicola* in rat population [1]. No nationwide or even statewide surveys on canine leptospirosis or maintenance host have been conducted since then. This study supports the conclusion that exposure to serovars *grippotyphosa* and *autumnalis* is common to household dogs rather than not present in this region and should be considered as a component of vaccines used in dogs. Where these serovars are known to be prevalent inclusion of serovars *pomona, grippotyphosa,* and *autumnalis* as part of canine leptospirosis vaccine should be considered for dogs of pure breed or nondescript mongrel at increased risk of exposure to this serovars.

The estimates on the population at risk were obtained from records on numbers of registered dogs from the veterinary dispensary, the National Animal Census 2007, Department of Animal Husbandry and Fisheries, Government of India; these estimates are based on the number of registered dogs in the veterinary dispensaries will provide the estimates of the proportion of the population at risk sampled for this study is likely to be less than stated in this survey.

The samples included in this study were collected over a one-year period during summer and winter. Secondary rainfall variations affecting survivability and transmission of leptospires, in combination with a short duration of titres after exposure, may have confounded these results. However, the summer and winter months in Tamilnadu typically have very different rainfalls, and the sampling period could be considered to cover the lowest risk period and the highest risk period of warm, wet weather. Further studies could more worthwhile for examining the seasonal variations in exposure.

References

[1] K. S. Venkataraman and S. Nedunchelliyan, "Epidemiology of an outbreak of leptospirosis in man and dog," *Comparative Immunology, Microbiology and Infectious Diseases*, vol. 15, no. 4, pp. 243–247, 1992.

[2] J. S. O'Keefe, J. A. Jenner, N. C. Sandifer, A. Antony, and N. B. Williamson, "A serosurvey for antibodies to Leptospira in dogs in the lower North Island of New Zealand," *New Zealand Veterinary Journal*, vol. 50, no. 1, pp. 23–25, 2002.

[3] F. Hill, "Infectious and parasitic disease of dogs in New Zealand," *Surveillance*, vol. 26, pp. 3–5, 1999.

[4] *The Index of Veterinary Specialties Annual*, UBM Medica, New Zealand, 2011.

[5] A. R. Bharti, J. E. Nally, J. N. Ricaldi et al., "Leptospirosis: a zoonotic disease of global importance," *Lancet Infectious Diseases*, vol. 3, no. 12, pp. 757–771, 2003.

[6] S. Faine, *Guidelines for the Control of Leptospirosis*, World Health Organization, Geneva, Switzerland, 1982.

[7] J. F. Prescott, R. L. Ferrier, and V. M. Nicholson, "Is canine leptospirosis under diagnosed in southern Ontario? In a case report and serological survey," *Canadian Veterinary Journal*, vol. 32, pp. 481–486, 1991.

[8] P. Rojas, A. M. Monahan, S. Schuller, I. S. Miller, B. K. Markey, and J. E. Nally, "Detection and quantification of leptospires in urine of dogs: a maintenance host for the zoonotic disease leptospirosis," *European Journal of Clinical Microbiology and Infectious Diseases*, vol. 29, no. 10, pp. 1305–1309, 2010.

[9] J. E. Stokes, J. B. Kaneene, W. D. Schall et al., "Prevalence of serum antibodies against six Leptospira serovars in healthy dogs," *Journal of the American Veterinary Medical Association*, vol. 230, no. 11, pp. 1657–1664, 2007.

[10] S. E. Heath and R. Johnson, "Clinical update: leptospirosis," *Journal of the American Veterinary Medical Association*, vol. 205, no. 11, pp. 1518–1523, 1994.

[11] H. L. B. M. Klaasen, M. J. C. H. Molkenboer, M. P. Vrijenhoek, and M. J. Kaashoek, "Duration of immunity in dogs vaccinated against leptospirosis with a bivalent inactivated vaccine," *Veterinary Microbiology*, vol. 95, no. 1-2, pp. 121–132, 2003.

[12] K. R. Harkin, Y. M. Roshto, J. T. Sullivan, T. J. Purvis, and M. M. Chengappa, "Comparison of polymerase chain reaction assay, bacteriologic culture, and serologic testing in assessment of prevalence of urinary shedding of leptospires in dogs," *Journal of the American Veterinary Medical Association*, vol. 222, no. 9, pp. 1230–1233, 2003.

[13] Z. J. Arent, S. Andrews, K. Adamama, C. Gilmore, D. Pardall, and W. A. Ellis, *Emergence of Novel Leptospira Serovars a Need for Adjusting Vaccination Policies for Dogs*, OIE Leptospirosis Reference Laboratory, Agri-Food and Biosciences Institute, Veterinary Sciences Division, Belfast, North Ireland, 2012.

[14] N. Birnbaum, S. C. Barr, S. A. Center, T. Schermerhorn, J. F. Randolph, and K. W. Simpson, "Naturally acquired leptospirosis in 36 dogs: serological and clinicopathological features," *Journal of Small Animal Practice*, vol. 39, no. 5, pp. 231–236, 1998.

[15] M. D. Miller, K. M. Annis, M. R. Lappin, and K. F. Lunn, "Variability in results of the microscopic agglutination test in dogs with clinical leptospirosis and dogs vaccinated against leptospirosis," *Journal of Veterinary Internal Medicine*, vol. 25, no. 3, pp. 426–432, 2011.

[16] J. E. Sykes, K. Hartmann, K. F. Lunn, G. E. Moore, R. A. Stoddard, and R. E. Goldstein, "ACVIM small animal consensus statement on leptospirosis diagnosis, epidemiology, treatment and prevention," *Journal of Veterinary Internal Medicine*, vol. 25, no. 1, pp. 1–13, 2011.

[17] J. G. Songer and A. B. Thiermann, "Leptospirosis: zoonoses update," *Journal of the American Veterinary Medical Association*, vol. 193, no. 10, pp. 1250–1254, 1988.

17

Occurrence of Ticks in Cattle in the New Pastoral Farming Areas in Rufiji District, Tanzania

Kamilius A. Mamiro,[1] **Henry B. Magwisha,**[1] **Elpidius J. Rukambile,**[1] **Martin R. Ruheta,**[2] **Expery J. Kimboka,**[3] **Deusdedit J. Malulu,**[4] **and Imna I. Malele**[4]

[1]*Central Veterinary Laboratory, TVLA, P.O. Box 9254, Dar Es Salaam, Tanzania*
[2]*Directorate of Veterinary Services, MLDF, P.O. Box 9152, Dar Es Salaam, Tanzania*
[3]*District Veterinary Office, P.O. Box 40, Utete, Rufiji, Tanzania*
[4]*Vector & Vector Borne Diseases Institute (VVBD), P.O. Box 1026, Tanga, Tanzania*

Correspondence should be addressed to Imna I. Malele; maleleimna@gmail.com

Academic Editor: Antonio Ortega-Pacheco

Ticks and tick-borne diseases plus trypanosomosis are a constraint to cattle rearing in Tanzania. Rufiji district was not known for important ticks infesting cattle because inhabitants were not engaged in keeping livestock. Not only has settlement of pastoralists and cattle in Rufiji increased the number of cattle but also cattle have been the source of bringing in and spreading of ticks. This study investigated tick species that have been introduced and managed to establish themselves in the new livestock farming areas in cattle in Rufiji. Tick distribution study was undertaken in three villages of Chumbi ward seasonally in 2009, 2011, and 2012. The identified ticks were *Amblyomma variegatum* (56.10%), *Rhipicephalus evertsi* (10.25%), *R. microplus* (27.40%), and *R. appendiculatus* (6.19%) out of 12940 ticks. Results indicate that ticks are present in the new livestock settlement areas. The occurrence of ticks is correlated with the recent settlement of cattle in the district.

1. Introduction

Ticks and tick-borne diseases and trypanosomosis and tsetse fly are major constraint to cattle rearing in Tanzania. Intensive tick surveys conducted between 1955 and 1961 provide the basic information on distribution of Tanzanian tick species. According to Yeoman and Walker [1], there are 8 tick genera with 60 identified species. However only 4 genera with 9 species, *Boophilus decoloratus*, *Rhipicephalus appendiculatus*, *Amblyomma variegatum*, *Rhipicephalus evertsi*, *Rhipicephalus microplus*, *Amblyomma lepidum*, *Rhipicephalus pravus*, *Amblyomma gemma*, and *Hyalomma albiparmatum*, characterize cattle tick population of Tanzania. The first 5 of these tick species are principle vectors of some of the most economically important tick-borne diseases of cattle in Tanzania.

Large numbers of indigenous cattle are mostly owned by pastoralists and agropastoralists and account for 98% of cattle population in the country. The grazing land for these animals in areas that is home to many pastoralists is no longer sufficient due to the increase in number of cattle and human population. As a result some of the pastoralists from these areas are currently migrating with their animals opting to settle in other areas of Tanzania where there is an ample grazing land for their animals. Such areas are in the eastern and southern part of Tanzania.

For many years, most areas in eastern Tanzania such as Rufiji district in Coast region have been keeping very few numbers of cattle. This is due to the fact that people living in these areas are not engaged in keeping livestock. Tick surveys conducted by Yeoman and Walker [1], provided information of tick distribution in few areas where very few numbers of cattle were being kept.

Settlement of pastoralists and their animals in some areas of Rufiji district in recent years has not only increased the number of cattle population but also the cattle have been the source for bringing in and spreading ticks of economic importance into the areas. The species of ticks that managed to establish themselves in these new areas together with tsetse fly species present transmit diseases to the animals. In this paper we present results of tick that has managed to establish themselves in the new livestock farming areas of Rufiji in cattle present in the areas.

2. Materials and Methods

2.1. Description of the Area. Rufiji is one of the six districts of Coast region covering an area of about 14,500 sq km. It lies between latitude 7.47–8.03°S and longitude 38.62–39.17°E with overall altitude of less than 500 metres above sea level. The climate is tropical with cool and dry season from June to September and hot and dry season from December to March. Long rainy season lasts from March to May and short rainy season from October to December. Short rains are unpredictable with variation from year to year. The overall mean temperature is 28°C.

Vegetation is characterized by tropical forests and grass-lands. The district has Rufiji River which is a prominent feature that divides the district into two halves. Furthermore Kilwa and Rufiji districts border Selous Game Reserve to the western part. Land utilized for grazing is estimated to be 90,000 ha out of 482,430 ha suitable for grazing.

2.2. Sample and Data Collections

2.2.1. Tick Collections. The district veterinary officer (DVO) assisted in providing information about areas where pastoral-ists from different areas of the country have settled with their animals. Longitudinal study was conducted seasonally in Chumbi ward in 2009, 2011, and 2012 for investigating ticks species. The ward was selected because of high density of cattle introduced from different areas of Tanzania compared to other wards in the district. Chumbi ward comprises three villages namely Chumbi, Kiwanga, and Muhoro.

Ticks were collected from 11 herds. One- to two-month visit intervals were made during the period of rainy season (March–May) and dry season (June–November). During each visit adult ticks were collected from 3-4 head of cattle randomly selected from the herd kraal after the consent was given by each owner in all villages. Collected ticks were preserved in 70% alcohol; however the collected immature stages, nymphs and larvae, were excluded from counting and identification of ticks. The adult ticks were identified in the laboratory according to published keys [2, 3] using a stereo microscope. As these animals were managed by the owners themselves, they were sometimes sprayed with acaricides for tick control.

2.2.2. Data Analysis. Collected data on identified tick species, season and village were entered into Microsoft excel software where they were coded before being analysed by statistical analysis software (SAS). A two-way ANOVA was conducted to detect the effect of season and village on the tick species. Ticks count was used as dependent variable while village, season, and tick species were used as independent variables. Means were separated at 95% confidence interval and the difference was considered significant at 5% in all statistical tests.

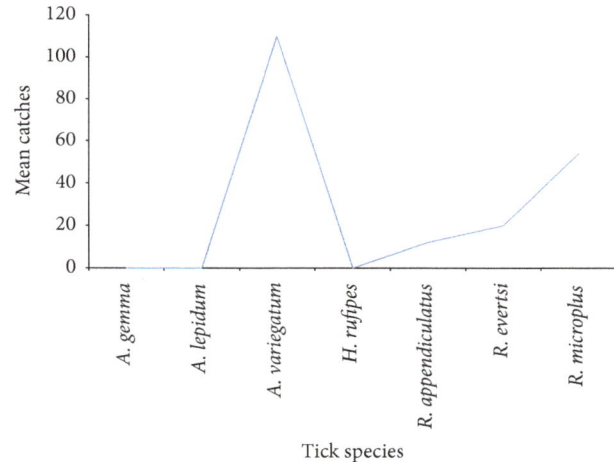

FIGURE 1: Mean ticks species for the villages of Rufiji district.

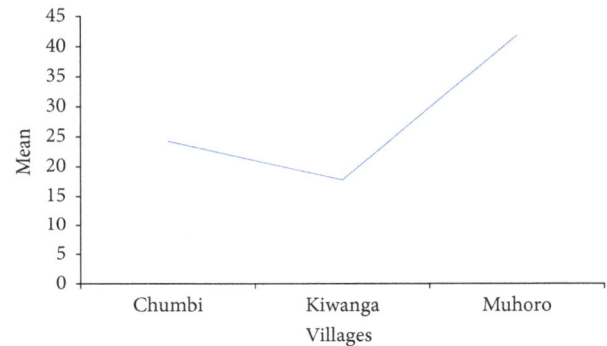

FIGURE 2: Mean ticks count from villages of Chumbi ward.

3. Results

Tick Species Collected and Identified. A total of 12,940 ticks were collected seasonally from cattle, between 2009, 2011, and 2012 which accounts to the overall mean tick collection of 27.99 ± 3.14. Mean catches for each species are shown in Figure 1. There was high significant difference between tick species ($P < 0.0001$).

The mean catch for *A. variegatum* was the highest (56.6%) followed by *R. microplus* (27.3%), *R. evertsi* (10.2%), and *R. appendiculatus* (6.1%). The less common species were *A. gemma* (0.02%), *Hyalomma rufipes* (0.02%), and *A. lepidum* (0.02%). Neither season ($P = 0.5981$) nor its interaction with species ($P = 0.7898$) and village ($P = 0.8650$) had significant effect on the mean tick count.

Villages had significant effect on the ticks species collected ($P = 0.0168$); ticks collected in Muhoro village were 50% of the total ticks (Figure 2). Further analysis of the interaction between species and villages showed high significant effect on the ticks count ($P = 0.0042$). *R. microplus* of Muhoro and Kiwanga villages was significantly different from the species collected from Chumbi village. *A. variegatum* collected in Kiwanga were significantly different from the

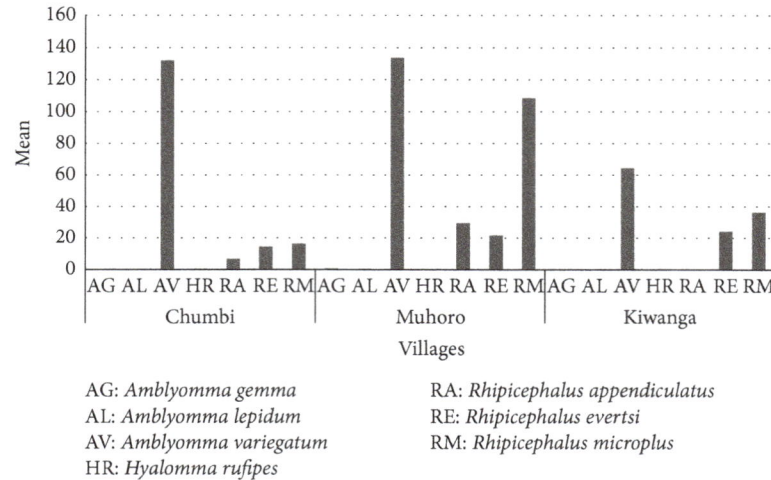

AG: *Amblyomma gemma*
AL: *Amblyomma lepidum*
AV: *Amblyomma variegatum*
HR: *Hyalomma rufipes*

RA: *Rhipicephalus appendiculatus*
RE: *Rhipicephalus evertsi*
RM: *Rhipicephalus microplus*

FIGURE 3: Mean tick species caught seasonally in the three villages of Chumbi ward.

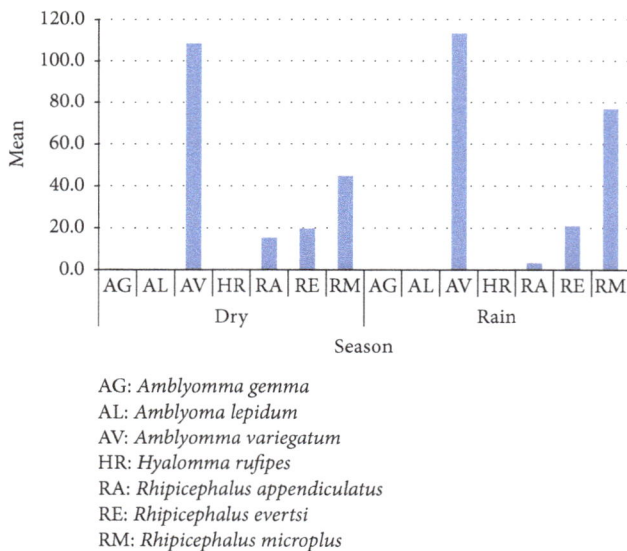

AG: *Amblyomma gemma*
AL: *Amblyoma lepidum*
AV: *Amblyomma variegatum*
HR: *Hyalomma rufipes*
RA: *Rhipicephalus appendiculatus*
RE: *Rhipicephalus evertsi*
RM: *Rhipicephalus microplus*

FIGURE 4: Mean tick species caught seasonally.

ticks of other villages. Figure 3 shows tick species found in each village. All tick species except *Hyalomma rufipes* were present in Muhoro village; again all tick species except *A. lepidum* were present in Chumbi village. *A. variegatum*, *R. evertsi*, and *R. microplus* were found in all three surveyed villages. *A. variegatum* was collected in all seasons in high numbers followed by *R. microplus* though the mean count of this species was high during the rainy season (Figure 4).

4. Discussion

4.1. Tick Species Collected and Identified. Seven tick species were encountered in the new cattle settlement areas of Rufiji, namely, *Amblyomma variegatum*, *Rhipicephalus (B) microplus*, *Rhipicephalus evertsi*, *Hyalomma rufipes*, *Amblyomma gemma*, *Amblyomma lepidum*, and *Rhipicephalus*

appendiculatus (Figure 1). These species are widely spread in other areas of Tanzania. More ticks were collected at Muhoro followed by Chumbi compared to Kiwanga. Their distribution and abundance in an area can be related to factors such as climate, vegetation, host density, and grazing habits [4].

The occurrence of these tick species in some areas of Rufiji district to which no livestock were kept before suggests that the species were introduced in these areas by the infested cattle and other livestock brought in by the pastoralists. It appears now that some of tick species introduced have managed to establish themselves, for instance, *Amblyomma variegatum*, which was collected from cattle in the widest range of habitats and assumed to be the most catholic tick species in Tanzania [5]; earlier documented reports indicate that the occurrences of the species in Lindi and areas of Rufiji were negligible with prevalence of 0–0.25. However in this study, the prevalence of *A. variegatum* was 56.10% for seasonal collection during the study period. In early 2007, the country saw a rapid increase in the number of livestock settled in Rufiji district, of the Coastal Region of Tanzania, following the evacuation of livestock from Usangu and Ihefu areas which were declared conservation areas and key water sources for hydroelectric power generation [6]. Many pastoralists opted to settle in the Coastal Region, which has a low human population density, hence ensuring ample grazing land for their animals. Settlement of pastoralists and their animals in the district has also been associated with pressures of land use in the northern circuit of the country [7] as a result; the animal populations in Rufiji district has increased rapidly as a result of this eviction from the wetland sources from 20,000 head of cattle in 2005/2006 to about 140,000 by mid 2008/2009. The updated tick occurrences reported by [5] were conducted between 1998 and 2001 as part of a robust integrated TTBD control regimen, in all 21 regions of the Tanzanian mainland and on Mafia Island in order to update the data on both tick distribution and TBD prevalence in preparation for a National TTBD control strategy based on present-day ecological and epidemiological knowledge of ticks. *A. variegatum* was collected in both seasons during this study (Figure 4).

A. gemma was reported to be restricted to central Tanzania, an arid/semiarid bushland/wooded and bushed grassland areas with shorter drought periods and bimodal rainfall [5]; however, during this study, it was found in Rufiji though in low numbers accounting to 0.02% of the total number of ticks collected.

R. microplus and R. evertsi were present on cattle during the collection schedules done during the dry season between June and November and rainy season between March and May (Figure 3). All of these species are important vectors of tick-borne disease pathogens reported in Tanzania [8] and elsewhere [9]. Although the study reported by [5] indicated that changing livestock policies, unrestricted livestock movement, and a continuous change in climatic/environmental conditions in Tanzania have brought about only limited changes in the distribution patterns of *R. appendiculatus*, *R. pravus,* and the three *Amblyomma* species investigated; it remains to be seen that the assumed limited changes in the long run coupled with environmental and/or climate changes will have an impact on the distribution of ticks as demonstrated in this study. Although posterior probability of occurrences of *R. appendiculatus* was 0–0.2 [5], in this study, the prevalence of 6.20% was recorded. The result indicates that *R. appendiculatus* can maintain itself under certain conditions and probably occur seasonally. The spread of *R. appendiculatus* (and ECF) from Lake Victoria basin southwards has also been linked before with migrant agropastoralists from the north-south movement from Sukuma land (Lake Victoria basin) to the Usangu plains (Southern highlands) and all the way to Mtwara [10, 11].

R. microplus is a normal species present in coastal areas of Tanzania [1, 4]. It seems that the coastal environment is favourable for this species to maintain itself. The coastal environment is also likely to be favourable for *A. variegatum* and *R. evertsi* which were encountered together with *R. microplus* (Figure 3) and are becoming common species infesting cattle in the pastoralist settlement areas. Earlier studies [12] reported that, except for extremely cold and dry areas, *Rhipicephalus (B) microplus* has extended its distribution range and is now present in all the northern regions of Tanzania and that high suitability is currently recorded for most of the previously nonoccupied areas. The temperature in Rufiji is around 28°C; hence it would support the existence of the species adapted to such temperatures and lower altitudes.

Rhipicephalus microplus occurs in areas with an estimated mean rainfall of 58 mm and there was no record of the species in Rufiji [12]; however in our study 27.4% were collected out of 12940 ticks. The very few numbers of *H. rufipes, A. gemma,* and *A. lepidum* collected (Figure 1) indicate that climatic conditions and probably other unknown factors in Rufiji district are not favourable for these species which were found infesting cattle introduced from other areas of Tanzania to be able to establish and adapt to the new climatic conditions.

4.2. Importance of Collected Ticks in Rufiji. *R. appendiculatus* collected in Rufiji transmits *Theileria parva* which is a causative agent of East Coast fever (ECF), whereas *Anaplasma marginale* causes anaplasmosis and is associated with *R.*

evertsi which was one of the ticks identified in the areas. Each of these two tick species are principal vectors of these diseases.

From the present surveys, ticks of cattle appear to be present in the new established cattle settlement areas of Rufiji. It is important for the livestock farmers to be aware and use effective chemicals and drugs to control the vectors. This study indicates that movement of animals in traditional pastoralist system is one of the factors for vector spread and establishment. Hence better land use and planning should be encouraged in order to mitigate factors behind movement of livestock in search of pastures as a result of overgrazing in former areas coupled with poor range land management which cannot support increasing number of cattle in the former pastoralist tradition areas.

Competing Interests

The authors declare no competing interests.

Authors' Contributions

Kamilius A. Mamiro, Henry B. Magwisha, Elpidius J. Rukambile, Martin R. Ruheta, Expery J. Kimboka, and Imna I. Malele designed the study. Kamilius A. Mamiro, Henry B. Magwisha, Elpidius J. Rukambile, Martin R. Ruheta, and Expery J. Kimboka carried the field work, Deusdedit J. Malulu analysed the data, Kamilius A. Mamiro, Henry B. Magwisha, and Imna I. Malele wrote the paper, and all authors read and edited the manuscript.

Acknowledgments

This work was funded by the Ministry of Livestock and Fisheries Development through ZARDEF fund. The authors acknowledge the assistance offered by CVL staff from Parasitology Department. They thank the District Veterinary Officer (DVO) from Rufiji District for support during the surveys.

References

[1] G. H. Yeoman and J. B. Walker, *The Ixodid Ticks of Tanzania,* Commonwealth Institute of Entomology, London, UK, 1967.

[2] M. H. Matthysse and M. H. Colbo, *Ticks of Uganda,* Entomological Society of America, College Park, Md, USA, 1987.

[3] A. R. Walker, L. J. L. Bouttonur, A. Camicus et al., "Ticks of domestic animals in Africa. A guide to identification of species," Bioscience Reports, Science, 2003.

[4] R. J. Tatchell and E. Easton, "Tick (Acari: Ixodidae) ecological studies in Tanzania," *Bulletin of Entomological Research,* vol. 76, no. 2, pp. 229–246, 1986.

[5] G. Lynen, P. Zeman, C. Bakuname et al., "Cattle ticks of the genera *Rhipicephalus* and *Amblyomma* of economic importance in Tanzania: distribution assessed with GIS based on an extensive field survey," *Experimental and Applied Acarology,* vol. 43, no. 4, pp. 303–319, 2007.

[6] J. A. Ngailo, "Assessing the effects of eviction on household food security of livestock keepers from the Usangu wetlands in SW

Tanzania," *Livestock Research for Rural Development*, vol. 23, no. 3, 2011.

[7] I. I. Malele, H. Nyingilili, and A. Msangi, "Factors defining the distribution limit of tsetse infestation and the implication for livestock sector in Tanzania," *African Journal of Agricultural Research*, vol. 6, no. 10, pp. 2341–2347, 2011.

[8] FAO, "Improvement of tick control in Tanzania," Tech. Rep. A.G. DP/URT/72/009, FAO, Rome, Italy, 1977.

[9] B. Minjauw and A. Mcleod, "Tick borne diseases and poverty. The impact of ticks and tick-borne diseases on the livelihood of small scale and marginal livestock owners in India and eastern and southern Africa," Research Report, DFID Animal Health Programme, Centre for Tropical Veterinary Medicine, University of Edinburgh, Edinburgh, UK, 2003.

[10] B. McCulloch, W. J. Kalaye, R. Tungaraza, B. J. Suda, and E. M. Mbasha, "A study of the life history of the tick *Rhipicephalus appendiculatus*—the main vector of East Coast fever—with reference to its behaviour under field conditions and with regard to its control in Sukumaland, Tanzania," *Bulletin of Epizootic Diseases of Africa*, vol. 16, no. 4, pp. 477–500, 1968.

[11] N. Ole-Lengisugi, "The livestock movements from Northern Tanzania southwards and their impact to poverty alleviation," Consultancy Report, Maasai Resource Centre for Indigenous Knowledge, 2000.

[12] G. Lynen, P. Zeman, C. Bakuname et al., "Shifts in the distributional ranges of *Boophilus* ticks in Tanzania: evidence that a parapatric boundary between *Boophilus microplus* and *B. decoloratus* follows climate gradients," *Experimental and Applied Acarology*, vol. 44, no. 2, pp. 147–164, 2008.

18

Phenotypic and Genotypic Characterization of Animal-Source *Salmonella* Heidelberg Isolates

Kristin A. Clothier[1,2] and Barbara A. Byrne[2,3]

[1]*California Animal Health & Food Safety Lab System, School of Veterinary Medicine, University of California, Davis, Davis, CA 95616, USA*
[2]*Departments of Pathology, Microbiology, and Immunology, School of Veterinary Medicine, University of California, Davis, Davis, CA 95616, USA*
[3]*Veterinary Medical Teaching Hospital, School of Veterinary Medicine, University of California, Davis, Davis, CA 95616, USA*

Correspondence should be addressed to Kristin A. Clothier; kaclothier@ucdavis.edu

Academic Editor: Antonio Ortega-Pacheco

Salmonella enterica serotype Heidelberg (*S.* Heidelberg) is frequently implicated in human foodborne *Salmonella* infections and often produces more severe clinical disease than other serotypes. Livestock and poultry products represent a potential risk for transmission to humans. The purpose of this study was to evaluate 49 *S.* Heidelberg veterinary isolates for exponential growth rate (EGR), PFGE pattern, and antimicrobial resistance to evaluate these parameters as mechanisms by which *S.* Heidelberg emerged as a virulent foodborne pathogen. Isolates were categorized by species of origin; clinical or environmental sources; and time frame of recovery. Growth rates were determined in nutrient media using serial dilutions and colony counts; PFGE was performed according to the CDC PulseNet protocol. Minimum inhibitory concentration and susceptibility determinations were performed against antimicrobials important in human medicine. Eighteen unique PFGE patterns were detected in the isolates tested. Antimicrobial resistance was significantly greater ($P < 0.05$) for ten of 15 drugs in clinical over environmental isolates; for four drugs between the time frames; and for ten drugs between species of origin. The large genetic diversity present in isolates of this serotype may convey competitive advantages to this organism, while the presence of antimicrobial resistance represents a potential zoonotic risk via animal-source food products.

1. Introduction

Salmonella is a major cause of foodborne outbreaks in the USA [1–4]. In 2012 alone, *Salmonella* was implicated in 25% of the 423 outbreaks associated with an infectious agent [2]. *S. enterica* serotype Heidelberg (*S.* Heidelberg) consistently ranks in the top ten serotypes detected from laboratory-confirmed *Salmonella* infections [2, 5–7]. Additionally, *S.* Heidelberg has been recovered from many livestock and poultry species posing risks for zoonotic transmission via food products [8–10].

Infections with *S.* Heidelberg are more likely to result in severe disease than other serotypes, emphasizing its pathogenic potential [7, 11, 12]. Recently, poultry products were implicated in *S.* Heidelberg outbreak that resulted in

634 illnesses involving people from 29 states [13]. While most foodborne *Salmonella* infections are self-limiting, 38% of patients in this outbreak required hospitalization [13]. Several published reports have documented a high prevalence of antimicrobial resistance in isolates of this serotype to a variety of drugs, further highlighting the potential health risk that *S.* Heidelberg represents [11, 14, 15].

Reasons for the emergence of *S.* Heidelberg as a virulent pathogen are unknown but may include phenotypic or genotypic changes over time that have enhanced fitness over other bacterial agents. Microbial growth rates are utilized in evaluating the effects of treatment on food products to determine the likelihood of risk reduction for specific interventions [16]. Higher growth rates decrease time needed to reach an infectious dose which may convey enhanced fitness to bacterial populations exhibiting them. Serotyping is essential part of *Salmonella* epidemiologic investigations; however, molecular subtyping methods can provide more insight into isolate relatedness within serotypes [17]. Pulse field gel electrophoresis (PFGE) is a highly robust method for assessing DNA similarity between isolates with high reproducibility between laboratories and is the preferred method for surveillance and outbreak investigations [18]. A standardized PFGE protocol published by CDC is widely used for foodborne *Salmonella* investigations [5, 19]. The purpose of the present study was to evaluate a panel of *S.* Heidelberg isolates recovered from veterinary clinical and environmental sources for exponential growth rate (EGR), PFGE pattern, and antimicrobial resistance over time and by source and species of origin to evaluate alterations in these parameters as mechanisms by which *S.* Heidelberg may have emerged as a highly virulent foodborne pathogen.

2. Materials and Methods

2.1. Bacterial Isolates. Forty-nine *S.* Heidelberg isolates were randomly selected for this study from the historical collection of bacteria recovered from samples submitted to the California Animal Health & Food Safety Lab System (CAHFS) from 1991 to 2013. Isolates had been stored at -70°C in preservation solution (Microbank, Pro-Lab Diagnostics, Austin, TX) or lyophilized for long-term storage as previously described [20]. Isolates were categorized according to animal species of origin (bovine [$n = 9$], chicken [$n = 34$], equine [$n = 2$], and turkey [$n = 4$]); associated history (recovered from clinical cases [$n = 21$] or environmental sources [$n = 28$]); and time frame of recovery (prior to 2006 [$n = 11$], 2006–2011 [$n = 12$], and 2012-2013 [$n = 26$]). Isolates from clinical cases were recovered from animals with diarrhea (chicken, bovine, and equine), nonenteric infections including peritonitis, pericarditis, hepatitis, pneumonia, and sepsis (chicken, turkey, and bovine), and gastrointestinal stasis (equine). Environmental sources consisted of drag swabs, fecal samples from animal lounging sites, rinse water, chicken fluff samples, and bedding.

2.2. EGR Determination. Bacterial isolates were recovered from long-term storage onto nutrient agar (5% sheep blood agar, SBA) and incubated at $35-37^\circ$C for 18–24 hours. Serotype identity was confirmed by biochemical and serological testing. Culture plates were assessed for purity and subcultured into liquid brain-heart infusion broth (BHI) incubated at $35-37^\circ$C for 18–24 hours prior to testing. Growth curve experiments were performed using published protocols [16]. Briefly, isolates were grown in flasks containing 150 mL of BHI incubated in ambient air at $35-37^\circ$C on a shaking incubator at 120 rpm. Aliquots were collected at 0, 2, 4, 6, and 8 hours of incubation and colony forming units per milliliter (cfu/mL) counts were determined using serial dilutions and culture plating on SBA. Exponential growth rates (EGR) *in vitro* were assessed utilizing published standard methods [21, 22] and calculated using $y = be^{Ax}$, where y is the final concentration of bacteria in the culture, b is the initial concentration in the culture, A is the exponential growth rate,

and x is the time of incubation. Summary statistics (mean, standard deviation [SD], and coefficient of variation [CV]) were calculated by species of origin, associated source, and time frame of recovery.

2.3. PFGE Testing. PFGE was performed according to the PulseNet protocol developed by the CDC utilizing digestion with *Xba*I (Promega) and analyzed using BioNumerics software (Applied Maths, Inc., Austin, TX) at the Laboratory for Molecular Typing, Cornell University. Isolates were considered identical if they differed by 0-1 bands, potentially related if they differed by 2-3 bands, and likely unrelated if they differed by >3 bands [17].

2.4. Antimicrobial Susceptibility Testing. Minimum inhibitory concentration (MIC) values were determined using microbroth dilution methods using TREK Sensititre (Thermo Fisher Scientific, Pittsburgh, PA) according to published criteria [23]. Testing was performed using the National Antimicrobial Resistance Monitoring System (NARMS) antimicrobial susceptibility panel. Susceptibilities were determined for each isolate against amoxicillin/clavulanic acid (AMC, 1/0.5–32/16 µg/mL), ampicillin (AMP, 1–32 µg/mL), azithromycin (AZI, 0.12–16 µg/mL), cefoxitin (FOX, 0.5–32 µg/mL), ceftiofur (TIO, 0.12–8 µg/mL), ceftriaxone (AXO, 0.25–64 µg/mL), chloramphenicol (CHL, 2–32 µg/mL), ciprofloxacin (CIP, 0.015–4 µg/mL), gentamicin (GEN, 0.25–16 µg/mL), kanamycin (KAN, 8–64 µg/mL), nalidixic acid (NAL, 0.5–32 µg/mL), streptomycin (STR, 32–64 µg/mL), sulfisoxazole (SUL, 16–256 µg/mL), tetracycline (TET, 4–32 µg/mL), and trimethoprim-sulfamethoxazole (SXT, 0.12/2.4–4/76 µg/mL). *Escherichia coli* American Type Culture Collection (ATCC) 25922, *E. coli* ATCC 35218, *Enterococcus faecalis* ATCC 29212, *Pseudomonas aeruginosa* ATCC 27853, and *Staphylococcus aureus* ATCC 29213 were used as quality control organisms. Susceptibility determinations were established using CLSI criteria where available [24]. Antimicrobials for which there are no CLSI interpretive criteria (AZI and STR) were evaluated using USDA NARMS guidelines [19]. Percent of resistant isolates was calculated as the number of isolates classified as "resistant" divided by the total number of isolates tested expressed as a percentage.

2.5. Statistical Analysis. Exponential growth was assessed for significant differences ($P < 0.05$) in mean rate between source, time frame of recovery, and species of origin using a one-way ANOVA. Percent of isolates resistant to an individual antimicrobial was assessed for statistically significant differences ($P < 0.05$) based on the null hypothesis that resistance was consistent between time frame of recovery, sample source, and species of origin using Fisher's exact test. Mode MIC value and range were determined for each antimicrobial by source, time frame, and species of origin; the nonparametric Kruskal-Wallis test was used to compare MICs for significant ($P < 0.05$) differences between groups for each of these categories. Statistical evaluations were performed using SAS Version 9.4 (SAS Institute, Inc., Cary, NC, USA).

TABLE 1: Summary statistics on exponential growth rate (EGR) measurements and number of unique PFGE patterns for *Salmonella* Heidelberg isolates by isolate source, time frame of recovery, and species of origin.

| | Exponential growth rate (EGR) | | | Number of unique PFGE patterns |
	Mean	SD	CV	
Isolate source				
Clinical ($n = 21$)	1.84	0.18	0.10	14
Environmental ($n = 28$)	1.90	0.13	0.07	8
Time frame of isolation				
Prior to 2006 ($n = 11$)	1.90	0.08	0.04	6
2006–2011 ($n = 12$)	1.88	0.09	0.05	9
2012-2013 ($n = 26$)	1.86	0.19	0.10	11
Species of origin				
Chicken ($n = 34$)	1.87	0.18	0.09	12
Bovine ($n = 9$)	1.83	0.06	0.03	6
Turkey ($n = 4$)	1.92	0.08	0.04	3
Equine ($n = 2$)	1.94	0.11	0.06	2

PFGE = pulse field gel electrophoresis; SD = standard deviation; CV = coefficient of variation.

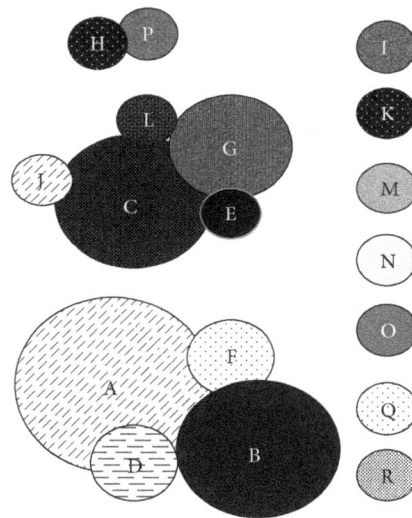

FIGURE 1: Relative relatedness (intersecting circles represent patterns that differ by ≤3 bands) and relative prevalence (size of circle denotes the frequency of identical patterns) of PFGE patterns determined for 49 *Salmonella* Heidelberg isolates recovered from CAHFS from 1991–2013. Letters designate individual PFGE patterns (A = 13, B = 9, C = 7, D = 2, E = 1, F = 2, G = 4, and H–R = 1 isolate each).

3. Results

3.1. EGR Determination.
Table 1 presents the summary statistics for EGR of these isolates by source, time frame of recovery, and species of origin, as well as the number of unique PFGE patterns for these criteria. The starting bacterial concentrations ranged from 7×10^1 to 4×10^4 cfu/mL and reached 2×10^8 to 8×10^9 cfu/mL after eight hours of incubation. EGR ranged from 1.151 to 2.105/hr. No significant differences in growth parameters were identified between time periods ($P = 0.65$), between species of origin ($P = 0.68$), or between clinical and environmental sources ($P = 0.19$).

3.2. PFGE Evaluation.
Eighteen distinct PFGE patterns were recognized in this group of isolates. Three patterns were identified more frequently than the others, primarily in environmental samples (A: $n = 13$ total, 8 from environmental samples; B: $n = 9$ total, 8 from environmental samples; C: $n = 7$ total, 6 from environmental samples). While these same three patterns were more commonly identified in samples from 2012-2013, eight other patterns were detected in this group as well. Figure 1 shows the relative relatedness (intersecting circles represent patterns that differ by ≤3 bands) of isolates determined by PFGE pattern analysis along with the relative prevalence of each pattern (size of circle). Isolates

(a)

(b)

(c)

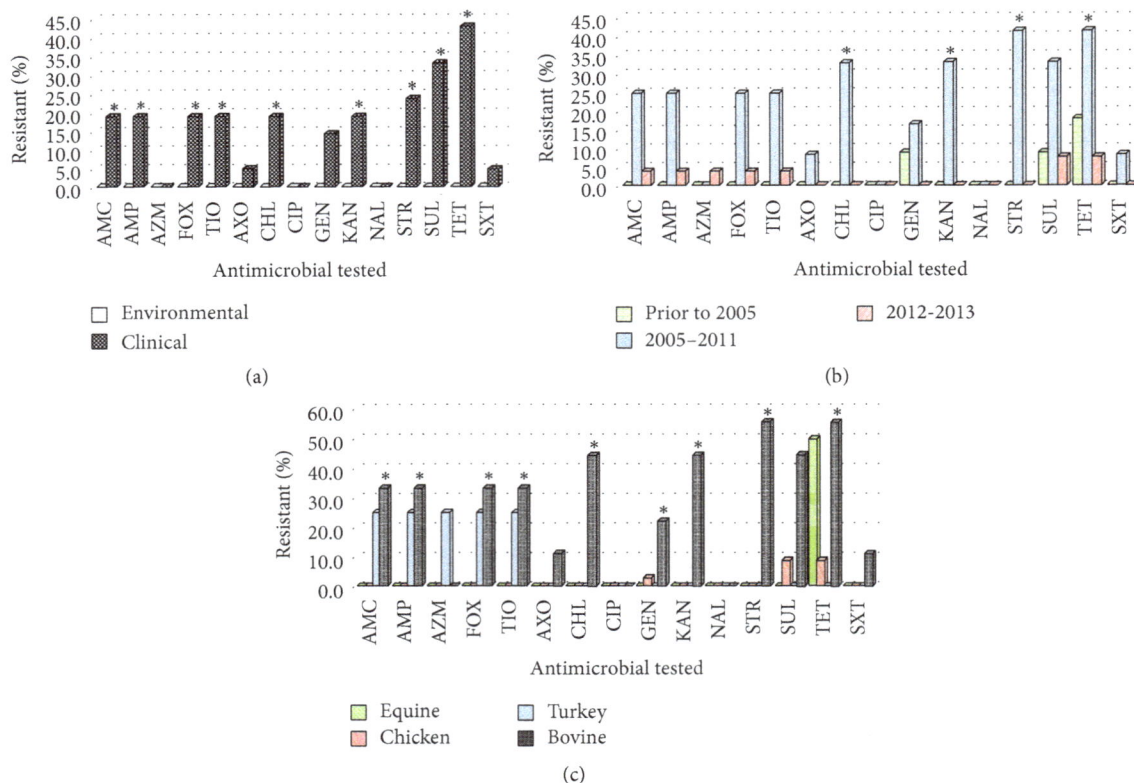

FIGURE 2: Percentage of resistance to the listed antimicrobials in *Salmonella* Heidelberg isolates from samples recovered (a) from environmental and clinical samples, (b) prior to 2006, 2006–2011, and 2012-2013, and (c) from equine, chicken, turkey, and bovine specimens. AMC = clavulanic acid/ampicillin, AMP = ampicillin, AZI = azithromycin, FOX = cefoxitin, TIO = ceftiofur, AXO = ceftriaxone, CHL = chloramphenicol, CIP = ciprofloxacin, GEN = gentamicin, KAN = kanamycin, NAL = nalidixic acid, STR = streptomycin, SUL = sulfisoxazole, TET = tetracycline, and SXT = trimethoprim/sulfamethoxazole; ∗ = significantly different ($P < 0.05$) percent of resistant isolates between (a) source, (b) time frame of recovery, and (c) species of origin.

clustered into three potentially related groups (2-3 bands different from one another) and into seven unique patterns (>3 bands different from one another) with a single isolate in each.

3.3. Antimicrobial Susceptibility Evaluation. The percentages of resistant isolates by source (panel (a)), time frame of recovery (panel (b)), and species of origin (panel (c)) are shown in Figure 2. There was significantly ($P < 0.05$) greater resistance in clinical isolates to AMC (19.0%), AMP (19.0%), FOX (19.0%), TIO (19.0%), AXO (19.0%), CHL (19.0%), KAN (19.0%), STR (23.8%), SUL (33.3%), and TET (42.9%) over environmental sources, which showed no resistance to any of the tested drugs. Antimicrobial resistance was significantly different ($P < 0.05$) between time frames of recovery for four compounds, with the greatest percent of resistant isolates for CHL (33.0%), KAN (33.0%), STR (41.7%), and TET (41.7%) in isolates recovered between 2005 and 2011.

Overall, resistance in these isolates was low for equine samples (one isolate to TET) and chicken samples (one isolate to GEN [2.9%], three isolates to SUL [8.8%], and three isolates to TET [8.8%]). One of the four turkey samples was

resistant to multiple drugs (AMC, AMP, AZI, FOX, and TIO). Statistically significant differences ($P < 0.05$) were identified between species of origin for AMC, AMP, FOX, TIO, AXO, CHL, KAN, STR, and TET, with bovine isolates exhibiting the highest percent of resistant isolates to these antimicrobials (AMC [33.3%], AMP [33.3%], FOX [33.3%], TIO [33.3%], AXO [33.3%], CHL [44.4%], KAN [44.4%], STR [55.6%], and TET [55.5%]).

3.4. MIC Results. Mode MIC values as well as the range of MICs for the isolates by source, time frame, and species of origin are presented in Table 2. Clinical isolates demonstrated significantly ($P < 0.05$) greater MICs for AMC, AMP, TIO, AXO, GEN, KAN, STR, SUL, and TET. Significant differences in MICs were identified between time frames for AXO, STR, and TET with a greatest percentage of isolates at the high end of the MIC range from 2005 to 2011 and between species for AMC, AMP, FOX, TIO, AXO, CIP, KAN, STR, and TET, in which equine and turkey isolates had the highest MICs for CIP while bovine isolates had the highest MIC for the remaining antimicrobials.

TABLE 2: Summary statistics of minimum inhibitory concentrations (MIC) values for S. Heidelberg isolates by source, time frame of recovery, and species of origin.

ABTC	MIC by source (μg/mL)		MIC by time frame (μg/mL)			MIC by species (μg/mL)			
	CLIN	ENV	<2006	2006–2011	2012-2013	BO	CH	TU	EQ[†]
	$n = 21$	$n = 28$	$n = 11$	$n = 12$	$n = 26$	$n = 9$	$n = 34$	$n = 4$	$n = 2$
AMC									
Mode	1/0.5[a]	1/0.5	1/0.5	1/0.5	1/0.5	1/0.5[c]	1/0.5	1/0.5	1/0.5
Range	1/0.5-32/16	1/0.5	1/0.5	1/0.5-32/16	1/0.5-32/16	1/0.5-32/16	1/0.5-2/1	1/0.5-32/16	1/0.5
AMP									
Mode	1[a]	1	1	1	1	1[c]	1	1	1
Range	1-32	1-2	1-2	1-32	1-32	1-32	1-2	1-32	1
AZI									
Mode	4	4	4	4	4	4	4	4	8
Range	2-16	2-8	4-8	2-8	2-16	2-8	2-8	4-16	4-8
FOX									
Mode	2	2	2	2	1	32[c]	2	2	4
Range	0.5-32	1-2	1-4	0.5-32	1-32	0.25-32	1-2	2-32	2-4
TIO									
Mode	1[a]	0.5	1	0.5	0.5	8[c]	0.5	1	1
Range	0.25-8	0.5-1	0.5-1	0.5-8	0.5-8	0.25-8	0.5-1	1-8	0.5-1
AXO									
Mode	0.25[a]	0.25	0.25[b]	0.25	0.25	0.25[c]	0.25	0.25	0.25
Range	0.25-64	0.25	0.25	0.25-64	0.25-32	0.25-64	0.25	0.25-32	0.25
CHL									
Mode	4	4	8	4	5	4	4	8	8
Range	4-32	4-8	4-8	4-32	4-16	4-32	4-8	4-16	4-8
CIP									
Mode	0.015	0.015	0.015	0.015	0.015	0.015[c]	0.015	0.015	0.03
Range	0.015-0.03	0.015	0.015-0.03	0.015	0.015-0.03	0.015	0.015	0.015-0.03	0.015-0.03
GEN									
Mode	0.5[a]	0.5	0.5	0.5	0.5	0.5	0.5	0.5	1
Range	0.5-16	0.25-8	0.5-16	0.5-16	0.25-8	0.5-16	0.25-16	0.5	0.5-1
KAN									
Mode	8[a]	8	8	8	8	8[c]	8	8	8
Range	8-64	8	8-32	8-64	8-32	8-64	8-32	8	8
NAL									
Mode	4	4	4	2	4	4	4	4	4
Range	2-4	2-4	2-4	2-4	2-4	2-4	2-4	2-4	2-4
STR									
Mode	32[a]	32	32[b]	32	32	32[c]	32	32	32
Range	32-64	32	32	32-64	32	32-64	32	32	32
SUL									
Mode	1[a]	1	1	1	1	1	1	1	128
Range	1-256	1-128	1-256	1-256	1-256	1-256	1-256	1	1-128
TET									
Mode	4[a]	4	4[b]	4	4	32[c]	4	4	32
Range	4-32	4	4-32	4-32	4-32	4-32	4-32	4	4-32
SXT									
Mode	0.12	0.12	0.12	0.12	0.12	0.12	0.12	0.12	0.12
Range	0.12-4	0.12-2	0.12	0.12-4	0.12-2	0.12-4	0.12-2	0.12	0.12

ABTC = antimicrobial tested; CLIN = clinical, ENV = environmental; CH = chicken; BO = bovine; EQ = equine; TU = turkey; AMC = amoxicillin-clavulanic acid, AMP = ampicillin, AZI = azithromycin, FOX = cefoxitin, TIO = ceftiofur, AXO = ceftriaxone, CHL = chloramphenicol, CIP = ciprofloxacin, GEN = gentamicin, KAN = kanamycin, NAL = nalidixic acid, STR = streptomycin, SUL = sulfisoxazole, TET = tetracycline, and SXT = trimethoprim/sulfamethoxazole; [†]Mode MIC was listed to the greater of the two values; [a]MIC values are significantly ($P < 0.05$) different between sources; [b]MIC values are significantly ($P < 0.05$) different between time frames; [c]MIC values are significantly ($P < 0.05$) different between species.

4. Discussion

Isolates studied in the present work demonstrated large genetic diversity, with seven PFGE patterns that had >3 band differences from all other patterns. Isolates are considered to be potentially closely related or share a common ancestor when pattern differences are consistent with a single genetic event, demonstrated by two to three band differences [17]. Pattern A, the most commonly identified pattern (n = 13), contained isolates from bovine, chicken, and turkey samples from clinical and environmental sources and from all three time frames. Patterns B (n = 9) and C (n = 7) were all from poultry sources but were also collected from all time frames and from clinical and environmental sources. Genetic variation such as that seen in these isolates can provide selective advantage, particularly during times of environmental stress [25]. Altered patterns of gene expression convey the ability to withstand stressful conditions such as extremes of heat and host immune response [25] which could provide competitive advantage to this serotype.

Bacterial exponential growth rates and the resultant doubling times are considered a species-specific characteristic under equivalent conditions; however, the acquired genes or mutations over time could provide additional advantage and alter exponential growth rate [22]. Reported doubling times in S. Typhimurium strains have been estimated at 27 to 30 minutes under nutrient-rich culture conditions [26, 27]. Doubling time for the isolates in this study was very consistent, ranging from 19.7 to 24.5 minutes for 47 of the 49 isolates studied, and differences over time or between sources were not identified. Although other serotypes were not investigated in the present work, it is possible that growth rates vary across *Salmonella* serotypes and faster growth rates may provide S. Heidelberg with a competitive advantage at similar infectious doses.

Four multidrug resistant (>5 drugs) isolates were identified in this collection (3 bovine animals recovered, 2006–2011, and 1 turkey recovered, 2012-2013; 8.2% of total tested). Isolates were resistant to AMC (n = 4), AMP (n = 4), FOX (n = 4), TIO (n = 4), CHL (n = 3, all bovine), KAN (n = 3, all bovine), STR (n = 3, all bovine), and TET (n = 3, all bovine). None of these isolates was recovered from animals with any herd or geographic relatedness. The presence of multidrug resistant isolates is of concern particularly to antimicrobials critical in the treatment of human infections. Antimicrobial resistance genes are most commonly carried on plasmids [7], and future testing for the presence of specific resistance genes as well as known plasmids may give more insight into the ecology of resistance found in these strains. Interestingly, all of the isolates recovered from animal environmental sources were susceptible to all antimicrobials tested, even those from sites containing feces from large numbers of animals (drag swabs, lounging areas). While antimicrobial use would be more likely in animals with clinical disease, particularly those with systemic symptoms, data on drug use for treatment or metaphylaxis in these animals was not provided. Consequently, establishing the risks of prior treatment on the presence of antimicrobial resistance was beyond the scope of this study.

Differences in MIC values even within the "susceptible range" can give early indications of trends toward resistance development and potential treatment failure [28]. Significant differences in MICs in this study closely followed those for percent of resistant isolates for many drugs; however, MICs for certain antimicrobials even within the susceptible range did demonstrate patterns for concern, specifically differences in ceftiofur (P = 0.043) and ciprofloxacin (P = 0.0008) between species and gentamicin (P = 0.025) between sources. Alterations in MIC of a single dilution are often considered biologically insignificant; however, epidemiologic studies on clinical treatment outcomes have determined that this may not be accurate. A study by Sakoulas et al. [29] identified a statistically significant difference (P < 0.02) in treatment success against methicillin-resistant S. *aureus* between vancomycin isolates with a MIC of ≤0.5 μg/mL and those with a MIC of 1-2 μg/mL even though the breakpoint for susceptible is ≤2 μg/mL. Assessments for MIC differences between groups can provide information that may not be evident when only looking at patterns of resistance.

Several limitations are evident in the present study, including the use of a convenience sample of isolates recovered in a single diagnostic laboratory system which would not be expected to represent the status of all S. Heidelberg isolates present in food-producing animals. Only two equine-source isolates were evaluated in this survey, limiting the value of conclusions about S. Heidelberg from this species. Additionally, the antimicrobials studied are important in human clinical use and not utilized in food-producing animals; consequently, the patterns found in these isolates may not fully demonstrate all resistance present in these bacteria.

Data from this work demonstrates that while growth rates were consistent within S. Heidelberg isolates from animals, genetic diversity was high which facilitate bacterial response to stress and agent survival. Although antimicrobial resistance was not widespread, the percent of resistance to a variety of drugs is of concern due to the risks of contamination of animal-source food products. Assessments for mechanisms of resistance were beyond the scope of this study, but future work investigating the presence of known resistance genes or acquired efflux mechanisms, particularly in the multidrug resistant isolates in this group, may reveal reasons for resistance development. Investigations on field isolates like those evaluated here can provide valuable insight into the potential risks from zoonotic pathogens which may be spread via animal food products.

Conflict of Interests

The authors have no conflict of interests regarding the publication of this paper.

Acknowledgments

The authors would like to recognize Dr. Bruce Charlton, Dr. Hailu Kinde, and Dr. Richard Breitmeyer for technical assistance on this study. The work was supported by the California Animal Health & Food Safety Lab System, School of

Veterinary Medicine, University of California, Davis, CA. The authors graciously acknowledge the Laboratory for Molecular Typing, Cornell University, Ithaca, NY, for performing the PFGE testing and the staff of the Veterinary Medical Teaching Hospital, UC Davis School of Veterinary Medicine, for performing the MIC testing.

References

[1] Centers for Disease Control and Prevention (CDC), *National Salmonella Surveillance Annual Report, 2011*, US Department of Health and Human Services, CDC, Atlanta, Ga, USA, 2013.

[2] Centers for Disease Control and Prevention (CDC), *Surveillance for Foodborne Disease Outbreaks, United States, 2012 Annual Report*, U.S. Department of Health and Human Services, CDC, Atlanta, Ga, USA, 2014.

[3] S. M. Crim, M. Iwamoto, J. Y. Huang et al., "Incidence and trends of infection with pathogens transmitted commonly through food—foodborne diseases active surveillance network, 10 US. Sites, 2006–2013," *Morbidity and Mortality Weekly Report*, vol. 63, no. 15, pp. 328–332, 2014.

[4] E. Scallan, R. M. Hoekstra, B. E. Mahon, T. F. Jones, and P. M. Griffin, "An assessment of the human health impact of seven leading foodborne pathogens in the United States using disability adjusted life years," *Epidemiology and Infection*, vol. 143, no. 13, pp. 2795–2804, 2015.

[5] P. S. Evans, Y. Luo, T. Muruvanda et al., "Complete genome sequences of *Salmonella enterica* serovar Heidelberg strains associated with a multistate food-borne illness investigation," *Genome Announcements*, vol. 2, no. 3, p. e01154-13, 2014.

[6] S. L. Foley, R. Nayak, I. B. Hanning, T. J. Johnson, J. Han, and S. C. Ricke, "Population dynamics of *Salmonella enterica* serotypes in commercial egg and poultry production," *Applied and Environmental Microbiology*, vol. 77, no. 13, pp. 4273–4279, 2011.

[7] A. M. Lynne, P. Kaldhone, D. David, D. G. White, and S. L. Foley, "Characterization of antimicrobial resistance in *Salmonella enterica* serotype heidelberg isolated from food animals," *Foodborne Pathogens and Disease*, vol. 6, no. 2, pp. 207–215, 2009.

[8] S. L. Foley and A. M. Lynne, "Food animal-associated *Salmonella* challenges: pathogenicity and antimicrobial resistance," *Journal of Animal Science*, vol. 86, no. 14, pp. E173–E187, 2008.

[9] S. L. Foley, A. M. Lynne, and R. Nayak, "*Salmonella* challenges: prevalence in swine and poultry and potential pathogenicity of such isolates," *Journal of Animal Science*, vol. 86, no. 14, pp. E149–E162, 2008.

[10] R. K. Gast, R. Guraya, J. Guard-Bouldin, P. S. Holt, and R. W. Moore, "Colonization of specific regions of the reproductive tract and deposition at different locations inside eggs laid by hens infected with *Salmonella* Enteritidis or *Salmonella* Heidelberg," *Avian Diseases*, vol. 51, no. 1, pp. 40–44, 2007.

[11] J. P. Folster, G. Pecic, A. Singh et al., "Characterization of extended-spectrum cephalosporin-resistant *Salmonella enterica* serovar Heidelberg isolated from food animals, retail meat, and humans in the United States 2009," *Foodborne Pathogens and Disease*, vol. 9, no. 7, pp. 638–645, 2012.

[12] M. Hoffmann, S. Zhao, Y. Luo et al., "Genome sequences of five *Salmonella enterica* serovar Heidelberg isolates associated with a 2011 multistate outbreak in the United States," *Journal of Bacteriology*, vol. 194, no. 12, pp. 3274–3275, 2012.

[13] Centers for Disease Control and Prevention (CDC), "Outbreak of *Salmonella* Heidelberg infections linked to a single poultry producer—13 states, 2012-2013," *Morbidity and Mortality Weekly Report*, vol. 62, no. 27, pp. 553–556, 2013.

[14] S. Zhao, D. G. White, S. L. Friedman et al., "Antimicrobial resistance in *Salmonella enterica* serovar Heidelberg isolates from retail meats, including poultry, from 2002 to 2006," *Applied and Environmental Microbiology*, vol. 74, no. 21, pp. 6656–6662, 2008.

[15] J. P. Folster, G. Pecic, R. Rickert et al., "Characterization of multidrug-resistant *Salmonella enterica* serovar Heidelberg from a ground Turkey-associated outbreak in the United States in 2011," *Antimicrobial Agents and Chemotherapy*, vol. 56, no. 6, pp. 3465–3466, 2012.

[16] V. K. Juneja and H. M. Marks, "Growth kinetics of *Salmonella* spp. pre- and post-thermal treatment," *International Journal of Food Microbiology*, vol. 109, no. 1-2, pp. 54–59, 2006.

[17] F. C. Tenover, R. D. Arbeit, R. V. Goering et al., "Interpreting chromosomal DNA restriction patterns produced by pulsed-field gel electrophoresis: criteria for bacterial strain typing," *Journal of Clinical Microbiology*, vol. 33, no. 9, pp. 2233–2239, 1995.

[18] M. Torpdahl, M. N. Skov, D. Sandvang, and D. L. Baggesen, "Genotypic characterization of *Salmonella* by multilocus sequence typing, pulsed-field gel electrophoresis and amplified fragment length polymorphism," *Journal of Microbiological Methods*, vol. 63, no. 2, pp. 173–184, 2005.

[19] National Antimicrobial Susceptibility Resistance Monitoring System (NARMS), *Retail Meat Report*, FDA, CDC, USDA, Silver Spring, Md, USA, 2011.

[20] R. D. Gitaitis, "Refinement of lyophilization methodology for storage of large numbers of bacterial strains," *Plant Disease*, vol. 71, no. 7, pp. 615–616, 1987.

[21] K. Todar, "The growth of bacterial populations," in *Todar's Online Textbook of Bacteriology*, K. Todar, Ed., pp. 1–4, 2012, http://textbookofbacteriology.net.

[22] F. Widdel, "Theory and measurement of bacterial growth," 2010, http://www.mpi-bremen.de/Binaries/Binary13037/Wachstums-versuch.pdf.

[23] Clinical and Laboratory Standards Institute, *Methods for Dilution Antimicrobial Susceptibility Tests for Bacteria That Grow Aerobically; Approved Standard—Ninth Edition*, M07-A9, vol. 32, no. 2, Clinical and Laboratory Standards Institute, Washington, DC, USA, 2012.

[24] Clinical Laboratory Standards Institute, "Performance Standards for Antimicrobial Susceptibility Testing; Twenty-Third Informational Supplement," M100-S23, Wayne, Pa, USA, 2013.

[25] P. L. Foster, "Stress responses and genetic variation in bacteria," *Mutation Research*, vol. 569, no. 1-2, pp. 3–11, 2005.

[26] C. Mims, N. Dimmock, A. Nash, and J. Stephen, *Mims Pathogensis of Infectious Disease*, Academic Press, London, UK, 4th edition, 1997.

[27] S.-Y. Zheng, B. Yu, K. Zhang et al., "Comparative immunological evaluation of recombinant *Salmonella* Typhimurium strains expressing model antigens as live oral vaccines," *BMC Immunology*, vol. 13, article 54, 2012.

[28] M. J. Murphy, *Clinical Pharmacokinetics*, American Society of Health-System Pharmacists, Bethesda, Md, USA, 5th edition, 2012.

[29] G. Sakoulas, P. A. Moise-Broder, J. Schentag, A. Forrest, R. C. Moellering Jr., and G. M. Eliopoulos, "Relationship of MIC and bactericidal activity to efficacy of vancomycin for treatment of methicillin-resistant *Staphylococcus aureus* bacteremia," *Journal of Clinical Microbiology*, vol. 42, no. 6, pp. 2398–2402, 2004.

19

Anthropozoonotic Endoparasites in Free-Ranging "Urban" South American Sea Lions (*Otaria flavescens*)

Carlos Hermosilla,[1] **Liliana M. R. Silva,**[1] **Mauricio Navarro,**[2,3] **and Anja Taubert**[1]

[1] *Institute of Parasitology, Justus Liebig University Giessen, 35392 Giessen, Germany*
[2] *Institute of Pathology, University Austral of Chile, Valdivia, Chile*
[3] *University of California Davis School of Veterinary Medicine, Sacramento, CA 95616, USA*

Correspondence should be addressed to Carlos Hermosilla; carlos.r.hermosilla@vetmed.uni-giessen.de

Academic Editor: Antonio Ortega-Pacheco

The present study represents the first report on the gastrointestinal endoparasite fauna of a free-ranging "urban" colony of South American sea lions (*Otaria flavescens*) living within the city of Valdivia, Chile. A total of 40 individual faecal samples of South American sea lions were collected during the year 2012 within their natural habitat along the river Calle-Calle and in the local fish market of Valdivia. Coprological analyses applying sodium acetate acetic formalin methanol (SAF) technique, carbol fuchsin-stained faecal smears and *Giardia/Cryptosporidium* coproantigen ELISAs, revealed infections with 8 different parasites belonging to protozoan and metazoan taxa with some of them bearing anthropozoonotic potential. Thus, five of these parasites were zoonotic (Diphyllobothriidae gen. sp., Anisakidae gen. sp., *Giardia*, *Cryptosporidium*, and *Balantidium*). Overall, these parasitological findings included four new parasite records for *Otaria flavescens*, that is, *Giardia*, *Cryptosporidium*, *Balantidium*, and *Otostrongylus*. The current data serve as a baseline for future monitoring studies on anthropozoonotic parasites circulating in these marine mammals and their potential impact on public health.

1. Introduction

The South American sea lions (*Otaria flavescens*, Carnivora: Otariidae) are common pinnipeds living along the eastern and western coasts of South America and are generally found in Peru, Chile, Argentina, and South Brazil [1–6]. Along the Chilean coastal shores, more than 200 colonies of free-ranging sea lions have been described. A vast amount of data on feeding ecology, reproduction, life history parameters, and population dynamics of these otariid species was published [7–16]. Several studies have also addressed aspects of the helminth fauna of South American sea lions, comprising single species records, taxonomy, and population studies of some parasitoses [5, 14–22]. However, very little is known on protozoan parasite infections of these free-ranging marine mammals.

Although their natural habitat is the marine environment, several pinniped and cetacean species are found in rivers containing fresh water. As such, a stable population of South American sea lions has been established within the city of Valdivia, Chile, resulting in permanent colonization for 20 years now. These animals have adapted extremely well not only to the fresh water of the river but also to human activities in the river Calle-Calle, such as regular ship- and boat-trafficking, rowing, kayaking, and sealing activities. This "urban" sea lion colony is allocated approximately 7 km upstream from the ocean shore and animals mainly feed on fish captured by themselves in the river (mainly carps, trouts, and salmons) or on remains of the local fish market. This unusual urban colony of South American sea lions consists of more than 72 individuals and is exclusively composed of males. The age of these animals varies from 2 to 15 years but some animals might be even older. Given that *O. flavescens* need to rest after swimming and diving activities, the sea lions in Valdivia utilize river floats, riverside piers, and footways along the river promenade as recreation areas with all of them being allocated in close proximity to inhabitants, tourists, domestic pets, or the local fish market. Since some of these animals

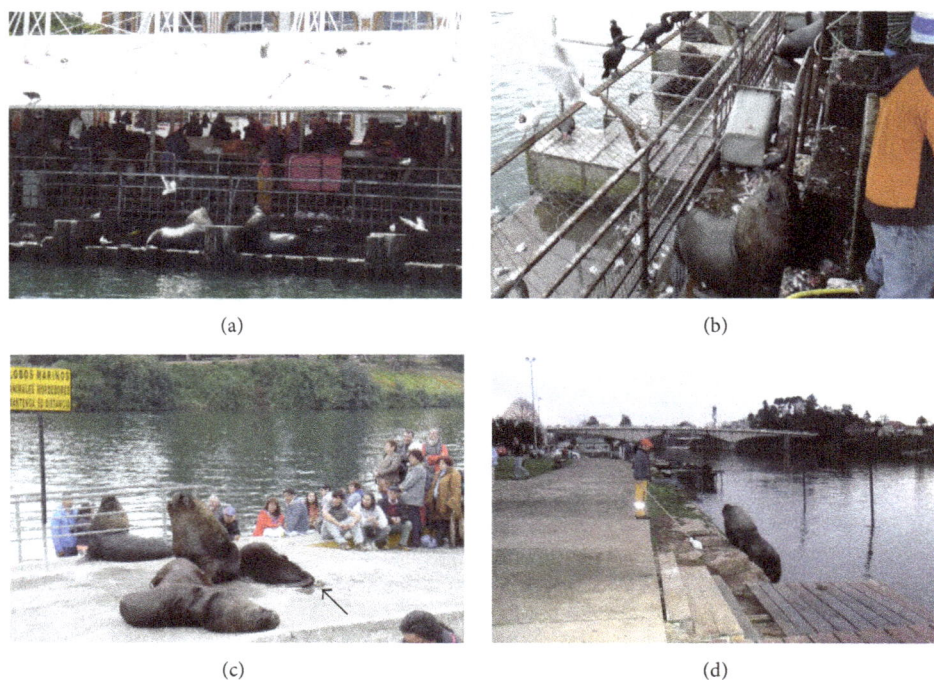

FIGURE 1: Illustration of urban South American sea lions (*Otaria flavescens*) in the city of Valdivia, Chile. (a) Sea lions on river shore of the fish market; (b) sea lions within the fish market premise in close contact to fisherman and sea products; (c) a group of sea lions at the promenade of the river surrounded by tourists despite the yellow signpost indicating the danger to get bitten by these wild animals (arrow indicates faecal contamination); (d) officer of the local "sea lion task force" using a stick with plastic bag fixed on the tip frightening an aggressive sea lion male to keep out of the promenade.

behave rather aggressive towards humans, animals, or even vehicles and additionally tend to expand their territory into the city center, the local city authorities have established a "sea lion task force" which should prevent the animals from harming humans and withhold them to premises alongside the river shore. However, given that these animals nowadays represent a tourist attraction, direct contacts of humans with these animals or their faeces as well as faecal contamination of the river water or the terrestrial environment cannot be avoided.

The present study therefore aimed to identify the actual gastrointestinal fauna in these free-ranging sea lions within their natural habitat in the river of the city of Valdivia, Chile, and to gain some insights in their potential zoonotic impact on public health issues.

2. Material and Methods

2.1. Study Area, Sample Collection, and Coproscopical Analyses. South American sea lions (*O. flavescens*) were studied along the shores of the river Calle-Calle of the city of Valdivia, Chile. The study area encompassed 3 km^2 and comprised river floats, riverside piers, footways along the river promenade, and the local fish market with all of them being allocated in close proximity of humans and domestic pets (Figures 1(a), 1(b), 1(c), and 1(d)). A total of 40 individual faecal samples were collected during the summer of 2012. Whenever defecation occurred, scat samples were immediately collected

and transferred into 2 mL plastic tubes (Eppendorf). The samples were fixed in 70% ethanol and stored at 4°C until further analysis. Parasitological analyses were conducted at the Institute of Parasitology, Justus Liebig University Giessen, Germany. Coproscopical analyses were performed by using the standard sodium acetate acetic acid formalin (SAF) technique [23]. The SAF technique was used for the detection of parasite eggs, cysts, sporocysts, and oocysts within faecal material in marine mammals as described elsewhere [24]. Additionally, a carbol fuchsin-stained faecal smear (CFS) [25] was carried out for the detection of *Cryptosporidium* oocysts. Moreover, coproantigen ELISAs (ProSpecT®, Oxoid) were performed for the detection of *Cryptosporidium* and *Giardia* antigens in faecal samples. The parasitological identification of eggs and cysts was based on morphological criteria referring to previous reports [24, 26, 27]. All sampling procedures were conducted in accordance with Institutional Ethic Commission of University Austral of Chile and the current Chilean Animal Law.

2.2. Molecular Analyses of Giardia-Positive Samples. *Giardia*-positive sea lion samples were further analyzed for the presence of *G. intestinalis* DNA by conventional and nested PCR detecting the beta-giardin gene (assemblage C). Genomic DNA was extracted from sea lion faecal material using the DNA extraction Stool Kit® (QIAGEN) according to the mammalian faecal protocol. Briefly, 1 mL of ethanol-fixed faeces was lysed in ASL buffer containing 30 glass beads

TABLE 1: Prevalence (in percentage) of parasitic infections in South American sea lions (*Otaria flavescens*), technique, and sample origin.

	Parasites	(%)	Technique	Material
Metazoan parasites	Anisakidae gen. sp.	21	SAF	Faeces
	Diphyllobothriidae gen. sp.	13	SAF	Faeces
	Trematoda indet.	2.5	SAF	Faeces
	Otostrongylus sp.	2.5	SAF	Faeces
Protozoan parasites	*Cryptosporidium*	10	CFS/coproELISA	Faeces
	Giardia	5.3	SAF/coproELISA	Faeces
	Isospora	5.3	SAF	Faeces
	Balantidium	2.5	SAF	Faeces

(4 mm diameter), under permanent stirring conditions. The DNA was thereafter purified using an anion exchange column (QIAGEN) and eluted in 100 μL of distilled water.

For the conventional *G. intestinalis*-PCR, the following specific oligonucleotide sequences were used: the forward oligonucleotide β-giardin G7F: 5′-AAGCCCGACGACCTC-ACCCGCAGTCG-3′ and the reverse oligonucleotide β-giardin G759R: 5′-GAGGCCGCCCTGGATCTTCGAGAC-GAC-3′ [28]. The PCR was performed in a total volume of 25 μL containing 5 μL faecal DNA sample, 5 μL faecal DNA (1 : 100), 1 μL βG7F oligonucleotides (10 μM), 1 μL βG759R oligonucleotides (10 μM), dNTPs 0.5 μL (10 μM), 0.5 μL Taq-polymerase (1 U/μL; PeqLab), and 14.5 μL H$_2$O. The following thermocycle profiles were used: 95°C for 5 min, 35 cycles at 95°C for 30 s, 65°C for 45 s, and 72°C for 1 min and 30 s followed by a final extension step at 72°C for 5 min and a final hold at 20°C. PCR amplificates were visualized in GelRed-stained 2% agarose gels (Biotium Incorporation).

In addition, a *G. intestinalis*-nested PCR was performed. For the nested PCR the following forward oligonucleotide sequences of βGiarF were used: 5′-GAACGAGATCGAGGT-CCG-3′ and reverse oligonucleotide sequence of βGiarR: 5′-CTCGACGAGCTTCGTTGTT-3′ [29]. The following thermocycle profiles for the nested PCR were used: 95°C for 5 min, 35 cycles at 95°C for 30 s, 50°C for 40 s, and 72°C for 1 min and 30 s followed by a final extension step at 72°C for 5 min. PCR amplificates were visualized using GelRed-stained 2% agarose gels as described above (Biotium Incorporation). Further cloning and sequencing were also performed.

3. Results

3.1. Parasite Infections. Parasitological analyses of faecal samples of South American sea lions revealed 8 different protozoan (4) and metazoan (4) taxa. The metazoan parasites consisted of trematodes (one species), cestodes (one species), and nematodes (two species). No acanthocephalan parasite eggs were found in the samples. A complete list of the parasite stages and their prevalence is given in Table 1. Illustrations of the parasitic stages are depicted in Figure 2.

The most prevalent metazoan parasites found in this "urban" sea lion colony were Anisakidae gen. sp. (21%) followed by Diphyllobothriidae gen. sp. (13%), Trematoda indet., and *Otostrongylus* sp. larvae (2.5%). The most prevalent protozoan parasites were *Cryptosporidium* (10%),

Giardia, and *Isospora* showing the same prevalence (5.3%). *Balantidium* infections were detected at lower prevalence (2.5%, Table 1). Within the metazoan endoparasites, the nematodes were the most rich in species (two species) followed by cestodes and trematodes with one species each. Referring to parasite genus level these parasitological findings included four new host records (*Cryptosporidium*, *Giardia*, *Balantidium*, and *Otostrongylus*) for *O. flavescens*. To our best knowledge, the genus *Balantidium* had only been described in fin whales (*Balaenoptera physalus*) from the North Atlantic [27]. All other protozoan parasites have already been reported for other marine mammals [4, 5, 17, 19, 20, 24, 30]. Some of the protozoan (3) and metazoan (2) endoparasite genera detected in sea lions bear an anthropozoonotic potential, such as *Cryptosporidium*, *Giardia*, *Balantidium*, Diphyllobothriidae gen. sp. (*Diphyllobothrium*), and Anisakidae gen. sp. (*Anisakis*, *Contracaecum*, and *Pseudoterranova*).

3.2. Molecular Analyses of Faecal Samples. Although sea lion faecal samples were immediately fixed in 70% ethanol after collection in the field in order to avoid DNA degradation, this goal was not successfully achieved. Thus no adequate *Giardia* DNA was possible to be extracted for further detailed molecular identification.

4. Discussion

Common collection methods for analyses of gastrointestinal parasites of wild sea lions generally rely on sections of accidentally stranded animals or on dead animals obtained from marine zoos [5, 14]. Several studies are restricted to the helminth parasite fauna of South American sea lions and include several single species records [4, 5, 15, 16, 18–22, 31]. Thus, protozoan endoparasites have rarely been considered. Conversely, by obtaining fresh faecal samples from resting sea lions, this record reveals unique insights into the actual gastrointestinal parasite fauna of free-ranging sea lions within their natural habitat.

In the present survey, 8 different parasite taxa were detected in individual sea lion faecal samples covering a respectable range of parasitic taxa. The parasitological diagnosis based on morphological criteria revealed as quite a challenge since very little data on parasitic eggs, larvae, cysts and oocysts for sea lions are available in literature. Thus, the photo galleries provided here might supply a supportive tool

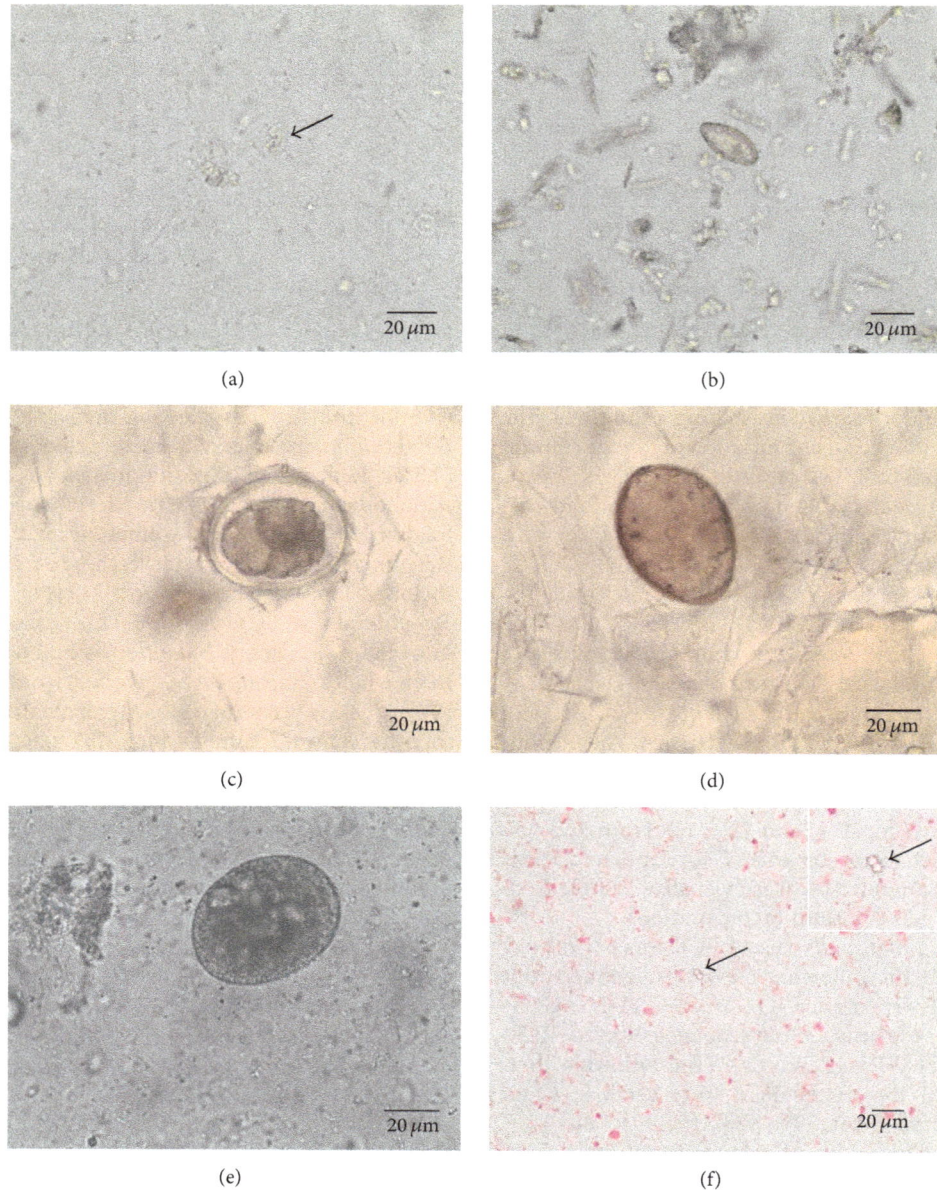

FIGURE 2: Parasite stages from faecal samples of urban South American sea lions (*Otaria flavescens*): (a) *Giardia* cyst (arrow), (b) Trematoda indet. egg, (c) Anisakidae gen. sp. egg, (d) Diphyllobothriidae gen. sp. egg, (e) *Balantidium* cyst, and (f) *Cryptosporidium* cysts (arrow).

for future parasitological research activities on sea lions and other marine mammals since many of the parasites described here infect a wide range of marine mammals, such as sea otters, seals, sea elephants, baleen, and toothed cetaceans [30].

The most prevalent parasitic stages found in the current study were eggs of Anisakidae gen. sp. However, owing to undistinguishable egg morphologies, characterization on species level was not possible. Based on parasite frequencies, these eggs most probably belong to the genera *Contracaecum*, *Pseudoterranova*, or *Anisakis* since these parasite species appear to be quite common in South American sea lions [5, 31]. Thus, South American sea lions are known

as definitive hosts for the zoonotic nematodes *Anisakis* spp., *Contracaecum ogmorhini*, and *Pseudoterranova cattani* [5, 31]. Ascarids parasitize either freely in the stomach or firmly attached, often as clusters, to the gastric mucosa [32]. Mucosal penetration via larvae [33] and adults [34] can cause severe ulcers, gastritis, and perforation [32]. Moreover, allergic reactions against epitopes of *Anisakis simplex* major allergen (Ani s1) have been reported to occur in humans after the reexposure to these parasites [35, 36]. The second most prevalent parasite species (13%) was Diphyllobothriidae gen. sp. Consistent to our findings, at least three different diphyllobothriid cestodes have previously been recorded in Chile, two freshwater species (*Diphyllobothrium latum* and

D. dendriticum) and one marine species (i.e., *Adenocephalus pacificus* (*Diphyllobothrium pacificum*)) [37, 38] and also in the intestine of stranded sea lions from Patagonia [5], but at a higher prevalence (26.8%). Diphyllobothriasis in sea lions generally is innocuous [32], but debilitation or even death of parasitized hosts might result in cases of high parasitic burdens. In addition, diphyllobothriasis also represents an important fish-borne zoonosis worldwide [39–43].

Overall, low prevalence of trematode and *Otostrongylus* sp. infections (both 2.5%) was diagnosed in the current study. Trematode infections in the pancreas and liver occur in almost all marine mammals by members of the genera *Campula, Zalophotrema, Oschmarinella*, and *Orthosplanchus*. Additionally, also the genera *Apophallus, Ascocotyle, Ogmogaster*, and *Pocitrema* have been reported as intestinal parasites of otariids [5, 44]. These may induce necrosis of the parenchymal tissue, chronic fibrotic hepatitis, enteritis [32], and even meningoencephalitis by aberrant trematode migrations [45]. Furthermore, the trematode genera *Pricetrema* and *Nanophyetes* have been reported to parasitize sea lions in the Northern hemisphere [46]. Whilst *Pricetrema* resides in the liver, *Nanophyetes* infects the small intestine.

Infections with the crenosomatid nematode *Otostrongylus* in pinnipeds are generally associated with respiratory clinical manifestations, primarily in young animals [47]. Adult *Otostrongylus* can obstruct the upper airways causing bronchitis and pneumonitis [47]. Interestingly, some sea lions of the current study showed strong coughing episodes, thereby expelling vast amount of mucus. Based on the current findings this might indicate the presence of clinical otostrongylosis within the Valdivian colony.

The parasitological findings of the study also included four new parasite host reports for *O. flavescens*, namely, *Cryptosporidium, Giardia, Balantidium*, and *Otostrongylus*, thereby providing a broader insight into the spectrum of parasitoses of this marine species. In addition, the protozoan parasites (i.e., *Cryptosporidium, Giardia*, and *Balantidium*) clearly bear zoonotic potential and are considered as typical water-borne/food-borne diseases. In consequence, the "urban" sea lion colony in Valdivia may function as relevant reservoir for these protozoans since the animals reside at the shore of the river and in close proximity to humans, pet animals, and especially in direct contact to the products of local fish market.

Within the genus *Balantidium*, *B. coli* is the only species of trichostome ciliates nowadays considered as pathogenic for mammals [48, 49]. Consistent with these findings, *Balatidium* infections in free-ranging fin whales (*Balaenoptera physalus*) from the North Atlantic Ocean were recently diagnosed [30], indicating that this terrestrial disease is circulating in the marine environment. More importantly, *B. coli* infections have been demonstrated in humans and pigs in Chile [50, 51]. As seen for balantidiasis, giardiasis and cryptosporidiosis have an almost cosmopolitan distribution. *Cryptosporidium* and *Giardia* are two common aethiological parasites of infectious enteritis in humans and animals [52, 53]. These enteric protozoans are usually transmitted by the faecal-oral route, following the ingestion of infective stages (oocysts or cysts). Moreover, marine mammals are well known as final hosts of *Giardia* and *Cryptosporidium* [24, 54–58]. Keeping in mind that the urban sea lion colony is close to populated riversides and that some touristic activities, such as "photos with sea lions" or "kayaking with sea lions," are becoming more popular, sea lions may become infected by human excretions or vice versa. As seen for giardiasis, *Cryptosporidium* infections can cause severe diarrhoea in terrestrial mammals; nonetheless, very little is known on the pathogenesis of cryptosporidiosis within the marine ecosystems [24, 55]. An essential component of the control of these diseases, from a public health perspective, is a better understanding of the sources and routes of transmission in different geographical regions [52].

Unfortunately, the current knowledge and understanding of the ecto- and endoparasite fauna (especially protozoan species) in free-ranging sea lions are still very scarce. Although some parasitoses, such as hookworm (e.g., *Uncinaria hamiltoni*) or ascarid (*Contracaecum ogmorhini, Pseudoterranova cattani*, and *Anisakis* spp.) [5], infections are discussed as pathogenic species for sea lions [32], the total parasite fauna of marine vertebrates has unfortunately not obtained sufficient attention, so far [24, 59].

In conclusion, this study adds some new anthropozoonotic parasite records to free-ranging sea lions and calls for more integrated research to avoid the exposure of humans and domestic animals with these parasites. In particular, regular monitoring programs should be established by local authorities for public health issues and for sea lion populations living in close proximity to human beings.

Competing Interests

The authors declare that they have no competing interests.

Acknowledgments

The authors are deeply thankful to Birgit Reinhardt, Agnes Mohr, and Christine Henrich (Institute of Parasitology, JLU Giessen) for their technical support in the coproscopical/molecular analyses and the coproELISAs performance of samples.

References

[1] R. Vaz-Ferreira, "*Otaria flavescens* (Shaw), South American sea lion," in *Mammals of the World*, Federal Aviation Administration, Ed., FAO Fisheries Series 5, pp. 447–495, Federal Aviation Administration, Rome, Italy, 1982.

[2] E. A. Crespo, *Dinámica Poblacional del Lobo Marino del sur Otaria flavescens (Shaw, 1800) en el Norte del Litoral Patagónico*, Universidad de Buenos Aires, Buenos Aires, Argentina, 1988.

[3] J. I. Túnez, H. L. Cappozzo, and M. H. Cassini, "Regional factors associated with the distribution of South American fur seals along the Atlantic coast of South America," *ICES Journal of Marine Science*, vol. 65, no. 9, pp. 1733–1738, 2008.

[4] F. J. Aznar, J. Hernández-Orts, A. A. Suárez, M. García-Varela, J. A. Raga, and H. L. Cappozzo, "Assessing host-parasite specificity through coprological analysis: a case study with species of *Corynosoma* (Acanthocephala: Polymorphidae) from

marine mammals," *Journal of Helminthology*, vol. 86, no. 2, pp. 156–164, 2012.

[5] J. S. Hernández-Orts, F. E. Montero, A. Juan-García et al., "Intestinal helminth fauna of the South American sea lion *Otaria flavescens* and fur seal *Arctocephalus australis* from northern Patagonia, Argentina," *Journal of Helminthology*, vol. 87, no. 3, pp. 336–347, 2013.

[6] E. M. Pereira, G. Müller, E. Secchi, J. Pereira Jr., and A. L. S. Valente, "Digenetic trematodes in South American sea lions from southern Brazilian waters," *Journal of Parasitology*, vol. 99, no. 5, pp. 910–913, 2013.

[7] E. A. Crespo, S. N. Pedraza, S. L. Dans et al., "Direct and indirect effects of the highseas fisheries on the marine mammal populations in the northern and central Patagonian coast," *Journal of Northwest Atlantic Fishery Science*, vol. 22, pp. 189–207, 1997.

[8] E. A. Crespo, A. Schiavini, F. Pérez, and H. L. Cappozzo, "Distribution, abundance and seasonal changes of South American fur seals, Arctocephalus australis, along the coasts of Argentina," in *Proceedings of the 13th Annual Conference of the European Cetacean Society*, Barcelona, Spain, 1999.

[9] M. Lima and E. Páez, "Demography and population dynamics of South American fur seals," *Journal of Mammalogy*, vol. 78, no. 3, pp. 914–920, 1997.

[10] M. K. Alonso, E. A. Crespo, S. N. Pedraza, N. A. García, and M. A. Coscarella, "Food habits of the South American sea lion, *Otaria flavescens*, off Patagonia, Argentina," *Fishery Bulletin*, vol. 98, no. 2, pp. 250–263, 2000.

[11] D. E. Naya, M. Arim, and R. Vargas, "Diet of South American fur seals (*Arctocephalus australis*) in Isla de Lobos, Uruguay," *Marine Mammal Science*, vol. 18, no. 3, pp. 734–745, 2002.

[12] A. A. Suarez, D. Sanfelice, M. H. Cassini, and H. L. Cappozzo, "Composition and seasonal variation in the diet of the South American sea lion (*Otaria flavescens*) from Quequén, Argentina," *Latin American Journal of Aquatic Mammals*, vol. 4, no. 2, pp. 163–174, 2005.

[13] H. L. Cappozzo and W. F. Perrin, "South American sea lion Otaria flavescens," in *Encyclopedia of Marine Mammals*, W. F. Perrin, B. Würsig, and J. G. M. Thewissen, Eds., Academic Press, London, UK, 2009.

[14] M. A. Sepúlveda, M. Seguel, M. Alvarado-Rybak, C. Verdugo, C. Muñoz-Zanzi, and R. Tamayo, "Postmortem findings in four south American sea lions (*Otaria byronia*) from an urban colony in Valdivia, Chile," *Journal of Wildlife Diseases*, vol. 51, no. 1, pp. 279–282, 2015.

[15] P. E. Cattan, B. B. Babero, and D. Torres, "The helminth fauna of CHIle: IV. Nematodes of the genera Anisakis Dujardin, 1845 and Phocanema Myers, 1954 in relation with gastric ulcers in a South American Sea Lion, Otaria byronia," *Journal of Wildlife Diseases*, vol. 12, no. 4, pp. 511–515, 1976.

[16] M. G. Nascimento and J. Carvajal, "Helminth parasites of the South American sea lion Otaria flavescens from the Gulf of Arauco, Chile," *Boletín chileno de Parasitología*, vol. 36, no. 3-4, pp. 72–73, 1981.

[17] J. A. Raga, M. Fernandez, J. A. Balbuena, and F. J. Aznar, "Parasites," in *Encyclopedia of Marine Mammals*, W. F. Perrin, H. G. M. Thewissen, and B. Würsing, Eds., pp. 821–830, Academic Press/Elsevier, San Diego, Calif, USA, 2nd edition, 2008.

[18] T. Southwell and A. J. Walker, "Notes on a larval cestode from a fur seal," *Annals of Tropical Medicine and Parasitology*, vol. 30, pp. 91–100, 1936.

[19] K. Zdzitowircki, "Corynosoma gibsoni sp. n., a parasite of Otaria flavescens (Shaw, 1980) from the Falkland Islands and a note on the occurrence of C. evae Zdzitowiecki 1984," *Acta Parasitologica Polonica*, vol. 31, pp. 29–32, 1980.

[20] K. Zdzitowircki, *Antartic Acanthocephala*, Synopses of the Antarctic Benthos, Koeltz Scientific Books, Koenigsein, Switzerland, 1991, Edited by J. W. Wägele and J. Sieg.

[21] G. Lauckner, "Diseases of mammalia: pinnipedia," in *Diseases of Marine Animals*, O. Kinne, Ed., pp. 683–793, Biologische Anstalt Helgoland, Hamburg, Germany, 1985.

[22] M. D. Dailey, "The distribution and intraspecific variation of helminth parasites in pinnipeds," in *Rapports et Proces-Verbaux des Réunions*, pp. 338–352, Conseil International pour l'Exploration de la Mer, Copenhagen, Denmark, 1975.

[23] J. Yang and T. Scholten, "A fixative for intestinal parasites permitting the use of concentration and permanent staining procedures," *American Journal of Clinical Pathology*, vol. 67, no. 3, pp. 300–304, 1977.

[24] S. Kleinertz, C. Hermosilla, A. Ziltener et al., "Gastrointestinal parasites of free-living Indo-Pacific bottlenose dolphins (*Tursiops aduncus*) in the Northern Red Sea, Egypt," *Parasitology Research*, vol. 113, no. 4, pp. 1405–1415, 2014.

[25] J. Heine, "An easy technique for the demonstration of Cryptosporidia in faeces," *Journal of Veterinary Medicine B Infectious Diseases Immunology Food Hygiene Veterinary Public Health*, vol. 29, no. 4, pp. 324–327, 1982.

[26] H. Mehlhorn and W. Peter, *Diagnose der Parasiten des Menschen Einschliesslich der Therapie Einheimischer und Tropisch Parasitosen*, Gustav Fisher, Stuttgart, Germany, 1983.

[27] R. C. Anderson, *Nematode Parasites of Vertebrates: Their Development and Transmission*, CABI Publishing, Cambridge, Mass, USA, 1992.

[28] S. M. Cacciò, M. De Giacomo, and E. Pozio, "Sequence analysis of the beta-giardin gene and development of a polymerase chain reaction-restriction fragment length polymorphism assay to genotype *Giardia duodenalis* cysts from human faecal samples," *International Journal for Parasitology*, vol. 32, no. 8, pp. 1023–1030, 2002.

[29] M. Lalle, E. Jimenez-Cardosa, S. M. Cacciò, and E. Pozio, "Genotyping of *Giardia duodenalis* from humans and dogs from Mexico using a β-giardin nested polymerase chain reaction assay," *Journal of Parasitology*, vol. 91, no. 1, pp. 203–205, 2005.

[30] C. Hermosilla, L. M. Silva, S. Kleinertz, R. Prieto, M. A. Silva, and A. Taubert, "Endoparasite survey of free-swimming baleen whales (*Balaenoptera musculus*, *B. physalus*, *B. borealis*) and sperm whales (*Physeter macrocephalus*) using non/minimally invasive methods," *Parasitology Research*, vol. 115, no. 2, pp. 889–896, 2016.

[31] M. George-Nascimento and J. Carvajal, "New records of anisakid nematodes from Chilean marine fauna (author's transl)," *Boletín Chileno de Parasitología*, vol. 35, no. 1-2, pp. 15–18, 1980.

[32] J. R. Geraci and D. J. St Aubin, "Effects of parasites on marine mammals," *International Journal for Parasitology*, vol. 17, no. 2, pp. 407–414, 1987.

[33] P. C. Young and D. Lowe, "Larval nematodes from fish of the subfamily anisakinae and gastro-intestinal lesions in mammals," *Journal of Comparative Pathology*, vol. 79, no. 3, pp. 301–313, 1969.

[34] G. McClelland, "Phocanema decipiens: pathology in seals," *Experimental Parasitology*, vol. 49, no. 3, pp. 405–419, 1980.

[35] R. M. Martínez-Aranguren, P. M. Gamboa, E. García-Lirio, J. Asturias, M. J. Goikoetxea, and M. L. S. Larruga, "In vivo and in vitro testing with rAni s 1 can facilitate diagnosis of Anisakis simplex allergy," *Journal of Investigational Allergology and Clinical Immunology*, vol. 24, no. 6, pp. 431–438, 2014.

[36] M. Garcia Alonso, M. L. Caballero, A. Umpierrez, M. Lluch-Bernal, T. Knaute, and R. Rodríguez-Pérez, "Relationships between T cell and IgE/IgG4 epitopes of the Anisakis simplex major allergen Ani s 1," *Clinical and Experimental Allergy*, vol. 45, no. 5, pp. 994–1005, 2015.

[37] P. Torres, S. Puga, L. Castillo, J. Lamilla, and J. Miranda, "Helmintos, myxozoos y microsporidios en músculos de peces comercializados frescos y su importancia como riesgo potencial para la salud humana en la ciudad de Valdivia, Chile," *Archivos de Medicina Veterinaria*, vol. 46, no. 1, pp. 83–92, 2014.

[38] P. Torres, V. Leyán, and S. Puga, "Prevalence, intensity, and abundance of infection and pathogenesis caused by diphyllobothriosis in vulnerable, native fish and introduced trout in Lake Panguipulli, Chile," *Journal of Wildlife Diseases*, vol. 48, no. 4, pp. 937–950, 2012.

[39] M. A. Curtis and G. Bylund, "Diphyllobothriasis: fish tapeworm disease in the circumpolar north," *Arctic Medical Research*, vol. 50, no. 1, pp. 18–24, 1991.

[40] T. Scholz, H. H. Garcia, R. Kuchta, and B. Wicht, "Update on the human broad tapeworm (genus diphyllobothrium), including clinical relevance," *Clinical Microbiology Reviews*, vol. 22, no. 1, pp. 146–160, 2009.

[41] E. J. Jenkins, J. M. Schurer, and K. M. Gesy, "Old problems on a new playing field: helminth zoonoses transmitted among dogs, wildlife, and people in a changing northern climate," *Veterinary Parasitology*, vol. 182, no. 1, pp. 54–69, 2011.

[42] J.-Y. Chai, K. D. Murrell, and A. J. Lymbery, "Fish-borne parasitic zoonoses: status and issues," *International Journal for Parasitology*, vol. 35, no. 11-12, pp. 1233–1254, 2005.

[43] R. Mercado, H. Yamasaki, M. Kato et al., "Molecular identification of the *Diphyllobothrium* species causing diphyllobothriasis in Chilean patients," *Parasitology Research*, vol. 106, no. 4, pp. 995–1000, 2010.

[44] J. S. Hernndez-Orts, F. E. Montero, E. A. Crespo, N. A. García, J. A. Raga, and F. J. Aznar, "A new species of ascocotyle (trematoda: Heterophyidae) from the South American sea lion, Otaria flavescens, off patagonia, Argentina," *Journal of Parasitology*, vol. 98, no. 4, pp. 810–816, 2012.

[45] D. Fauquier, F. Gulland, M. Haulena, M. Dailey, R. L. Rietcheck, and T. P. Lipscomb, "Meningoencephalitis in two stranded California sea lions (*Zalophus californianus*) caused by aberrant trematode migration," *Journal of Wildlife Diseases*, vol. 40, no. 4, pp. 816–819, 2004.

[46] R. K. Stroud and M. D. Dailey, "Parasites and associated pathology observed in pinnipeds stranded along the Oregon coast," *Journal of Wildlife Diseases*, vol. 14, no. 3, pp. 292–298, 1978.

[47] J. G. Elson-Riggins, L. Al-Banna, E. G. Platzer, and I. Kaloshian, "Characterization of *Otostrongylus circumlitus* from Pacific harbor and northern elephant seals," *Journal of Parasitology*, vol. 87, no. 1, pp. 73–78, 2001.

[48] F. Ponce-Gordo, F. Fonseca-Salamanca, and R. A. Martínez-Díaz, "Genetic heterogeneity in internal transcribed spacer genes of *Balantidium coli* (Litostomatea, Ciliophora)," *Protist*, vol. 162, no. 5, pp. 774–794, 2011.

[49] J. M. Hassell, D. P. Blake, M. R. Cranfield et al., "Occurrence and molecular analysis of *Balantidium coli* in mountain gorilla (*Gorilla beringei beringei*) in the Volcanoes National Park, Rwanda," *Journal of Wildlife Diseases*, vol. 49, no. 4, pp. 1063–1065, 2013.

[50] H. Palomino and R. Donckaster, "Clinical and epidemiological study of a case of human balantidiasis," *Boletin Chileno de Parasitologia*, vol. 26, no. 1, pp. 44–45, 1971.

[51] T. Letonja, A. Henríquez, G. Reyes, and L. Zapata, "Prevalence of *Balantidium coli* infections in swine from Santiago, Chile (author's transl)," *Boletin Chileno de Parasitologia*, vol. 30, no. 3-4, pp. 88–89, 1975.

[52] H. Abeywardena, A. R. Jex, and R. B. Gasser, "A perspective on cryptosporidium and giardia, with an emphasis on bovines and recent epidemiological findings," *Advances in Parasitology*, vol. 88, pp. 243–301, 2015.

[53] M. Bouzid, K. Halai, D. Jeffreys, and P. R. Hunter, "The prevalence of Giardia infection in dogs and cats, a systematic review and meta-analysis of prevalence studies from stool samples," *Veterinary Parasitology*, vol. 207, no. 3-4, pp. 181–202, 2015.

[54] H. Mehlhorn and G. Piekarski, *Grundriss Der Parasitenkunde: Parasiten des Menschen und der Nutztiere*, vol. 516, Gustav FIsher, Stuttgart, Germany, 1998.

[55] J. M. Hughes-Hanks, L. G. Rickard, C. Panuska et al., "Prevalence of *Cryptosporidium* spp. and *Giardia* spp. in five marine mammal species," *Journal of Parasitology*, vol. 91, no. 5, pp. 1225–1228, 2005.

[56] R. C. A. Thompson, C. S. Palmer, and R. O'Handley, "The public health and clinical significance of Giardia and Cryptosporidium in domestic animals," *Veterinary Journal*, vol. 177, no. 1, pp. 18–25, 2008.

[57] A. Reboredo-Fernández, H. Gómez-Couso, J. A. Martínez-Cedeira, S. M. Cacciò, and E. Ares-Mazás, "Detection and molecular characterization of *Giardia* and *Cryptosporidium* in common dolphins (*Delphinus delphis*) stranded along the Galician coast (Northwest Spain)," *Veterinary Parasitology*, vol. 202, no. 3-4, pp. 132–137, 2014.

[58] C. Hermosilla, L. M. Silva, R. Prieto, S. Kleinertz, A. Taubert, and M. A. Silva, "Endo- and ectoparasites of large whales (Cetartiodactyla: Balaenopteridae, Physeteridae): Overcoming difficulties in obtaining appropriate samples by non- and minimally-invasive methods," *International Journal for Parasitology: Parasites and Wildlife*, vol. 4, no. 3, pp. 414–420, 2015.

[59] J. B. Oliveira, J. A. Morales, R. C. González-Barrientos, J. Hernández-Gamboa, and G. Hernández-Mora, "Parasites of cetaceans stranded on the Pacific coast of Costa Rica," *Veterinary Parasitology*, vol. 182, no. 2–4, pp. 319–328, 2011.

20

Subcutaneous Implants of a Cholesterol-Triglyceride-Buprenorphine Suspension in Rats

M. Guarnieri,[1] C. Brayton,[2] R. Sarabia-Estrada,[1] B. Tyler,[1] P. McKnight,[3] and L. DeTolla[4]

[1]*Johns Hopkins School of Medicine, Department of Neurological Surgery, Baltimore, MD, USA*
[2]*Johns Hopkins School of Medicine, Department of Molecular and Comparative Pathobiology, Baltimore, MD, USA*
[3]*George Mason University, Fairfax, VA, USA*
[4]*University of Maryland School of Medicine, Departments of Pathology, Medicine, Epidemiology and Public Health and the Program of Comparative Medicine, Baltimore, MD, USA*

Correspondence should be addressed to M. Guarnieri; mguarnieri@comcast.net

Academic Editor: Vito Laudadio

A Target Animal Safety protocol was used to examine adverse events in male and female Fischer F344/NTac rats treated with increasing doses of a subcutaneous implant of a lipid suspension of buprenorphine. A single injection of 0.65 mg/kg afforded clinically significant blood levels of drug for 3 days. Chemistry, hematology, coagulation, and urinalysis values with 2- to 10-fold excess doses of the drug-lipid suspension were within normal limits. Histopathology findings were unremarkable. The skin and underlying tissue surrounding the drug injection were unremarkable. Approximately 25% of a cohort of rats given the excess doses of 1.3, 3.9, and 6.5 mg/kg displayed nausea-related behavior consisting of intermittent and limited excess grooming and self-gnawing. These results confirm the safety of cholesterol-triglyceride carrier systems for subcutaneous drug delivery of buprenorphine in laboratory animals and further demonstrate the utility of lipid-based carriers as scaffolds for subcutaneous, long-acting drug therapy.

1. Introduction

The challenge of providing long-acting drug therapy to laboratory animals has been managed by adding drugs to the feed or water supplies [1, 2]. The utility of this method decreases when the mixture may be released inadvertently to the environment, or the drug is regulated, such as controlled substance. Feed-based drugs also may have limited postsurgical applications because pain can suppress appetite. Alternative approaches have focused on long-acting drug implants made by combining a drug with biodegradable envelops composed of lipids or polymers.

Polymers have been studied as drug carriers for neurooncology [3]. Side effects generally have been modest and localized when the polymer is implanted into neural tissue [4]. Less is known about biodegradable polymers for subcutaneous (SC) delivery of chemotherapy.

Moderate to severe inflammatory reactions have been reported for SC implants of polymer-opiate constructs [5–10].

We investigated the properties of lipid-based delivery vehicles. Cholesterol, triglycerides, and phospholipids have been widely used as drug-carriers [11]. Kent described an implantable cholesterol matrix that delivered large molecules such as insulin and growth hormone [12]. Grant and coworkers demonstrated that a phospholipid-morphine liposome had prolonged activity and greater safety in mice than the free drug [13]. Liposomal strategies have been refined for the delivery of several opiates [14]. Pontani and Misra described a cholesterol-triglyceride matrix for the long-term delivery of drugs to treat chronic pain and opiate addiction [15]. The cholesterol-triglyceride vehicle appeared to provide a promising carrier to examine the delivery of antibiotics, anti-inflammatory drugs, and analgesics in surgically treated animals. To investigate the safety of this system we chose buprenorphine as a model drug. It has a high therapeutic index [16] and is a front-line analgesic for animals [17, 18].

The present report describes bioequivalence studies demonstrating that a 0.65 mg/kg dose of a lipid-buprenorphine suspension provides blood concentrations of drug greater than 0.7 ng/mL for 2-3 days. This concentration has been associated with clinically effective analgesia in mice, dogs, and humans [19–23]. A standard analgesiometric test confirmed the efficacy of the intended 0.65 mg/kg dose. Safety studies used a Target Animal Safety (TAS) trial format [24, 25]. Surgically treated male and female rats were injected with multiple overdoses of the drug suspension and monitored for adverse events (AE). The trials included clinical tests, histopathology studies, and clinical observations. The results described in the present report, when taken together with a previous report on the safety of a lipid-buprenorphine suspension in mice [26], provide further evidence that SC drug implants using lipid envelopes increase options for long-term drug therapy in rats. A preliminary account of this research has been published [27].

2. Methods

2.1. Animals and Husbandry. Studies were approved by the Johns Hopkins Institutional Animal Care and Use Committee. The protocol complies with the National Institutes of Health Guide for the Care and Use of Laboratory Animals and the requirements of the Association for the Assessment and Accreditation of Laboratory Animal Care International Program. Guidelines for TAS studies specify a minimum number of three animals per group. Four rats were used in TAS studies to account for potential morbidity during jugular vein phlebotomy. Fischer F344/NTac rats, 6–8 weeks old (male 160–180 g; female 120–130 g), were obtained from Taconic Farms (Hudson NY) and housed in an environmentally controlled room which maintained the temperatures of 20 to 26°C. Monthly health surveillance was conducted by a soiled-bedding sentinel system. Sentinel rats were considered negative for pneumonia virus of mice, reovirus, Sendai virus, lymphocytic choriomeningitis virus, rat coronavirus, sialodacryoadenitis virus, rat parvovirus, Kilham rat virus, Toolan H1 parvovirus, rat theilovirus, cilia-associated respiratory bacillus, *Pneumocystis carinii, Mycoplasma pulmonis,* and pinworms throughout the study.

The facility maintained a relative humidity of 30 to 70% with a 12-hour light cycle with lights on from 6 AM–6 PM. Animals were ear tagged and group housed (up to 3 per cage) during the quarantine and acclimation period based on sex. The rats were quarantined and acclimated for six days prior to dosing. No disease-related signs were noted during the quarantine/acclimation period. Prior to being placed on test, a Clinical Veterinarian approved the animals for study use. All rats appeared normal prior to dosing. The animals assigned to the two TAS trials were randomized by body weight into four groups per trial of 4 male and 4 female rats using random numbers generated by Excel (Microsoft Corp., Redmond, WA). The weight of each animal was within 10% of the mean weight of the group. On allocation and dosing, rats

in the bioequivalence, efficacy, 4-day, and 12-day TAS trials were individually housed in ventilated microisolator cages throughout the study. Cages were changed daily to reduce redosing by coprophagy. Studies used soft fiber bedding from Carefresh Natural Bedding (Ferndale, WA) to house the rats. Animals were provided ad libitum with access to drinking water (Baltimore City Water System, Baltimore, MD) in disposable water bottles. The animals were provided ad libitum with access to Harlan TEKLAD Certified Global Rodent Diet 2016C (Harlan TEKLAD, Indianapolis, IN). Rats were provided with enrichment devices of polycarbonate red tubes (Bio Services, Uden, The Netherlands).

2.2. Experimental Design. The intended label dose of 0.65 mg/kg, which provides 2-3 days of clinically significant blood levels of drug, was established in bioequivalence trials and efficacy studies to be described using male and female rats. Single- and repeat-dose TAS trials were performed using excess amounts of the intended dose. In both safety trials, the lowest dose of drug tested was twofold greater than the intended label dose of 0.65 mg/kg. In the single-dose phase of the trials, 4 groups of 8 rats (4 male, 4 female) were dosed after surgery (described below) with 0.0 (vehicle control), 1.3 (2x), 3.9 (6x), or 6.5 (10x) mg/kg drug suspension of buprenorphine on day 0. The volumes of the vehicle control, 2x, 6x, and 10x doses were 1.0, 0.2, 0.6, and 1.0 mL, respectively. As shown in Table 1, blood and urine samples were collected at day 2. On day 4 animals were euthanized and blood and urine collected. In the repeat-dose trials, 4 groups of 8 rats (4 male, 4 female) were dosed after surgery with the vehicle control or drug suspensions containing 1.3, 3.9, or 6.5 mg/kg of buprenorphine on day 0 and following anesthesia on days 4 and 8. Surgery was not repeated on days 4 and 8. Blood and urine samples were collected at day 6. Blood, urine, and histopathology studies were conducted on tissues collected following euthanasia on day 12 (Table 1).

2.3. Surgery. A surgical procedure was performed to mimic the implantation of an implantable pump or a telemetry device. Each rat was anesthetized by isoflurane gas at approximately 3% with an oxygen flow rate of 1% during the procedure. The duration of the anesthesia exposure was approximately 2 minutes. Following induction of anesthesia, the scapular surface (between the shoulder blades) was shaved, washed with ethanol, and then coated with Betadine. The animal was transferred to a clean procedural area where it was assessed to ensure a deep surgical plane of anesthesia using the toe pinch method. Once deep anesthesia was verified, breathing rate and capillary fill rate were documented. Clean, sterilized forceps were used to gently grasp the skin, and then clean, sterile scissors were used to make a 4-5 mm incision through the skin only. Bone and muscle were not penetrated. The clean, sterile scissors were used to separate the skin 2 cm rostral and distal, and 2 cm lateral in the subcutis, and create a subcutaneous pocket (approximately 2 × 4 cm). The incision was then apposed and stapled using a 9 mm Autoclip® (Kent Scientific, Torrington, CT).

TABLE 1: Dose, analyses, and histopathology schedules for TAS Trials 1 and 2.

(a) TAS Trial 1: single dose

Trial days	1	2	3	4
Anesthesia	+			
Surgery	+			
Drug or negative control dose	+			
Hematology		+		+
Chemistry		+		+
Urinalysis		+		+
Weight		+		+
Observed AM		+	+	+
Observed PM	+	+	+	
Histopathology				+

(b) TAS Trial 2: repeat dose

Trial days	1	2-3	4	5	6	7	8	9–11	12
Anesthesia	+		+				+		
Surgery	+								
Drug or negative control dose	+		+				+		
Hematology					+				+
Chemistry					+				+
Urinalysis					+				+
Weight			+		+		+		+
Observed AM		+	+	+	+	+	+	+	+
Observed PM	+	+	+	+	+	+	+	+	
Histopathology									+

2.4. Drug Delivery.

The buprenorphine-free control suspension consisted of cholesterol and glycerol tristearate (96 : 4) suspended in medium-chain triglyceride oil (8 mg/100 uL). The drug suspension consisted of buprenorphine, cholesterol, and glycerol tristearate, suspended in a medium-chain triglyceride oil (8 mg/100 uL), trade name Animalgesics for Mice. Control and drug suspensions were supplied by Animalgesic Labs (Millersville, MD). To limit stress associated with constraining conscious animals for SC injections, each rat was injected with the designated dose of test article or buprenorphine-free control suspension following surgery before they recovered from anesthesia in the single-dose trial. In the repeat-dose trial, rats were injected with drug following surgery and under anesthesia on day 0 and under anesthesia on days 4 and 8. The dose was administered SC on the middorsal area about 1 cm rostral to the surgical incision using a 25 G needle (BD, Franklin, NJ) attached to a 1 mL BD tuberculin syringe. Following dose administration, animals were transferred to a clean cage on a heating pad until recovered. Once the rat regained consciousness and demonstrated normal movement and the absence of signs of distress, it was returned to its home cage.

2.5. Bioavailability.

Male and female rats were provided with a single dose of drug and sampled at time intervals from 8 hours to 9 days to measure blood concentrations of buprenorphine. Rat blood samples were obtained from technician-restrained, unanesthetized animals by jugular vein phlebotomy. One mL disposable syringes with 20-gauge needles were used to collect approximately 0.4 mL of blood. The sample was immediately transferred to BD tubes containing dipotassium EDTA. The samples were stored on ice for approximately 1 hour and then centrifuged to collect plasma. The plasma was stored at −20°C until it was thawed for analysis. Buprenorphine plasma concentrations were measured by the McWhorter School of Pharmacy, Samford University (Birmingham, AL), using a Shimadzu LC-20AD (Columbia, MD) and mass spec Applied Biosystems 4000 QTrap (Carlsbad, CA) assay requiring 0.25 mL of plasma. The sensitivity of the assay was 0.5 ng/mL. Mean concentration-time data was used for the pharmacokinetic analysis. Noncompartmental-analyses module in Phoenix WinNonlin version 5.3 (Princeton NJ) was used to assess the area under the curve (AUC) and the maximum plasma concentration (Cmax) time at which the Cmax is realized (Tmax). Cmax and Tmax were the observed values. The AUC was calculated by the log-linear trapezoidal rule to the end of the sample collection (AUClast) [28].

2.6. Efficacy.

Studies were conducted with 18 F344 female rats at two dose levels: 0.65 and 1.3 mg/kg. Rats were injected with vehicle, 0.65, and 1.3 mg/kg dose of drug and tested for their tail flick response using a 55°C water bath. Tests were conducted by a female veterinarian who was blinded to the treatment group. Female rats were used because mu opioid agonists such as morphine appear to be less sensitive in female than male rats [29, 30]. The rats were injected with drug or vehicle on day 0 and examined for 5 days to monitor tail flick reaction times [31]. The rats were housed 3 per cage and cages were changed daily.

2.7. Clinical Observations. During the course of this study, animals were observed at the cage level once daily by a single observer prior to 9 AM for morbidity, mortality, and signs of pain or stress: abnormal breathing, tremors, ocular discharge, facial signs (squinting, eyes closed), posture, and movement and overall appearance including condition of the hair coat and grooming. Incision sites were examined at the 9 AM time for bleeding, swelling, or signs of infection. Because pica was not expected, methods to measure it, such as kaolin intake, were not used. Animals received "hands-on" detailed clinical observations once daily by a single observer after 2 PM for abnormal clinical signs (ocular discharge, motor activity, and signs of pain or distress). Incision sites were examined again at this time for bleeding, swelling, and signs of infection. Body surface was inspected for skin lesions. The process used to observe and record nausea-related behaviors has been published [27]. Briefly, observers noted in comments on the report form of hair loss and the presence of lesions as evidence of excessive grooming or self-gnawing behavior. They did not grade the amount of hair loss or the degree of biting. We considered any reports of hair loss or lesions on the paws to be signs of nausea-related behavior, and we recorded the number of rats of each sex in each experimental group that showed these signs during each observation period [27].

The observers were blinded to the treatment group. Approximately 38,000 data points were recorded in the two trials. In addition, the observers could add comments to each chart. The two male observers were Certified (AALAS) Lab Animal Technologist and Technician.

2.8. Body Weights. Weights of individual animals were taken for randomization (prior to study start), at midpoints (day 2 and day 6) and endpoints (day 4 and day 12) of the safety trials by an observer blinded to the dose.

2.9. Clinical Pathology. Blood and urine samples were collected at the mid- and endpoint of the each TAS trial. Blood was collected in the morning via jugular vein puncture. Approximately 0.5 ml of blood was collected for the midpoint clinical pathology studies. The midpoint sample was transferred to a collection tube containing dipotassium EDTA. Approximately 0.5 mL of the endpoint sample was transferred to a collection tube containing dipotassium EDTA, and 1 mL was transferred to a collection tube containing sodium citrate for coagulation factor measurements. The samples were refrigerated before analyses. The hematology examination included red blood cell (RBC) count, hemoglobin, hematocrit, mean corpuscular volume, mean corpuscular hemoglobin, mean corpuscular hemoglobin concentration, platelet count, white blood cell (WBC) count, differential blood cell count, and blood smear. Clinical chemistry tests

included glucose, urea nitrogen, creatinine, total protein, albumin, globulin (as calculation), total cholesterol, alanine aminotransferase, alkaline phosphatase, aspartate aminotransferase, calcium, sodium, potassium, chloride, and phosphate. In the two TAS trials, coagulation factor measurements were prothrombin time, activated partial thromboplastin time, and fibrinogen. Because of the amount of blood needed, coagulation factors were analyzed only on endpoint days 4 and 12. Expressed urine samples were collected in the afternoon on a clean surface and pipetted into a sterile Eppendorf tube. Urine dip sticks (Bayer Multistix 10 SG Reagent Strips, Romeoville, IL) were read manually. These tests measured pH, appearance, color, protein, glucose, bilirubin, and blood.

2.10. Necropsy. After the final collection of blood and urine specimens on endpoint days 4 and 12, animals were humanely euthanized using CO_2 inhalation, followed by a thoracotomy. Death was confirmed by cessation of heart rate. A comprehensive necropsy was then performed for each animal. Once the lungs were examined and weighed they were inflated with formalin to ensure proper fixation. Tissues were placed in an individually labeled container containing 10% neutral-buffered formalin, with the exception of testes (males) and eyes with optic nerves, which were preserved in modified Davidson's fixative. For short term studies, testes and eyes with optic nerves were transferred from the modified Davidson's solution to 70% ethanol 1-2 days following collection. The transfer was performed and documented by the histology lab. Containers were labeled with study number, date, group number, and animal number.

Organ weights included adrenal, brain, epididymis, heart, kidney, liver, lung, ovaries, spleen, testes, thyroid with parathyroid, and uterus with cervix. According to TAS protocols, histopathology studies were performed on the vehicle control animals and the animals given the highest dose of drug in the single- and repeat-dose trials, Table 1. Unless significant pathology was observed at the highest doses, slides from the two lower doses were not examined. Slides from the vehicle control animals and both doses in the long-term study were examined. Thirty-three tissues were harvested for histopathology examination of organs including the dorsal skin surrounding the injection site: adrenal gland, large intestine, colon, small intestine (jejunum, ileum, and duodenum), large intestine (cecum), liver, bone with bone marrow, femur, urinary bladder, lung, spinal cord with spine, brain (cerebrum, midbrain, cerebellum, and medulla/pons), lymph nodes including submandibular superficial cervical collected with salivary glands from the neck, mesenteric and pancreaticoduodenal collected with mesentery and pancreas, spleen, epididymis (males), mammary glands (females), stomach, eyes with optic nerve, ovaries (females), ventral skin, gall bladder, pancreas, heart, and parathyroid gland. Parathyroid glands were evaluated when present in the plane of section of the thyroid gland, thyroid (with parathyroid), testis (male), kidneys, and skeletal muscle (biceps femoris).

2.11. Statistics. A comprehensive statistical analysis (mean, standard deviations, N) was conducted for group mean body

TABLE 2: (a) Rat plasma concentrations of buprenorphine with single dose of lipid-buprenorphine suspension. (b) Pharmacokinetics of lipid-bound buprenorphine in male and female rats.

(a)

Dose (n = 3/sex)		0 Hrs	6 hrs (day 0)	24 hrs (day 1)	48 hrs (day 2)	72 hrs (day 3)	96 hrs (day 4)	168 hrs (day 7)	216 hrs (day 9)
0.65 mg/kg	♂	0	1.9 ± 1.2*	3.4 ± 0.8*	1.9 ± 1.2*	0.6 ± 0.2	0.4 ± 0.1	0	0
	♀	0	1.2 ± 0.3*	1.8 ± 0.8*	1.2 ± 0.3*	0.7 ± 0.1	0.3 ± 0	2.3 ± 3*	0
1.35 mg/kg	♂	0	1.9 ± 0.8*	5.4 ± 2.1*	6.6 ± 2.4*	5.1 ± 2.1*	3.5 ± 1.2*	No test	No test
	♀	0	4.9 ± 3.0*	9.6 ± 3.3*	7.0 ± 1.5*	7.4 ± 5.3*	1.6 ± 0.6*		

Asterisk signifies clinically significant drug concentrations, defined as greater than 0.75 ng/mL of plasma buprenorphine.

(b)

Dose	Sex	AUClast hr*ng/mL	Cmax ng/mL	Tmax hr
0.65 mg/kg	Male	154.2	3.4	24
	Female	99.7	1.8	24
1.35 mg/kg	Male	459	6.6	48
	Female	517.2	9.6	24

TABLE 3: Mean effects of drug on tail flick measurements at 55°C in female rats.

Dose	Time (days)				
	1	2	3	4	5
	Thermal latency in seconds				
Control	4.7 ± 2.0	6.5 ± 1.2	7.8 ± 1.5	7.1 ± 0.4	6.0 ± 0.9
0.65 mg/kg	16 ± 2.0*	27 ± 7.6*	24 ± 2.3*	22 ± 6.3*	19.4 ± 2.9*
1.3 mg/kg	13 ± 6.8*	26 ± 6.0*	27 ± 14*	25 ± 7.4*	17.6 ± 4.1*

*$P > 0.05$ for drug versus vehicle group, $n = 6$.

weight data comparing treated groups to the control group of each sex using one-way Analysis of Variance (ANOVA). An additional zero-inflated Poisson regression was conducted to estimate the dose and sex differences over time for pica behavior [32]. The zero-inflated Poisson regression model provides robust estimates and hypothesis tests for count data with a predominance of zeros. Statistical analyses (mean, standard deviations, N) were conducted for organ weight and clinical pathology data comparing treated groups to the control group using one-way Analysis of Variance (ANOVA). Additionally, Dunnett's t-test was used for control versus treated group comparisons [33].

3. Results

3.1. Bioequivalence and Efficacy Studies.
The bioavailability of buprenorphine and its pharmacokinetic profile in male and female rats at defined time points following a single SC injection of the test article was examined. As shown in Table 2(a), a single dose of 0.65 mg/kg provided at least 2 days of clinically significant drug concentrations, defined as greater than 0.75 ng/mL of plasma buprenorphine. A single female had a significant concentration of plasma buprenorphine at day 7. Table 2(a) also shows the concentrations of blood present in rats dosed with 1.3 mg/kg of drug.

Both male and female rats had clinically relevant plasma concentrations of buprenorphine throughout the 4 days of the single-dose and repeat-dose trials in which the lowest dose evaluated for adverse effects was 1.35 mg/kg (Table 2(a)). The estimated values for the AUC, Tmax, and Cmax are given in Table 2(b). Tmax for female rats in both dose groups was 24 hours. Tmax for male rats in the 1.3 mg/kg dose group moved to 48 hours based on a slightly greater mean blood concentration of buprenorphine on day 2. Cmax values in the 0.65 mg/kg group were 3.4 and 1.8 ng/mL for male and female rats, respectively. The estimated Cmax values for male and female rats in the 1.3 mg/kg dose group were 2-fold greater in male rats and 5-fold greater in females. The data in Table 3 shows that the extended release preparation of buprenorphine provided significant analgesic effects ($P > 0.05$) at 0.65 and 1.3 mg/kg dose.

3.2. Clinical Observations.
All rats survived to the scheduled termination date in both trials. Rats dosed with the test article on average appeared with slightly slower movement scores when compared with the vehicle control rats on study day 0, approximately 5 hours after dose administration. Minor wounds on the front paw or wrists associated with excess grooming and self-gnawing were noted in the drug treated animals in both trials. Excessive grooming and self-gnawing

TABLE 4: Signs of nausea-related behavior in single- and repeat-dose trials.

Group 4♀, 4♀	Observation of biting or self-licking											
	Day											
	1	2	3	4	5	6	7	8	9	10	11	12
Single dose												
0.0				*								
1.3		1♀	1♀	*								
3.9	1♂	1♂ 1♀	1♂ 2♀	*								
6.5			1♂ 1♀	*								
Repeat doses				*2nd dose*				*3rd dose*				
0.0							1♂			2♂		*
1.3	1♂	1♂	1♂	2♂ 1♀	2♂ 1♀	2♂	2♂ 1♀	1♂ 1♀	1♂	2♂ 1♀	2♂	*
3.9	1♀	1♀	1♀		1♀	4♂		1♂	1♂			*
6.5					1♀		1♂ 1♀		2♂ 1♀			*
Cumulative %	5	8	25	9	16	19	19	9	16	13	6	

*No observation.

behavior were not observed during the morning observation period that was given to each animal. This behavior was inferred by the absence of hair and the presence of a wound on the paw. The observer noted the findings as a comment on the animal's chart. The amount of hair loss and the degree of biting were not graded. There was no evidence of an open wound. These nausea-related signs were seen in the PM observation cycle when the animals were physically handled during an examination of the surgery site and monitoring of the entire skin surface for lesions.

Signs of nausea-related behavior were first noted in one male animal 1 day after an analgesic injection of 3.9 mg/kg, in the single-dose trial, Table 4. A single male rat in the 1.3 mg/kg dose group exhibited the behavior on day 2 and on day 3. The rats in the 3.9 mg/kg dose group showed an increasing incidence over time of the behavior and had the highest cumulative number of animals exhibiting the signs with $n = 1$ on day 1, $n = 2$ on day 2, and $n = 3$ on day 3. The highest dose group of 6.5 (10x) mg/kg exhibited a delayed onset and a lower incidence of the behavior compared to the 3.9 mg/kg (6x) group ($n = 2$ on day 3). A similar pattern was seen in the repeat-dose trial. Overall, by day 3, self-licking or paw biting was seen in 6 (25%) of the animals in the drug treated groups (beta = 1.01, SE = 0.41, and $P = 0.01$). The behavior consistently focused on the forepaws. Male and female rats exhibited similar rates of these types of behavior (beta = −0.406, SE = 0.65, and $P = 0.53$). Three of the animals in the vehicle control group of the repeat-dose trial exhibited this behavior. No signs of pain or distress were noted in the animals.

3.3. Weight Changes. All males and one female rat treated with 3.9 mg/kg buprenorphine lost weight between days 0 and 4 in the single-dose trial (Table 5). Two of the male

rats treated with 3.9 mg/kg of buprenorphine continued to lose weight during the course of the study, while the other two gained weight between days 2 and 4 and had an overall weight gain during the course of the study. All female rats treated with 3.9 mg/kg buprenorphine lost weight between days 2 and 4, but only two of them had an overall weight loss during the course of the study. All male rats treated with 6.5 mg/kg buprenorphine lost weight between days 0 and 2, while all females treated with the same dosage gained weight. Alternatively, all female rats treated with 6.5 mg/kg buprenorphine lost weight between days 2 and 4, while all males treated with the same dosage gained weight. As shown in Table 5, a similar pattern of weight changes was seen in the repeat-dose trial. Male rats in the 6.5 mg/kg dose group treated with 3 doses in 8 days gained the least amount of weight by day 12. Female rats in the 1.3 mg/kg repeat-dose group showed the least weight gain. Overall, there were no significant changes in body weights between the vehicle control and drug treated rats.

There were no significant changes in organ weight measurements with increasing doses of drug in either male or female rats in the single-dose trial. Organ weights for livers of males in the 3.9 mg/kg and 6.5 mg/kg groups in the repeat-dose trial showed significant post hoc differences when compared to the vehicle control group, but no treatment-related effects were seen upon microscopic examination of the tissues. Organ weight measurements for brain, heart, kidneys, spleen, and thyroid remained essentially unchanged. Increasing doses of drug also had no effects on the weights for epididymis and testes in males and uterus in females. The average weight of adrenal glands in male rats increased from a control value of 0.050 to 0.074 g in the highest dose group. The change was not seen in female rats. Average liver weights decreased in drug treated male and female rats. There were no

TABLE 5: Mean Body Weight Gains (BWG) for male and female rats in repeat dose trial.

Dose mg/kg	BWG Day 0–4	BWG Day 4–6	BWG Day 6–8	BWG Day 8–12	BWG Day 0–12
Male					
Control					
Mean	10.9	4.2	−4.1	10.9	22.0
SD	1.5	1.8	6.1	0.9	6.1
1.3					
Mean	2.5	6.9	−1.3	11.9	20.1
SD	1.5	2.5	3.9	5.6	7.3
3.9					
Mean	0.3	7.1	−1.1	13.2	19.6
SD	2.4	1.4	2.5	2.0	3.0
6.5					
Mean	−0.7	5.6	−2.7	8.6	11.0
SD	1.5	1.9	4.2	3.9	7.5
Female					
Control					
Mean	2.1	2.2	−1.2	6.4	9.6
SD	2.1	2.4	3.0	1.2	2.0
1.3					
Mean	−1.9	2.0	−3.4	6.7	3.4
SD	0.3	0.9	3.5	1.4	5.1
3.9					
Mean	−3.2	3.8	−2.7	6.7	4.6
SD	1.5	2.6	1.2	5.4	6.3
6.5					
Mean	−1.5	3.4	−1.8	7.0	7.0
SD	3.5	1.9	2.7	5.8	6.2

significant weight changes in the organs, other than the liver, of the rats in the long-term study.

3.4. Clinical Laboratory Studies. Semiquantitative (dipstick) tests of expressed urine in the single-dose trial detected urine protein in 11 (34%) and 16 (50%) of 32 rats on day 2 and day 4, respectively. In the repeat-dose trial, protein was detected in all animals in both day 6 and day 12 samples. The finding did not correlate with the dose group or sex. In the single-dose trial trace amounts of blood were detected in 21 (66%) and 10 (31%) rats on day 2 and day 4, respectively. In the repeat-dose trial, blood was detected in 7 (22%) rats on day 6 and 2 (6%) rats on day 12. In both trials, values varied from trace to moderate levels. The findings did not correlate with sex or dose group. Tests for glucose and bilirubin were negative for all samples. Appearance, pH, and color were normal in all samples in both trials.

Coagulation factor tests were performed on blood from day 4 of the single-dose trial and day 12 from the repeat-dose trial. Prothrombin time, activated partial thromboplastin time, and fibrinogen levels were normal in all dose groups in male and female rats.

Average differences in values between control and drug groups were noted in 9 of 14 hematology values and 14 of 16 clinical chemistry parameters in one or both TAS trials. These parameters were examined to determine whether changes with drug treatment varied or increased with increasing dose in male or female rats. In numerous cases, differences between control values and values from animals seen at 1.3 mg/kg dose levels were not seen in the 3.9 and 6.5 mg/kg dose levels. When differences were noted between the controls and the animals receiving drug-challenges, the changing values remained within the normal range or equaled values in the control group.

RBC values consistently decreased in day 4 and day 12 endpoint collections compared to the day 2 and day 6 midpoint values in all groups. This change was attributed to blood loss due to the previous blood collection. There was a slight increase in WBC counts after phlebotomy, an increase that we have observed in mouse phlebotomy [34]. Among the RBC indices there were no significant differences between the control groups and the animals in the 6.5 mg/kg dose groups. This indicates that the differences noted per group and sexes were random. There was no evidence of leucopenia or cytosis. Absolute values for nucleated WBCs were unremarkable, including neutrophils, eosinophils, and basophils.

Alanine aminotransferase and aspartate aminotransferase are sensitive yet modestly specific indicators of hepatocyte damage. Elevations in these serum or plasma enzyme activities are expected in drug-induced hepatotoxicity. In the present study, the enzyme levels in the drug groups closely resembled control values, even at the highest levels of drug tested. In several groups, they were modestly decreased. Serum alkaline phosphatase (ALP) can be altered by physiologic or pathologic changes in various tissues including kidney, hepatobiliary, intestine, and bone. In the present study, ALP values decrease significantly with increasing dose challenges. Sustained decreased levels of ALP have been associated with loss of appetite and fasting.

Cholesterol, BUN, creatinine, and calcium levels show small but inconsistent, and not significant, changes between the drug and control groups. The values in the drug and control groups remain within established laboratory normal values. Electrolyte levels were unremarkable: chloride, sodium, and potassium. As shown in Table 6, total protein levels on average were decreased in the highest dose group compared to controls. The decrease was not significant in the 1.3 and 3.9 mg/kg dose groups. The decrease in total protein levels appeared entirely related to decreased albumin levels with increasing drug exposure, Table 6. Primary factors affecting albumin synthesis include protein and amino acid nutrition, colloidal osmotic pressure, the action of certain hormones, and disease states. Fasting or a protein-deficient diets cause a decrease in albumin synthesis as long as the deficiency state is maintained. In the long-term study BUN values were decreased in the 1.3 mg/kg group compared to the 0.65 mg/kg group and the vehicle controls, 13.3 ± 1.0, 15.5 ± 1.0 and 16.5 ± 1.3 mg/dL, respectively.

TABLE 6: Decreasing plasma protein levels (mean ± SD) in combined male and female groups with increasing doses of drug.

Day	Dose(s)	Buprenorphine dose group			
		Control	1.3 mg/kg	3.9 mg/kg	6.5 mg/kg
		Total protein g/dL			
2	1	5.9 ± 0.3	5.9 ± 0.2	5.7 ± 0.3	5.4 ± 0.4
4	1	5.7 ± 0.3	5.6 ± 0.1	5.6 ± 0.4	5.5 ± 0.2
6	2	5.8 ± 0.4	5.6 ± 0.2	5.5 ± 0.3	5.4 ± 0.2
12	3	5.8 ± 0.4	5.6 ± 0.5	5.5 ± 0.4	5.6 ± 0.1
		Albumin g/dL			
2	1	3.2 ± 0.2	3.1 ± 0.2	2.9 ± 0.2	2.8 ± 0.2
4	1	3.0 ± 0.2	3.0 ± 0.1	3.0 ± 0.2	2.9 ± 0.1
6	2	3.2 ± 0.3	3.1 ± 0.1	2.8 ± 0.2	2.7 ± 0.1
12	3	3.2 ± 0.2	3.2 ± 0.3	2.95 ± 0.2	2.8 ± 0.1

3.5. Histopathology. The single-dose study reported a macroscopic observation of the thymus of one male rat in the control dose group presenting as "discolored red." Microscopically, this presented with hemorrhage and was considered an incidental finding, possibly related to terminal cardiocentesis. No other microscopic changes were observed.

In the repeat-dose trial, macroscopic observations during necropsy included reddened mandibular lymph node in one vehicle control female and one male rat treated with 6.5 mg/kg, subcutaneous hemorrhage below the injection site in one female and two males treated with 6.5 mg/kg, fluid filled uterus in one female treated with 1.3 mg/kg, thickened skin lateral to the site of injection in one female treated with 6.5 mg/kg, and 8 × 5 × 4 mm nodule on the median lobe of the liver in one female in the 6.5 mg/kg dose group. Although organ weights for livers of males in the 3.9 mg/kg and 6.5 mg/kg groups in the repeat-dose trial showed significant post hoc differences when compared to the vehicle control group, no treatment-related effects were seen upon microscopic examination of the tissues. Inflammatory changes (granulocytic infiltration and mixed cell infiltrates) and hemorrhage were commonly seen at increased severity at or near the dorsal skin injection sites in rats in the 6.5 mg/kg dose group. Similar changes were seen in the vehicle control group. No other microscopic changes were observed.

4. Discussion

The objective of this study was to evaluate the safety of a lipid suspension of buprenorphine for delivery of postprocedural pain relief in F344 rats. Blood level measurements demonstrated that a single 0.65 mg/kg SC dose of a cholesterol-triglyceride buprenorphine suspension provided significant blood concentrations of drug for at least two days (Table 2(a)). Following declining mean plasma concentrations of drug on days 3 and 4, a single female rat in this dose group had an elevated blood concentration at day 7. This secondary peak may be attributed to redosing by coprophagy. Studies have shown that more than 75% of an initial dose of buprenorphine is excreted unmetabolized within one week [35]. Tmax for the intended dose of 0.65 mg/kg was 24 hours in male and female rats. The estimated AUC for the female rats given single 0.65 mg/kg was about 60% the value for male rats given the same dose but slightly greater than males when given the 1.3 mg/kg dose (Table 2(b)). A comparison of the parameters between the two dose groups is difficult because little is known about the pharmacokinetics of SC lipid drug delivery systems. Blood was not collected after day 4 from the rats in the 1.3 mg/kg test group to limit potential morbidity associated with jugular phlebotomy.

Efficacy studies using a potentially painful stimulus confirmed that a 0.65 mg/kg dose in male and female rats provided analgesia for at least three days (Table 4). Reviews of the specificity of these tests have demonstrated that thermal sensitivity tests provide a good predictor of clinical efficacy in humans [17, 36]. High thermal latency measurements at days 4 and 5 at the 0.65 mg/kg dose level are somewhat surprising because bioequivalence tests on a separate cohort of male and female rats at this dose level (Table 3) demonstrated that mean blood levels of buprenorphine dropped below 0.4 mg/mL by day 4. Yet, the results are consistent with the studies of an extended release buprenorphine depot in human volunteers showing blood level decreases of drug below 0.75 mg/ml at the end of the first week and significant clinical effects maintained for almost 6 weeks [37]. Buprenorphine and its metabolite norbuprenorphine are rapidly converted to glucuronide conjugates in rats [38]. Both conjugates have biologic activity [39] and may be relatively undetected in standard LC/MS assays.

A standard safety trial format in the present study used excess dose challenges to monitor adverse effects that might occur in real world situations where the animal was given a repeat dose of the drug or had morbidities that could enhance drug toxicity. Opiates as a class have been associated with respiratory deficiency. Studies in rats have demonstrated that compared to morphine, fentanyl, and methadone there is a ceiling effect on the action of buprenorphine [40, 41]. The present study demonstrates that prolonged buprenorphine therapy in a lipid envelop can be safely tolerated in young adult F344 rats, but the effects on other species, older animals, and transgenic rats remain unknown.

Decreasing efficacy, tolerance, and hyperalgesia have been attributed to opiates including buprenorphine [42,

43]. Studies have illustrated a complex association between experimental designs, chronic drug therapy, and hyperalgesia [44]. No significant signs of locomotor activity or hyperalgesia were observed in the studies described here. Of interest, questions concerning the clinical significance of "hyperalgesia" appear to have been mooted by the studies of chronic buprenorphine therapy using transdermal skin patches. In all cases, reported hyperalgesic signs have been minimal in rats and humans [45–48].

In 1977, Cowan et al. described the first report of buprenorphine-induced "nausea" in rats: increased stereotyped licking and biting movements [49]. Mitchell and coworkers demonstrated the association of nausea with pica by spinning rats to induce motion sickness [50]. Yamamoto et al. demonstrated that radiation sickness induced pica [51]. Takeda and coworkers confirmed the association by treating rats with opiate inhibitors to prevent nausea [52]. De Jonghe et al. demonstrated that pica in rats is an adaptive response to nausea [53]. Drugs that block mu receptors such as methylnaltrexone can be used to block the emetic effects of opiates in humans and pica in rats [54].

The two TAS trials at 1.3, 3.9, and 6.5 mg/kg doses, which were conducted on soft bedding, reduced a risk of intestinal blockage and allowed a prospective determination of the rate of emetic behavior. As shown in Table 5, the observed cumulative rate of nausea signs in the 4-day, single-dose trial increased to 25%. The observed cumulative rate was 19% in the 12-day repeat-dose trial. The animals were identified by the observers in the PM observation cycle who examined the dorsal skin surfaces of the paws. The actual rate in the 4-day trial may have been higher because animals were removed from the study before the PM observation. The rate did not increase in the 12-day trial with increasing doses of drug. In both trials, the behavior was self-limiting and produced no apparent lasting consequences. This incidence is similar to the incidence of nausea-related behavior reported in human patients treated with opiate therapies [55].

Weight loss has been cited as a deterrent to the use of postsurgical buprenorphine analgesia, and it has been linked to significant morbidity secondary to gastrointestinal blockage associated with hardwood bedding [56, 57]. A number of reports between 2000 and 2010 described weight loss in rats treated with buprenorphine without reference to the bedding used in the experiment [58], or they report using hardwood bedding without reference to previous reports associating hardwood bedding with pica [39]. Previous studies have demonstrated that the risk of pica-related gastric distress can be controlled by the appropriate choice of bedding [59]. The studies reported here confirm this observation.

5. Conclusion

There do not appear to be clinically significant treatment-related effects following repeated subcutaneous injections of an extended release lipid suspension of buprenorphine at 1.3 mg/kg, 3.9 mg/kg, or 6.5 mg/kg dose. Although several clinical pathology findings exceeded normal limits and urinalysis results showed abnormal parameters, there were no correlated changes or findings in body weights, clinical observations, organ weights, or microscopic evaluation of tissues.

Disclosure

M. Guarnieri owns a significant financial interest in Animalgesic Labs.

Conflicts of Interest

The authors declare that they have no conflicts of interest.

Acknowledgments

The authors acknowledge the support of Dr. Rana Rais for the analyses of the pharmacokinetic parameters and Dr. Greg Gorman for the analyses of plasma buprenorphine. Funding for this research was supplied by the Maryland Biotechnology Center Biotechnology Development Awards, Maryland Industrial Partnerships (MIPS), and by Animalgesic Labs.

References

[1] K. S. P. Abelson, K. R. Jacobsen, R. Sundbom, O. Kalliokoski, and J. Hau, "Voluntary ingestion of nut paste for administration of buprenorphine in rats and mice," *Laboratory Animals*, vol. 46, no. 4, pp. 349–351, 2012.

[2] M. J. Molina-Cimadevila, S. Segura, C. Merino, N. Ruiz-Reig, B. Andrés, and E. de Madaria, "Oral self-administration of buprenorphine in the diet for analgesia in mice," *Laboratory Animals*, vol. 48, no. 3, pp. 216–224, 2014.

[3] B. Tyler, S. Wadsworth, V. Recinos et al., "Local delivery of rapamycin: a toxicity and efficacy study in an experimental malignant glioma model in rats," *Neuro-Oncology*, vol. 13, no. 7, pp. 700–709, 2011.

[4] R. J. Tamargo, J. I. Epstein, C. S. Reinhard, M. Chasin, and H. Brem, "Brain biocompatibility of a biodegradable, controlled-release polymer in rats," *Journal of Biomedical Materials Research*, vol. 23, no. 2, pp. 253–266, 1989.

[5] T. S. Clark, D. D. Clark, and R. F. Hoyt Jr., "Pharmacokinetic comparison of sustained-release and standard buprenorphine in mice," *Journal of the American Association for Laboratory Animal Science*, vol. 53, no. 4, pp. 387–391, 2014.

[6] E. T. Carbone, K. E. Lindstrom, S. Diep, and L. Carbone, "Duration of action of sustained-release buprenorphine in 2 strains of mice," *Journal of the American Association for Laboratory Animal Science*, vol. 51, no. 6, pp. 815–819, 2012.

[7] P. L. Foley, H. Liang, and A. R. Crichlow, "Evaluation of a sustained-release formulation of buprenorphine for analgesia in rats," *Journal of the American Association for Laboratory Animal Science*, vol. 50, no. 2, pp. 198–204, 2011.

[8] L. Divincenti Jr., L. A. D. Meirelles, and R. A. Westcott, "Safety and clinical effectiveness of a compounded sustained-release formulation of buprenorphine for postoperative analgesia in New Zealand white rabbits," *Journal of the American Veterinary Medical Association*, vol. 248, no. 7, pp. 795–801, 2016.

[9] E. A. Nunamaker, D. F. Stolarik, J. Ma, A. S. Wilsey, G. J. Jenkins, and C. L. Medina, "Clinical efficacy of sustained-release buprenorphine with meloxicam for postoperative analgesia in

Beagle dogs undergoing ovariohysterectomy," *Journal of the American Association for Laboratory Animal Science*, vol. 53, no. 5, pp. 494–501, 2014.

[10] E. A. Nunamaker, L. C. Halliday, D. E. Moody, W. B. Fang, M. Lindeblad, and J. D. Fortman, "Pharmacokinetics of 2 formulations of buprenorphine in macaques (macaca mulatta and macaca fascicularis)," *Journal of the American Association for Laboratory Animal Science*, vol. 52, no. 1, pp. 48–56, 2013.

[11] D. K. Mishra, V. Dhote, P. Bhatnagar, and P. K. Mishra, "Engineering solid lipid nanoparticles for improved drug delivery: promises and challenges of translational research," *Drug Delivery and Translational Research*, vol. 2, no. 4, pp. 238–253, 2012.

[12] J. S. Kent, "Cholesterol matrix delivery system for sustained release of macromolecules," US Patent 4,452, 7755, June 1984.

[13] G. J. Grant, K. Vermeulen, M. I. Zakowski, M. Stenner, H. Turndorf, and L. Langerman, "Prolonged analgesia and decreased toxicity with liposomal morphine in a mouse model," *Anesthesia and Analgesia*, vol. 79, no. 4, pp. 706–709, 1994.

[14] L. J. Smith, B. K. Kukanich, L. A. Krugner-Higby, B. H. Schmidt, and T. D. Heath, "Pharmacokinetics of ammonium sulfate gradient loaded liposome-encapsulated oxymorphone and hydromorphone in healthy dogs," *Veterinary Anaesthesia and Analgesia*, vol. 40, no. 5, pp. 537–545, 2013.

[15] R. B. Pontani and A. L. Misra, "A long-acting buprenorphine delivery system," *Pharmacology, Biochemistry and Behavior*, vol. 18, no. 3, pp. 471–474, 1983.

[16] M. Guarnieri, C. Brayton, L. DeTolla, N. Forbes-McBean, R. Sarabia-Estrada, and P. Zadnik, "Safety and efficacy of buprenorphine for analgesia in laboratory mice and rats," *Lab Animal*, vol. 41, no. 11, pp. 337–343, 2012.

[17] J. V. Roughan and P. A. Flecknell, "Buprenorphine: a reappraisal of its antinociceptive effects and therapeutic use in alleviating post-operative pain in animals," *Laboratory Animals*, vol. 36, no. 3, pp. 322–343, 2002.

[18] N. M. Gades, P. J. Danneman, S. K. Wixson, and E. A. Tolley, "The magnitude and duration of the analgesic effect of morphine, butorphanol, and buprenorphine in rats and mice," *Contemporary Topics in Laboratory Animal Science*, vol. 39, no. 2, pp. 8–13, 2000.

[19] N. Schildhaus, E. Trink, C. Polson et al., "Thermal latency studies in opiate-treated mice," *Journal of Pharmacy and Bioallied Sciences*, vol. 6, no. 1, pp. 43–47, 2014.

[20] P. L. Foley, "Current options for providing sustained analgesia to laboratory animals," *Lab Animal*, vol. 43, no. 10, pp. 364–371, 2014.

[21] M. Guarnieri, C. Brayton, L. Detolla, N. Forbes-Mcbean, R. Sarabia-Estrada, and P. Zadnik, "Safety and efficacy of buprenorphine for analgesia in laboratory mice and rats," *Lab Animal*, vol. 41, no. 11, pp. 337–343, 2012.

[22] I. Park, D. Kim, J. Song et al., "Buprederm™, a new transdermal delivery system of buprenorphine: pharmacokinetic, efficacy and skin irritancy studies," *Pharmaceutical Research*, vol. 25, no. 5, pp. 1052–1062, 2008.

[23] K. Pieper, T. Schuster, O. Levionnois, U. Matis, and A. Bergadano, "Antinociceptive efficacy and plasma concentrations of transdermal buprenorphine in dogs," *Veterinary Journal*, vol. 187, no. 3, pp. 335–341, 2011.

[24] Guidance for Industry (GFI#61)—FDA Approval of Animal Drugs for Minor Uses and for Minor Species, Target Animal Safety and Effectiveness Protocol Development and Submission, 2008, https://www.fda.gov/Drugs/GuidanceComplianceRegulatoryInformation/Guidances/default.htm.

[25] *Guidelines of Target Animal Safety for Pharmaceuticals, VICH Topic GL43*, European Medicines Agency Veterinary Medicines and Inspections, 2006.

[26] K. A. Traul, J. B. Romero, C. Brayton et al., "Safety studies of post-surgical buprenorphine therapy for mice," *Laboratory Animals*, vol. 49, no. 2, pp. 100–110, 2015.

[27] A. Cowan, R. Sarabia-Estrada, G. Wilkerson, P. McKnight, and M. Guarnieri, "Unanticipated adverse events associated with an extended-release buprenorphine toxicity study in Fischer 344 rats," *Lab Animal*, vol. 45, no. 1, pp. 28–34, 2016.

[28] R. Rais, A. Jančařík, L. Tenora et al., "Discovery of 6-diazo-5-oxo-l-norleucine (DON) prodrugs with enhanced CSF delivery in monkeys: a potential treatment for glioblastoma," *Journal of Medicinal Chemistry*, vol. 59, no. 18, pp. 8621–8633, 2016.

[29] A. C. Barrett, C. D. Cook, J. M. Terner, R. M. Craft, and M. J. Picker, "Importance of sex and relative efficacy at the μ opioid receptor in the development of tolerance and cross-tolerance to the antinociceptive effects of opioids," *Psychopharmacology*, vol. 158, no. 2, pp. 154–164, 2001.

[30] R. E. Bartok and R. M. Craft, "Sex differences in opioid antinociception," *Journal of Pharmacology and Experimental Therapeutics*, vol. 282, no. 2, pp. 769–778, 1997.

[31] P. J. Tiseo, E. B. Geller, and M. W. Adler, "Antinociceptive action of intracerebroventricularly administered dynorphin and other opioid peptides in the rat," *Journal of Pharmacology and Experimental Therapeutics*, vol. 246, no. 2, pp. 449–453, 1988.

[32] D. Lambert, "Zero-inflated poisson regression, with an application to defects in manufacturing," *Technometrics*, vol. 34, no. 1, pp. 1–14, 1992.

[33] IBM Knowledge Center, https://www.ibm.com/support/knowledgecenter/SSLVMB_20.0.0/com.ibm.spss.statistics.help/aalg_post.hoc_equalvar_dunnett_2tailed.htm.

[34] N. Forbes, C. Brayton, S. Grindle, S. Shepherd, B. Tyler, and M. Guarnieri, "Morbidity and mortality rates associated with serial bleeding from the superficial temporal vein in mice," *Lab Animal*, vol. 39, no. 8, pp. 236–240, 2010.

[35] R. B. Pontani, N. L. Vadlamani, and A. L. Misra, "Disposition in the rat of buprenorphine administered parenterally and as a subcutaneous implant," *Xenobiotica*, vol. 15, no. 4, pp. 287–297, 1985.

[36] A. C. Thompson, M. B. Kristal, A. Sallaj, A. Acheson, L. B. E. Martin, and T. Martin, "Analgesic efficacy of orally administered buprenorphine in rats: methodologic considerations," *Comparative Medicine*, vol. 54, no. 3, pp. 293–300, 2004.

[37] S. C. Sigmon, D. E. Moody, E. S. Nuwayser, and G. E. Bigelow, "An injection depot formulation of buprenorphine: extended biodelivery and effects," *Addiction*, vol. 101, no. 3, pp. 420–432, 2006.

[38] A. Bulka, P. F. Kouya, Y. Böttiger, J.-O. Svensson, X.-J. Xu, and Z. Wiesenfeld-Hallin, "Comparison of the antinociceptive effect of morphine, methadone, buprenorphine and codeine in two substrains of Sprague-Dawley rats," *European Journal of Pharmacology*, vol. 492, no. 1, pp. 27–34, 2004.

[39] S. M. Brown, M. Holtzman, T. Kim, and E. D. Kharasch, "Buprenorphine metabolites, buprenorphine-3-glucuronide and norbuprenorphine-3-glucuronide, are biologically active," *Anesthesiology*, vol. 115, no. 6, pp. 1251–1260, 2011.

[40] L. Chevillard, B. Mégarbane, P. Risède, and F. J. Baud, "Characteristics and comparative severity of respiratory response to

toxic doses of fentanyl, methadone, morphine, and buprenorphine in rats," *Toxicology Letters*, vol. 191, no. 2-3, pp. 327–340, 2009.

[41] A. Dahan, A. Yassen, H. Bijl et al., "Comparison of the respiratory effects of intravenous buprenorphine and fentanyl in humans and rats," *British Journal of Anaesthesia*, vol. 94, no. 6, pp. 825–834, 2005.

[42] L. I. Curtin, J. A. Grakowsky, M. Suarez et al., "Evaluation of buprenorphine in a postoperative pain model in rats," *Comparative Medicine*, vol. 59, no. 1, pp. 60–71, 2009.

[43] C. W. Berthold III and J. M. Moerschbaecher, "Tolerance to the effects of buprenorphine on schedule-controlled behavior and analgesia in rats," *Pharmacology, Biochemistry and Behavior*, vol. 29, no. 2, pp. 393–396, 1988.

[44] E. P. Wala and J. R. Holtman Jr., "Buprenorphine-induced hyperalgesia in the rat," *European Journal of Pharmacology*, vol. 651, no. 1–3, pp. 89–95, 2011.

[45] K. Böhme, B. Heckes, and K. Thomitzek, "Application of a seven-day buprenorphine transdermal patch in multimorbid patients on long-term ibuprofen or diclofenac," *MMW Fortschritte der Medizin*, vol. 152, no. 4, pp. 125–132, 2011 (German).

[46] N. Griessinger, R. Sittl, and R. Likar, "Transdermal buprenorphine in clinical practice—a post-marketing surveillance study in 13179 patients," *Current Medical Research and Opinion*, vol. 21, no. 8, pp. 1147–1156, 2005.

[47] I. Park, D. Kim, J. Song et al., "Buprederm™, a new transdermal delivery system of buprenorphine: pharmacokinetic, efficacy and skin irritancy studies," *Pharmaceutical Research*, vol. 25, no. 5, pp. 1052–1062, 2008.

[48] J. Pergolizzi, R. H. Böger, K. Budd et al., "Opioids and the management of chronic severe pain in the elderly: consensus statement of an international expert panel with focus on the six clinically most often used world health organization step III opioids (Buprenorphine, Fentanyl, Hydromorphone, Methadone, Morphine, Oxycodone)," *Pain Practice*, vol. 8, no. 4, pp. 287–313, 2008.

[49] A. Cowan, J. C. Doxey, and E. J. R. Harry, "The animal pharmacology of buprenorphine, an oripavine analgesic agent," *British Journal of Pharmacology*, vol. 60, no. 4, pp. 547–554, 1977.

[50] D. Mitchell, J. D. Laycock, and W. F. Stephens, "Motion sickness-induced pica in the rat," *The American Journal of Clinical Nutrition*, vol. 30, no. 2, pp. 147–150, 1977.

[51] K. Yamamoto, N. Takeda, and A. Yamatodani, "Establishment of an animal model for radiation-induced vomiting in rats using pica," *Journal of Radiation Research*, vol. 43, no. 2, pp. 135–141, 2002.

[52] N. Takeda, S. Hasegawa, M. Morita, and T. Matsunaga, "Pica in rats is analogous to emesis: an animal model in emesis research," *Pharmacology, Biochemistry and Behavior*, vol. 45, no. 4, pp. 817–821, 1993.

[53] B. C. De Jonghe, M. P. Lawler, C. C. Horn, and M. G. Tordoff, "Pica as an adaptive response: Kaolin consumption helps rats recover from chemotherapy-induced illness," *Physiology and Behavior*, vol. 97, no. 1, pp. 87–90, 2009.

[54] H. H. Aung, S. R. Mehendale, J.-T. Xie, J. Moss, and C.-S. Yuan, "Methylnaltrexone prevents morphine-induced kaolin intake in the rat," *Life Sciences*, vol. 74, no. 22, pp. 2685–2691, 2004.

[55] R. Aparasu, R. A. McCoy, C. Weber, D. Mair, and T. V. Parasuraman, "Opioid-induced emesis among hospitalized nonsurgical patients: effect on pain and quality of life," *Journal of Pain and Symptom Management*, vol. 18, no. 4, pp. 280–288, 1999.

[56] H. M. Bender, "Pica behavior associated with buprenorphine administration in the rat," *Laboratory Animal Science*, vol. 48, no. 1, article 5, 1998.

[57] C. Jacobson, "Adverse effects on growth rates in rats caused by buprenorphine administration," *Laboratory Animals*, vol. 34, no. 2, pp. 202–206, 2000.

[58] M. P. Brennan, A. J. Sinusas, T. L. Horvath, J. G. Collins, and M. J. Harding, "Correlation between body weight changes and postoperative pain in rats treated with meloxicam or buprenorphine," *Lab Animal*, vol. 38, no. 3, pp. 87–93, 2009.

[59] P. Jablonski, B. O. Howden, and K. Baxter, "Influence of buprenorphine analgesia on post-operative recovery in two strains of rats," *Laboratory Animals*, vol. 35, no. 3, pp. 213–222, 2001.

21

Tamoxifen Promotes Axonal Preservation and Gait Locomotion Recovery after Spinal Cord Injury in Cats

Braniff de la Torre Valdovinos,[1] **Judith Marcela Duenas Jimenez,**[2]
Ismael Jimenez Estrada,[3] **Jacinto Banuelos Pineda,**[4] **Nancy Elizabeth Franco Rodriguez,**[1]
Jose Roberto Lopez Ruiz,[5] **Laura Paulina Osuna Carrasco,**[5]
Ahiezer Candanedo Arellano,[5] **and Sergio Horacio Duenas Jimenez**[5]

[1]*Department of Computer Science, CUCEI, Universidad de Guadalajara, Avenida Revolucion No. 1500 Building M, Laboratory 212,*
  44430 Guadalajara, JAL, Mexico
[2]*Department of Physiology, CUCS Universidad de Guadalajara, Sierra Mojada 950, Building P Third Floor,*
  44290 Guadalajara, JAL, Mexico
[3]*Department of Physiology Biophysics and Neurosciences, Centro de Investigacion y Estudios Avanzados IPN,*
  Avenida Instituto Politecnico Nacional 2508, 07360 Mexico City, DF, Mexico
[4]*Department of Veterinary and Medicine, CUCBA Universidad de Guadalajara, Camino Ing. Ramon Padilla Sanchez 2100,*
  45110 Zapopan, JAL, Mexico
[5]*Department of Neuroscience, CUCS Universidad de Guadalajara, Sierra Mojada 950, Building P Third Floor,*
  44290 Guadalajara, JAL, Mexico

Correspondence should be addressed to Sergio Horacio Duenas Jimenez; sduenas@cucs.udg.mx

Academic Editor: Vito Laudadio

We performed experiments in cats with a spinal cord penetrating hemisection at T13-L1 level, with and without tamoxifen treatment. The results showed that the numbers of the ipsilateral and contralateral ventral horn neurons were reduced to less than half in the nontreated animals compared with the treated ones. Also, axons myelin sheet was preserved to almost normal values in treated cats. On the contrary, in the untreated animals, their myelin sheet was reduced to 28% at 30 days after injury (DAI), in both the ipsilateral and contralateral regions of the spinal cord. Additionally, we made hindlimb kinematics experiments to study the effects of tamoxifen on cat locomotion after the injury: at 4, 16, and 30 DAI. We observed that the ipsilateral hindlimb angular displacement (AD) of the pendulum-like movements (PLM) during gait locomotion was recovered to almost normal values in treated cats. Contralateral PLM acquired similar values to those obtained in intact cats. At 4 DAI, untreated animals showed a compensatory increment of PLM occurring in the contralateral hindlimb, which was partially recovered at 30 DAI. Our findings indicate that tamoxifen exerts a neuroprotective effect and preserves or produces myelinated axons, which could benefit the locomotion recovery in injured cats.

1. Introduction

Thoracolumbar penetrating spinal cord injury (SCI) often produces motor and sensory alterations in hindlimbs [1]. Promising pharmacological treatments and treadmill locomotion training are used for inducing restoration of locomotion and spinal reflexes after contusive, compressive lesions or by a penetrating SCI [2–4]. Locomotion disturbances occur in concordance with the type of injury and the spinal cord area suffering the trauma [5, 6].

Axonal and neuronal death is an important secondary effect after a penetrating injury in brain and spinal cord lesions [7, 8]. Tamoxifen has been shown to be an effective treatment to brain and spinal cord injuries; it has been proposed as an inflammatory response modulator and participates in locomotion recovery after a SCI [2, 8, 9]. Tamoxifen is a selective estrogen receptor modulator (SERM) acting on α- and β-estrogen receptors; also, it is been shown to prevent demyelination and promote differentiation to oligodendrocytes from multipotential cells in the cerebral cortex [7]. It is unknown whether tamoxifen exerts neuroprotective effects in cats after a SCI.

In this study, experiments were made on cats with a T13-L1 level spinal cord hemisection and the effects of tamoxifen were assessed by evaluating the survival of neurons in the spinal cord, axonal myelin preservation, or remyelination and by analyzing the kinematic angular displacement of both hindlimbs during unrestricted gait.

2. Material and Methods

2.1. Subjects and Ethics Statement. Adult male cats were used in this study (Laboratory Animal Center of the Guadalajara University, 3.5–4 kg, $n = 9$). All the procedures described here were performed with the guidelines contained in the National Institutes of Health Guide for the Care and Use of Laboratory Animals (USA) and with the ethical considerations stipulated in the experimental animal treatment on the Official Mexican Norm (NOM-062-ZOO-1999). Experiments were approved by the ethics committee for research and biosafety (Universidad de Guadalajara).

2.2. General Procedures for Surgery and Spinal Cord Injury. Cats were divided in three groups: intact (INT, $n = 3$), injured and treated with tamoxifen (IWT, $n = 3$), and injured without tamoxifen (IWOT, $n = 3$). A prophylactic antibiotic treatment was given (Gentamicin 2 mg/kg i.m.). For preventing pain, Ketoprofen (2.5 mg/kg i.m.) was administered two days before the spinal cord hemisection. The cats were anesthetized with Ketamine (10 mg/kg i.p.) and Xylazine (1 mg/kg i.p.) for performing spinal cord injury. The dorsal surface of the T12 vertebra was exposed and the apophysis was removed with a surgical gouge. A microdrill was used for opening the right lamina, and a surgical blade (HERGOM® number 11) for hemisecting the spinal cord segment. After surgery, a drop of medical grade cyanoacrylate was applied on the dura mater and bone wax was used to cover the vertebra. Animals were treated for three days with postoperative antibiotics (Gentamicin 2 mg/kg i.m.). IWT cats received tamoxifen (1 mg/kg i.p.) at days 0, 1, and 2 DAI (days after injury). Animals had free access to water and food and were housed one per cage (1 m height × 1 m wide × 1 m tall) to allow them to move freely. Room temperature was maintained at 25-26°C.

2.3. Kinematic Analysis. Prior to the surgery, animals were trained to walk through a transparent acrylic passway (200 cm long × 50 cm high × 20 cm width) daily during one week, in order to record a basal walk kinematic in cats. Video contrasting dots were placed in the iliac crest, hip (i.e., greater trochanter), knee, ankle (i.e., lateral malleolus), and fifth metatarsal phalangeal joints. The marks were placed in both hindlimbs and videotaped with a 30-frame-per-second video camera (SONY FDR-AX100). "Total video converter" (Shareware®) was used for decomposing the video into individual frames and the Cartesian coordinates of each joint mark were determined by the Image J software (Scion Corporation, NIH). Subsequently, the joint mark coordinates were introduced in a LabView® environment computer program (developed in CINVESTAV, IPN, México) [10]. Line graphs were constructed to illustrate the hindlimb movements from at least 3 consecutive strides. The computer program also calculates the hip and knee joint angles in a movement sequence executed by the ipsilateral and contralateral hindlimbs during strides. The joint angular displacement (JAD) was calculated from the difference between the maximum and minimal angular values of each stride. In addition, hindlimb PLM was analyzed by determining the angle between a line drawn from the iliac crest to the ankle and the y-axis (Figure 1). Control kinematics data was obtained prior to spinal cord injury in all subjects; subsequently, the experimental values were acquired at 4, 16, and 30 DAI in IWT and IWOT groups. All data were normalized and were graphically represented as a percent of the angular displacement.

2.4. Tissue Preparation. At 30 DAI cats were deeply anesthetized (pentobarbital euthanasia dose 50 mg/kg i.m.) and intracardially perfused with 500 mL of 0.1 M phosphate buffered saline (PBS) containing 0.5 mL of heparin (1000 U.I./mL), followed by 500 mL of a fixative solution (4% paraformaldehyde in 0.1 M PBS). The spinal cord segment T13-L1 was extracted and placed in the fixative solution during 24 hours and then washed in 0.1 M PBS for another 24 hours. The spinal cord segment was cryoprotected in 0.1 M PBS containing 30% of sucrose and 30% ethylene glycol for 72 hours. Subsequently, the spinal cord segment was divided in three regions: (1) injury site (IS), (2) cuts initiating 200 μm rostral from the injury site (RFI), and (3) cuts initiating caudally from the injury site (CFI). The tissue was embedded in Leica® Tissue Freezing Medium and representative 15 μm thick coronal cuts of each section were obtained from the T13-L1 segment using a Leica CM1850 cryostat.

2.5. Histology and Myelin Staining. Nine coronal cuts were placed per each slide; two slides per section were stained and analyzed. A Hematoxylin and Eosin (H&E) staining protocol was used for evaluating the histopathology status (observing whether Wallerian degeneration occurred; and the lesion similarity) of the spinal cord in INT, IWT, and IWOT cats. Hematoxylin solution was used for 5 minutes per slide and alcoholic Eosin Y solution (0.5% eosin in 90% ethanol) for 30 seconds; slides were washed with tap water for 5 minutes after staining. Toluidine blue staining protocol was used for assessing myelin thickness after SCI in all groups. O-Toluidine hydrochloride solution (3% o-toluidine in 0.1 M acetate-acetic buffer pH 5.0) was used for 5 minutes per slice; 2-minute washing was performed with tap water. Subsequently, an ethanol dehydration protocol was applied and the slices were mounted with Entellan®.

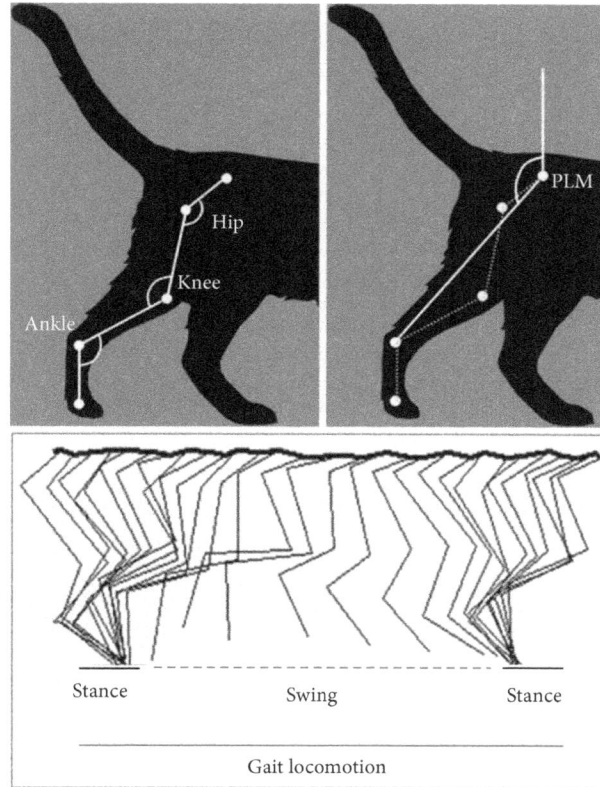

FIGURE 1: Diagram illustrating the experimental arrangement. Figure shows a schematic representation of the hip, knee, ankle, and pendulum like-movement (PLM) angles as well as the swing and stance step phases.

2.6. Axonal and Myelin Morphometric Analysis. The ventral white matter was visualized with light microscopy (Olympus, BX51W1) and photographed with a high resolution camera (Canon EOS Rebel T3). A 300 μm^2 square microscopic field was delimited for establishing a qualitative white matter axon observation using the Portable Olympus® Image Pro plus software V 6.0. The myelin area was determined in axons from the ventral white matter (cat 1, $n = 30$; cat 2, $n = 20$; cat 3, $n = 30$, per analyzed section); the inclusion criterions were maximum diameter of 15 μm and a round-like morphology. This study was performed using an image software analyzer (Motic Images Plus 2.0). The axonal myelin area was determined by establishing a perimeter trace around the outer myelin sheet and a second perimeter trace around the inside myelin sheet. The area between perimeters was calculated subtracting their respective area values.

2.7. Immunohistochemistry and Cell Count. Spinal cord tissue was pretreated with a PBS solution containing 0.3% X-100 Triton at 26°C for 30 minutes. The nonspecific antigen binding sites were blocked by a 10% normal goat serum for 1 hour at room temperature. The sections were incubated for 18 hours with the primary antibody at 4°C: anti-FOX3 for neurons, previously known as NeuN [11] (Abcam 104225, 1:1000). The slices were washed between incubations (three times) in PBS for 10 min. After primary antibody, the slices were incubated with the goat polyclonal secondary antibody:

anti-IgG Alexa fluor 488 conjugated anti-rabbit (invitrogen A-11008, 1:1000) during 2 hours at room temperature. After the secondary antibody, tissues were incubated with 4,6-diamidino-2-phenylindole (DAPI) (Molecular Probes® D3571, 1:100) for 5 minutes. Slices were washed in PBS for 10 minutes. Nine coronal cuts per slide were placed manually, and three slides were evaluated in each level (cat 1: 18 cuts for RFI, 18 cuts for IS, and 18 cuts for CFI; cat 2: 18 cuts for RFI, 18 cuts for IS, and 18 cuts for CFI; cat 3: 18 cuts for RFI, 18 cuts for IS, and 18 cuts for CFI); the ethanol dehydration protocol was applied and sealed with Entellan. Neurons were counted using a digital image software (Portable Olympus Image Pro plus software V 6.0), adapted to a fluorescence microscope. Six microscopic fields (500 μm^2) were studied in the dorsal horn (DH; Rexed lamina I and II), ventral horn (VH; Rexed lamina VIII and IV), and periaqueductal zone (PAZ; Rexed lamina X), ipsilateral and contralateral to the injury. The total studied area was equivalent to 1.62 mm^2.

2.8. Statistics. All data is expressed as mean ± SD. Neurons ($n = 18$ cuts per slide) and myelin morphometric ($n = 30$) data was analyzed using a nonparametric Kruskal-Wallis test and Mann-Whitney U test for multiple comparisons. Kinematic assessment was analyzed using a nonparametric Friedman test followed by Wilcoxon post hoc test for multiple specific comparisons. A $p < 0.05$ value was considered for establishing statistical significance. IBM SPSS (release 20.0.0)

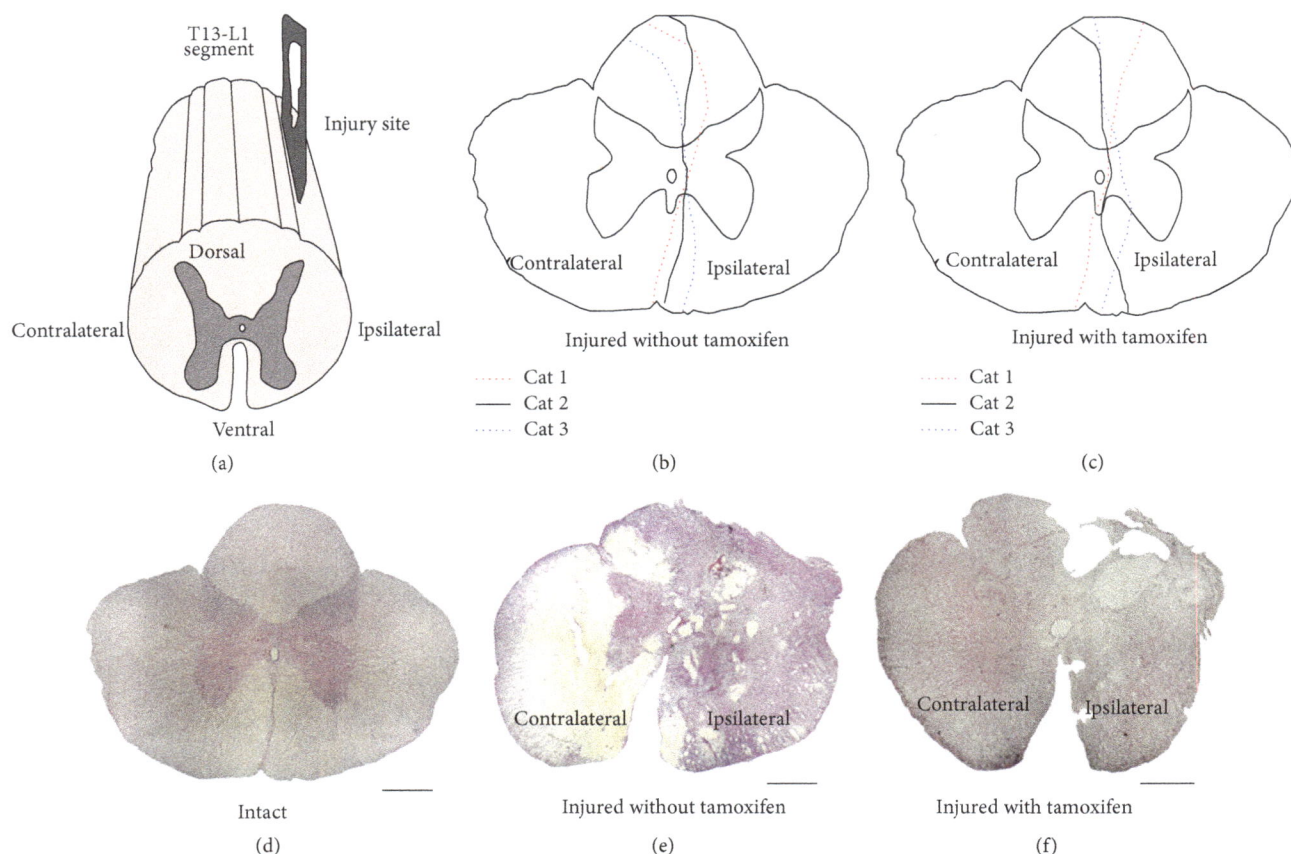

FIGURE 2: Representative T13-L1 microscopy images stained with H&E in coronal cuts (20 μm thick) and schematic illustrations showing the lesion extension size. (a) Schematic diagram T13-L1 segment; (b) schematic diagram illustrating the lesion extension size for each one of the three cats injured without tamoxifen group; black continuous line represents cat 1, red circular dotted line cat 2, and blue oval dotted line cat 3; (c) schematic diagram showing lesions extensions in each one of the cats in the injured with tamoxifen group, lines as indicated. (d) Spinal cord coronal cut from an intact cat. (e) Spinal cord coronal cut from an injured cat without tamoxifen. (f) Spinal cord cut from an injured cat with tamoxifen; scale bar: 500 μm.

software was used for statistical tests and graphs were made using statistical software (GraphPad Prism 6.0).

3. Results

3.1. Tamoxifen Preserved the Contralateral Spinal Cord Tissue, in Similarly Injured Cats.

A schematic drawing of the spinal cord damage for treated and untreated cats is illustrated in Figures 2(b) and 2(c). The spinal cord slices from intact cats show defined borders between gray and white matter. The gray matter showed a purple homogeneous color definition (basophilic staining, Figure 2(d)). Considerable damage, involving a large portion of the ipsilateral white and gray matter, is observed in the IWOT spinal cord tissue. The border between white and gray matter disappeared; the contralateral white matter showed hypochromic staining and the gray matter has poor basophilic and eosinophilic staining features showing abnormal characteristics (Figure 2(e)). In IWT cats, the ipsilateral side of the spinal cord has basophilic staining characteristics. Also tissue hallows as well as poor

delimitation of white and gray matter were observed. In contrast, the contralateral side has preserved normal characteristics (Figure 2(f)).

3.2. Histological Analysis of White Matter Ventral Axons.

A qualitative assessment of the ventral white matter axons was made. Symmetrical axon morphology and a purple homogeneous color definition were observed in intact white matter, and there is no tissue inflammation or hollows (Figures 3(a), 3(f), and 3(k)). At the IS in the IWOT cats, axons in the ventral white matter of the ipsilateral side appeared with spheroid morphology (Figure 3(g)). In the contralateral side, a hypochromic staining with Wallerian degeneration characteristics was observed (Figure 3(i)). In IWT cats, axons appeared with a clearly defined morphology which was similar to INT cats axons at the ipsi- and contralateral side (Figures 3(h) and 3(j)). Similar normal stained characteristics were observed in CFI (Figures 3(l)–3(o)). At RFI, Wallerian degeneration was not observed in IWT or IWOT (Figures 3(b)–3(e)).

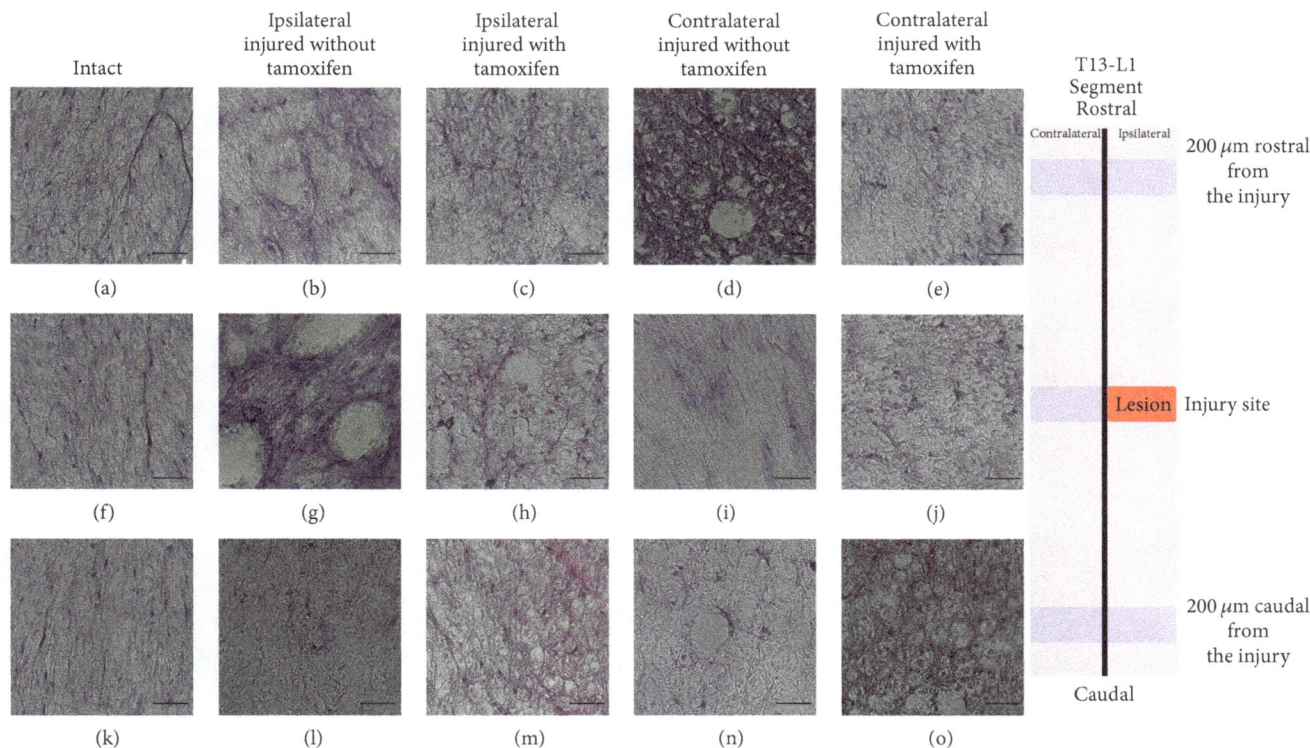

FIGURE 3: Illustrates ventral T13-L1 axons using H&E staining. ((a)–(o)) exhibits ventral axons of the white matter of the intact, injured treated with tamoxifen, and injured without tamoxifen cats in the ipsilateral and contralateral sides. ((a), (f), and (k)) Intact cat, ((b), (g), and (l)) ipsilateral side coronal cuts in an injured cat without tamoxifen, ((c), (h), and (m)) ipsilateral side coronal cuts from an injured cat treated with tamoxifen, ((d), (i), and (n)) contralateral coronal cuts obtained in an injured cat without tamoxifen, and ((e), (j), and (o)) contralateral coronal cut obtained from an injured with tamoxifen cat.

3.3. Tamoxifen Favored Ventral Axons Myelin Recovery of Injured Cats.

Myelin in INT, IWT, and IWOT ventral axons is illustrated in Figures 4(a)–4(o); intact axon myelin thickness in ventral axons was considered as 100%. Ipsilateral IS axonal myelin was reduced to $29.7 \pm 2.4\%$ in IWOT cats; in IWT cats, myelin was reduced to $64 \pm 2.0\%$ with a significant differences between groups ($p < 0.001$) (Figure 4(q)). Contralateral side myelin was reduced to $28.7 \pm 6.7\%$ in IWOT cats and to $65 \pm 11.06\%$ in IWT cats ($p < 0.001$). Similar results were obtained in the RFI and CFI regions (Figures 4(p) and 4(r), resp.). IWT and IWOT groups showed significant ipsilateral and contralateral statistical changes in the myelin percentages in comparison with INT cats. These changes occurred in IS, RFI, and CFI regions (Figures 4(p)–4(r)). Although the previously mentioned results were normalized to percentage values, real myelin thickness values are presented in the present work (Table 4).

3.4. Tamoxifen Effect on Neuronal Survival after Injury.

FOX-3/DAPI positive cells were counted for evaluating spinal cord neuronal survival in INT, IWO, and IWT cats. At 30 DAI, an increase of the neuronal survival in tamoxifen treated cats was observed, particularly in the ventral zone (Figures 5(a)–5(r)). The number of neurons in INT, IWT, and IWOT groups in ipsilateral and contralateral side at the IS, RFI, and CFI regions is plotted in Figure 6. At 30 DAI, VH neurons decreased in IS, RFI, and CFI regions on both sides in IWT and IWOT cats. The number of ipsilateral and contralateral neurons was partially recovered by tamoxifen treatment (Table 1, Figures 6(c), 6(f), and 6(i)). Spinal cord damage reduced PAZ neurons in all studied regions, in treated and untreated cats (Table 1, Figures 6(b), 6(e), and 6(h)). DH neurons quantities did not change in the IS and the CFI site, in ipsilateral or contralateral spinal cord. This partial neuronal preservation occurred in treated and untreated cats (Figures 6(d) and 6(g)). It is important to mention that DH neurons were significantly reduced in the RFI region in untreated cats but recovered in treated cats in ipsilateral and contralateral spinal cord regions (Figure 6(a)).

3.5. Tamoxifen Treatment Induces a Recovery in the Hindlimb Gait Locomotion after Injury.

Gait locomotion was evaluated in IWT and IWOT cats before and after SCI. Three consecutive ipsilateral hindlimb (IHL) and contralateral hindlimb (CHL) strides were recorded (Figure 7). In normal stepping cats, the IHL and CHL executed symmetrical steps with well-defined stance and swing phases (Figures 7(a) and 7(h)). In contrast, at 4 DAI, IHL exhibited asymmetrical steps and limb dragging in both IWT and IWOT cats (Figures 7(b) and 7(c)). At 16 DAI, we observed that IWT and IWOT cats

TABLE 1: Number of FOX-3/DAPI positive cells.

Site	Ipsilateral									Contralateral								
	INT			IWOT			IWT			INT			IWOT			IWT		
	DH	PAZ	VH	DH	PAZ	VH	DH	PAZ	VH	DH	PAZ	VH	DH	PAZ	VH	DH	PAZ	VH
	n = 18	n = 18	n = 18	n = 18	n = 18	n = 18	n = 18	n = 18	n = 18	n = 18	n = 18	n = 18	n = 18	n = 18	n = 18	n = 18	n = 18	n = 18
200 μm RFI	59 ± 1	33.8 ± 1.4	15.9 ± 0.1	34.7 ± 6.3	12.5 ± 2.1	6.3 ± 1.2	58.7 ± 8	17 ± 1.6	13.1 ± 3	58 ± 0.5	32.1 ± 1.3	15 ± 1	38.5 ± 2.3	4 ± 2.3	6.2 ± 1.5	60.4 ± 10.2	4.9 ± 2.8	11.8 ± 3.4
IS	62.3 ± 0.8	32.4 ± 1.2	15.4 ± 1.1	33.6 ± 10.5	10.3 ± 2.4	5.3 ± 1.7	48.5 ± 11.9	13.72 ± 4.4	12.8 ± 2.5	63.1 ± 1	31.4 ± 1.6	16 ± 0.8	39.9 ± 10.4	16 ± 8.4	5.5 ± 0.6	46.2 ± 12	14.9 ± 2.5	12.6 ± 3.1
200 μm CFI	58.6 ± 1.2	33.5 ± 1.1	16 ± 0.4	41.1 ± 4.4	15.5 ± 5.3	6.7 ± 0.7	50.3 ± 9.5	13.1 ± 6.1	11.7 ± 4.7	61 ± 0.6	33.1 ± 2	17 ± 1	50.1 ± 8.8	16.4 ± 4	7.2 ± 0.8	57.8 ± 5.5	13.4 ± 4.7	12.7 ± 4

INT, intact; IWOT, injured without tamoxifen; IWT, injured with tamoxifen; DH, dorsal horn; PAZ, periaqueductal zone; VH, ventral horn; RFI, rostral from injury; IS, injury site; CFI, caudal from injury.

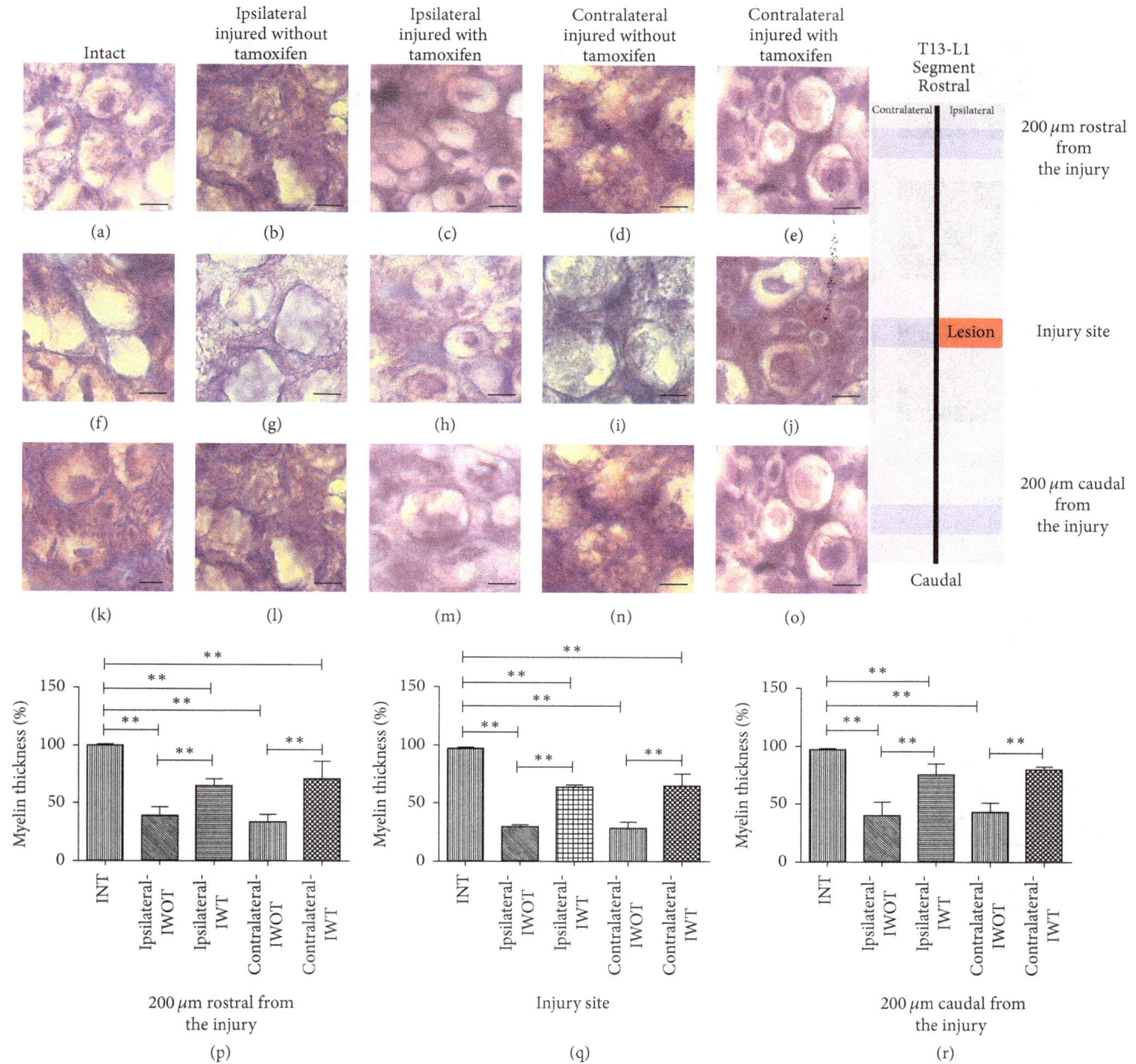

FIGURE 4: Myelin sheet of T13-L1 ventral axons is illustrated using Toluidine Blue staining. ((a), (f), and (k)) Axons in coronal cuts from an intact cat, ((b), (g), and (l)) ipsilateral axons from an injured cat without tamoxifen, ((c), (h), and (m)) ipsilateral axons from an injured cat with tamoxifen, ((d), (i), and (n)) contralateral axons in a cat without tamoxifen, and ((e), (j), and (o)) contralateral axons in a cat with tamoxifen. Graphs: ordinates exhibit the myelin thickness percentage from ventral zone axons; abscise different studied groups. (p) Myelin axon thickness valued at 200 μm rostral from the injury, (q) axon myelin thickness valued in the injury site, (r) axon myelin thickness valued 200 μm caudal from the injury situ, $^{**}p < 0.001$; scale bar: 5 μm. Schematic diagram illustrates in site the rostral and caudal zones to value myelin thickness. The black horizontal line over the bars indicates a statistical significant difference between referred groups.

partially recovered their gait locomotor movements (Figures 7(d) and 7(e)). At 30 DAI, treated and untreated cats ILH showed a normal stepping sequence, indicating complete gait locomotion recovery (Figures 7(f) and 7(g)). At 4 DAI, IWOT cats exhibited an altered stride and oscillatory-like hip movements (as a compensatory process for maintaining gait locomotion and avoiding animal downfall) (Figure 7(i)).

Stride alteration continued at 16 DAI (Figure 7(k)) and partial locomotion recovery is observed at 30 DAI (Figure 7(m)). In IWT cats, a locomotion recovery was observed at day 16 and it was clearly maintained until 30 DAI (Figures 7(l)–7(n)). The hip angular displacements in the IHL and CHL in IWT and IWOT cats are illustrated in Figure 8. Ipsilateral hip AD values in both groups of animals (IWT and IWOT

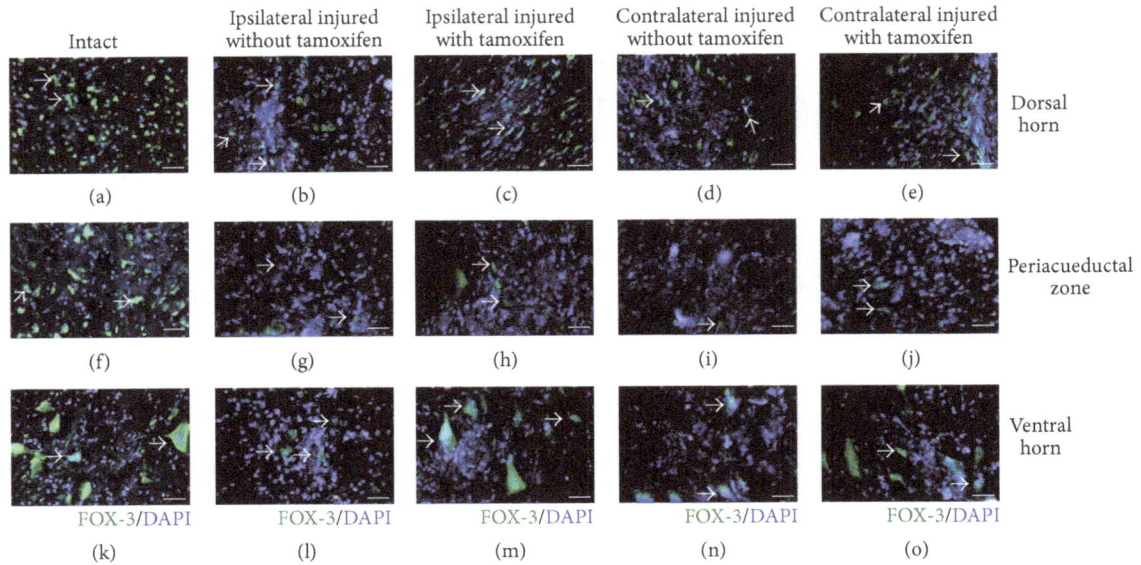

FIGURE 5: Microscopy images of FOX-3/DAPI positive cells in the dorsal horn, periaqueductal zone, and ventral horn, at T13-L1 spinal cord injury site. Dorsal horn neurons: ((b) and (c)) ipsilateral side, ((d) and (e)) contralateral side: (a) intact cat, (b) injured untreated cat, (c) injured treated cat, (d) injured untreated cat, and (e) injured treated cat. Periaqueductal Zone Neurons: ((g) and (h)) ipsilateral side and ((i) and (j)) contralateral side. (f) Intact cat, (g) injured cat without tamoxifen, (h) injured cat with tamoxifen, (i) injured cat without tamoxifen, and (j) injured cat with tamoxifen. Neurons in the ventral horn: ((l) and (m)) ipsilateral side and ((n) and (o)) contralateral side. (k) Intact cat, (l) injured cat without tamoxifen, (m) injured cat with tamoxifen, (n) injured cat without tamoxifen, and (o) injured cat with tamoxifen, scale bar 150 μm; FOX-3 neurons in green, cell nuclei in blue.

cats) decreased approximately by 40% at 4 DAI but returned to their base values at 16 and 30 DAI (Figure 8(a) and Table 2). Whereas the IWOT cat contralateral hip exhibited a significant decrement in JAD values (nearly 50%) at 4 and 16 DAI, recovery was attained at 30 DAI. In contrast, the contralateral hip of IWT cats showed a considerable increment in JAD values (nearly to 150%; Table 2) at 4 and 16 DAI and recovered their base values at 30 DAI (Tables 2 and 3, Figure 8(b)). At 4 and 16 DAI, the ipsilateral knee of IWOT cats exhibited a statistically significant decrease in JAD values, approximately 50%, whereas the knee joint of IWT cats showed an increment in JAD values of approximately 50%. Both groups (IWT and IWOT cats) returned to their base values at 30 DAI (Figure 8(c)). No significant changes were observed in the contralateral knee (Tables 2 and 3, Figure 8(d)). In hindlimb PLM, both ipsi- and contralateral HAD values recovered faster in cats treated with tamoxifen, as compared to nontreated animals. At 4 DAI, IHL angular displacement values showed a statistically significant decrease in both, IWT and IWOT groups. IWT cat's pendulum-like movement values showed partial recovery at 16 DAI and nearly a 100% recovery at 30 DAI. At 30 DAI, pendulum-like movement of IWOT cats recovered by nearly 90% (Tables 2 and 3, Figure 8(e)). At 4 and 16 DAI, IHL angular displacement values in IWOT cats increased by 50% and 20%, respectively. At 30 DAI, angular displacement values were nearly recovered to 100%. In IWT cats, no differences occurred in the contralateral PLM (Tables 2 and 3, Figure 8(f)).

4. Discussion

The penetrating injury applied in our model produced a degeneration process characterized by spheroid axons and tissue hollows occurring in ipsilateral as well as in the contralateral side of the injury. A Wallerian degenerative process seems to be occurring on both sides in accordance with previous results, reporting an axonal Wallerian degeneration after a spinal cord injury [12, 13].

Tamoxifen is SERM acting on the β-estradiol estrogen receptors (ER) [14, 15]. It has clinical therapeutic uses in human breast cancer treatment. In addition, it produces neuronal protection after brain penetrating injury [16] and reduces microglia reactivity [17]. In rats, tamoxifen reduces the inflammatory process after a spinal cord injury [8] and the neuronal death [9]. These effects could be attributed to its actions on glial and neuronal ER. Further experiments studying tamoxifen's effects on neural inflammation process, neurotrophic factors, and inflammatory interleukins would be required for comparing tamoxifen's effects in cats to those observed in rats.

Contusion impact in a cat's spinal cord produces an altered axonal morphology [18]. In our study, tamoxifen reduced spheroid axons in the ipsilateral spinal cord in IWT cats, recovering a quasi-normal morphology. The contralateral axons in the IWT group were partially preserved. This preservation could be favored by an inhibition of the glutamate excitotoxicity after the injury and also by an attenuation of inflammatory mediated damage [8, 19].

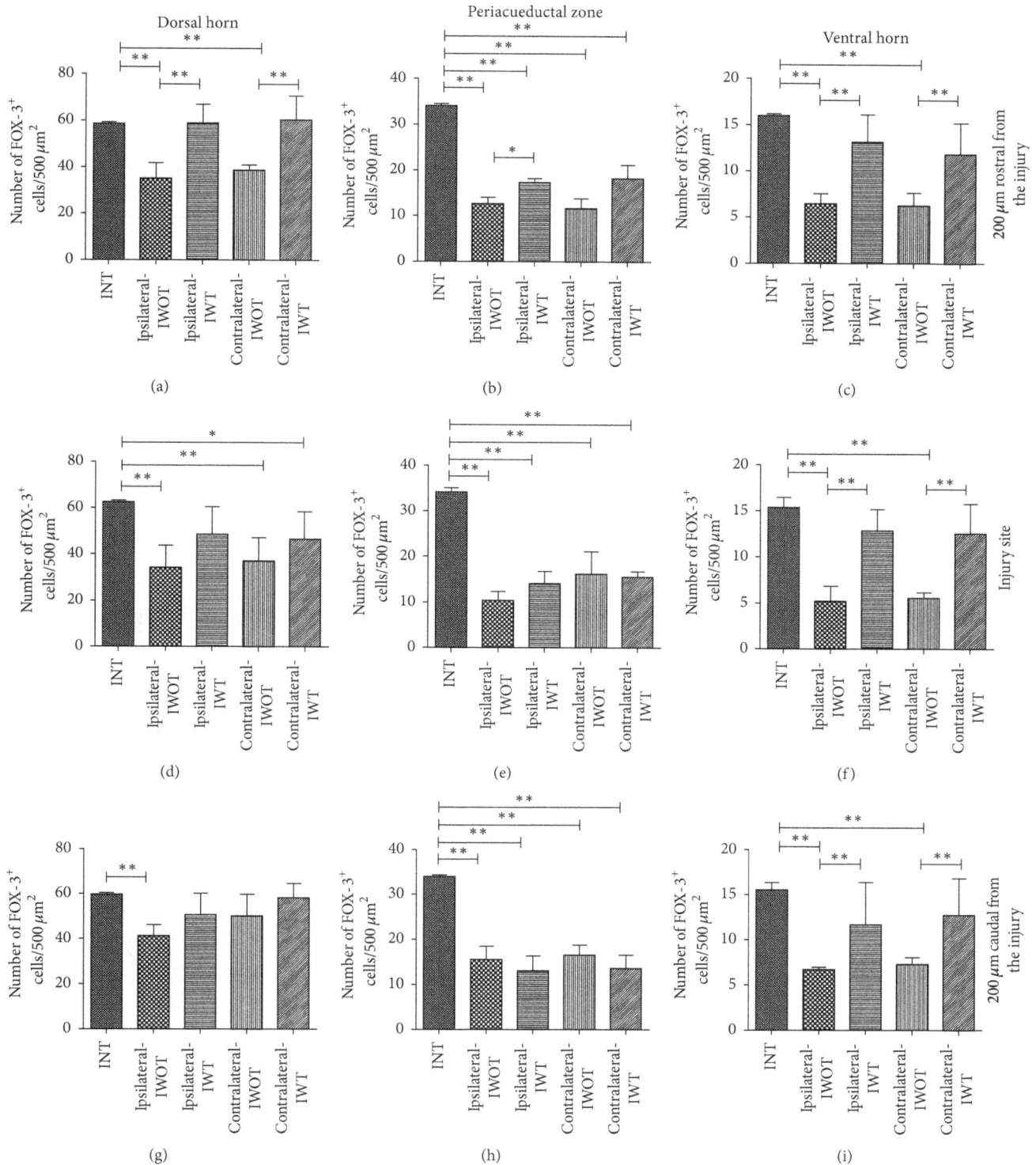

FIGURE 6: Number of counted neurons at the studied sites, graphs ordinates exhibited the number of FOX-3/DAPI positive cells and abscise different groups: intact, injured with tamoxifen, and injured without tamoxifen cats. Number of neurons 200 μm rostral from the injury site: (a) dorsal horn, (b) periaqueductal zone, and (c) ventral horn. Number of neurons in the injury site: (d) dorsal horn, (e) periaqueductal zone, and (f) ventral horn. Number of neurons counted 200 μm caudal from the injury: (g) dorsal horn, (h) periaqueductal zone, and (i) ventral horn; $^{**}p < 0.001$, $^{*}p < 0.05$. Schematic diagram illustrates rostral, injury site and caudal zones. The black horizontal line over bars indicates a statistically significant difference between referred groups.

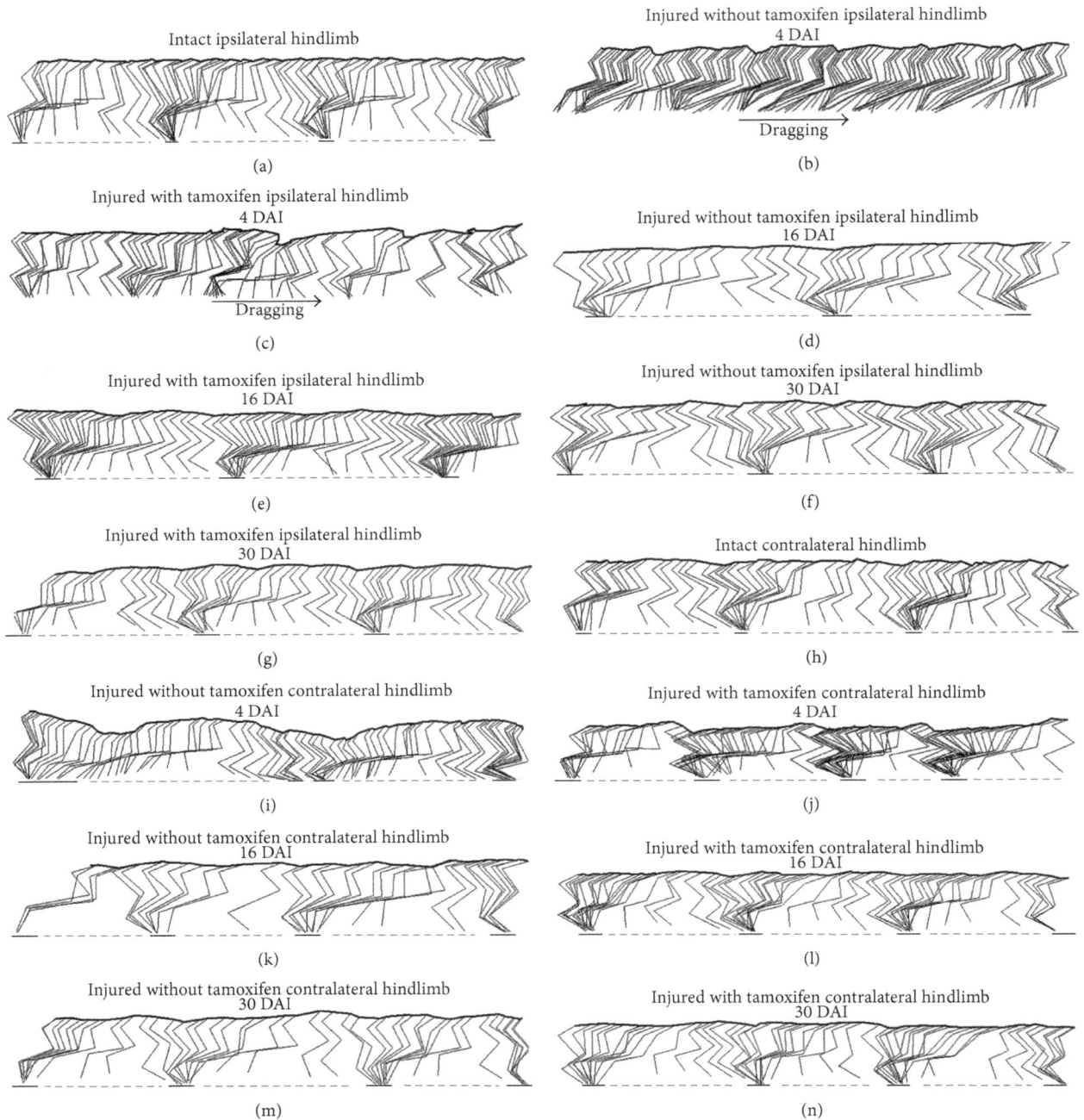

FIGURE 7: Stick figures illustrating both cat hindlimb during overground locomotion in intact and in spinal hemisected cats treated with tamoxifen. ((a)–(n)) Stick figures illustrating gait locomotion in intact cat and after 4, 16, and 30 DAI: in treated and untreated cats. (a) Ipsilateral hindlimb during locomotion in a intact cat. (b) Ipsilateral hindlimb during locomotion in an untreated cat at 4 DAI; arrow shows dragging during forward displacement. (c) Ipsilateral hindlimb locomotion in treated cat, at 4 DAI. (d) Ipsilateral hindlimb locomotion in an untreated cat, at 16 DP. (e) Ipsilateral hindlimb, in treated cat, at 16 DAI. (f) Ipsilateral hindlimb in an untreated cat at 30 DAI. (g) Ipsilateral hindlimb locomotion in treated cat, at 30 DAI. (h) Contralateral hindlimb locomotion in an intact cat. (i) Contralateral hindlimb locomotion in an untreated cat, at 4 DAI. (j) Contralateral hindlimb in treated cat, at 4 DAI. (k) Contralateral hindlimb locomotion in an untreated cat, at 16 DAI. (l) Contralateral hindlimb in treated cat, at 16 DAI. (m) Contralateral hindlimb locomotion in a untreated cat, at 30 DAI. (n) Contralateral hindlimb locomotion in treated cat, at 30 DAI.

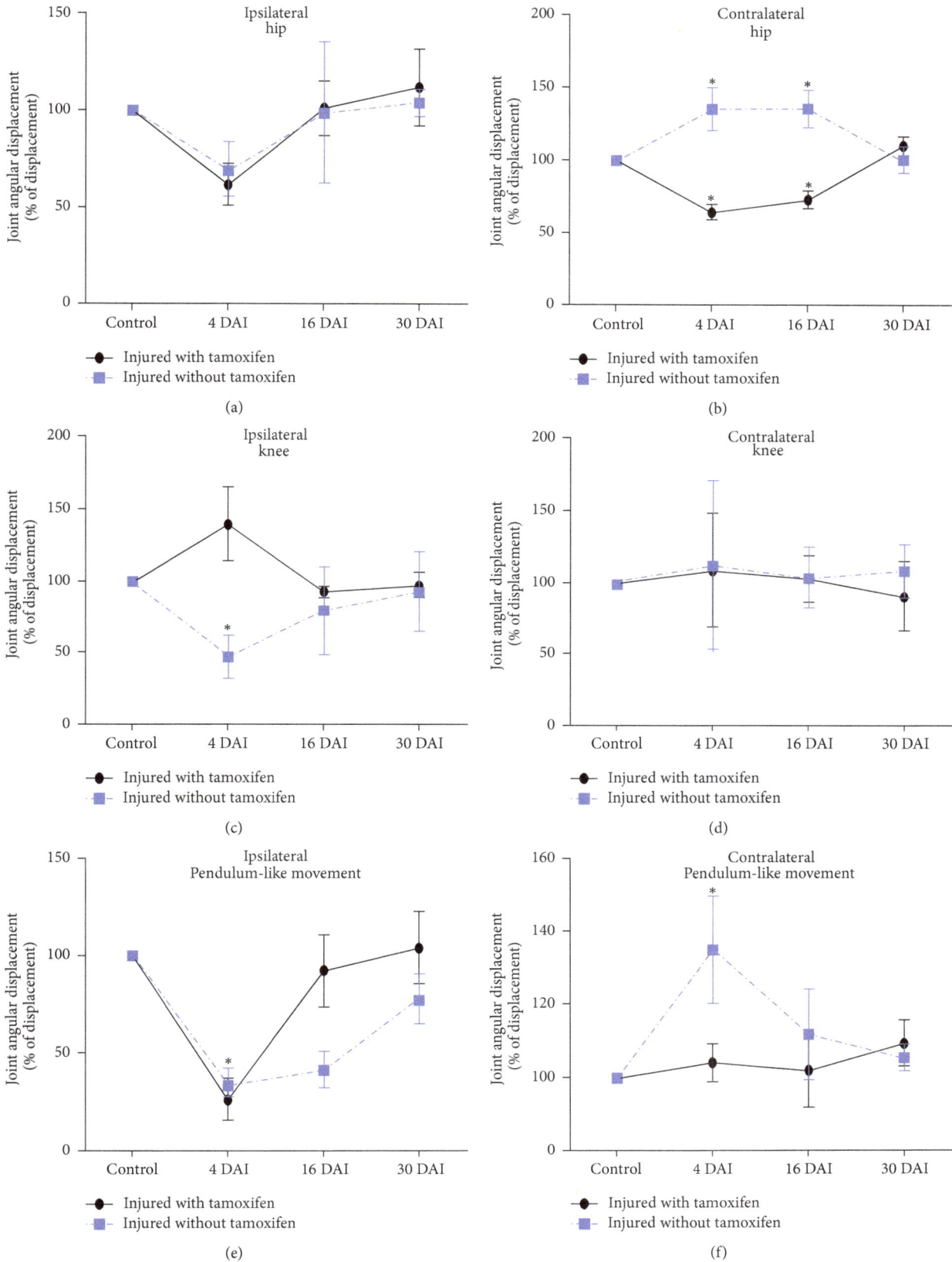

FIGURE 8: Graphs exhibit hip, knee joints, and the hindlimb pendulum-like movement angular displacement during stride. Movement changes in percent at different times (4, 16, and 30 DAI) comparing the respective angles and pendulum-like movement previous to the injury (control). ((a) and (b)) Hip angular displacement, ((c) and (d)) knee angular displacement, and ((e) and (f)) pendulum-like movement angular displacement; $^{*}p < 0.05$.

TABLE 2: Comparison of the ipsilateral hindlimb angular displacement to control during locomotion at 4, 16, and 30 DAI.

| | | IHL | | | | | | | | | | | |
| | Control | 4 DAI | | | | 16 DAI | | | | 30 DAI | | | |
Joint	INT	IWOT	p value	IWT	p value	IWOT	p value	IWT	p value	IWOT	p value	IWT	p value
Hip	100	69.8 ± 14.5	NS	62.2 ± 10.8	NS	99.0 ± 36.2	NS	101.3 ± 14	NS	104.1 ± 7.1	NS	112.1 ± 20	NS
Knee	100	46.6 ± 14.7	$^*p < 0.05$	140.3 ± 25.8	NS	80.2 ± 3.8	NS	92.6 ± 3.3	NS	92.7 ± 28	NS	98 ± 8.9	NS
Ankle	100	106.8 ± 35.8	NS	155.5 ± 47.8	$^*p < 0.05$	131.3 ± 19	NS	92.23 ± 31	NS	138.3 ± 16.1	NS	94.7 ± 22.3	NS
PLM	100	35.2 ± 7	$^*p < 0.05$	26.7 ± 10.1	$^*p < 0.05$	41.4 ± 9.6	$^*p < 0.05$	92.8 ± 18.3	NS	77.6 ± 12.8	NS	104 ± 18.9	NS

LH, ipsilateral hindlimb; NS, not significant; INT, intact; IWT, injured with tamoxifen; IWOT, injured without tamoxifen; DAI, days after injury; * denotes $p < 0.05$.

TABLE 3: Comparison of the contralateral hindlimb angular displacement to control during locomotion at 4, 16, and 30 DAI.

Joint	Control INT	4 DAI				CHL 16 DAI				30 DAI			
		IWOT	p value	IWT	p value	IWOT	p value	IWT	p value	IWOT	p value	IWT	p value
Hip	100	135.5 ± 14.2	*p < 0.5	64.09 ± 5.07	*p < 0.05	135.8 ± 12.8	*p < 0.05	73.2 ± 6.1	*p < 0.05	100.7 ± 8.6	NS	110.5 ± 6.5	NS
Knee	100	112.5 ± 59.2	NS	109.1 ± 39.9	NS	103.8 ± 21	NS	103.6 ± 16.5	NS	108.9 ± 18.8	NS	90.96 ± 24.8	NS
Ankle	100	140.7 ± 18	NS	127.3 ± 41.3	NS	149.7 ± 53.2	NS	105.6 ± 36.5	NS	180.7 ± 80.6	NS	99.3 ± 18.5	*p < 0.05
PLM	100	135.25 ± 14.8	*p < 0.05	104.23 ± 5.1	NS	112 ± 12.5	NS	102.1 ± 10.1	NS	105.7 ± 3.6	NS	109.6 ± 6.3	NS

CHL, contralateral hindlimb; NS, not significant; INT, intact; IWT, injured with tamoxifen; IWOT, injured without tamoxifen; DAI, days after injury; * denotes p < 0.05.

TABLE 4: Myelin thickness in micrometers.

	Ipsilateral						Contralateral					
	INT n = 30	IWT n = 30	IWOT n = 30	INT vs IWT	INT vs IWOT	IWOT vs IWT	INT n = 30	IWT n = 30	IWOT n = 30	INT vs IWT	INT vs IWOT	IWOT vs IWT
200 µm RFI	39 ± 11.3 µm	22 ± 5.7 µm	13.7 ± 5.8 µm	$p < 0.001$	$p < 0.001$	$p < 0.001$	38 ± 5.6 µm	23.5 ± 8 µm	10.8 ± 4 µm	$p < 0.001$	$p < 0.001$	$p < 0.001$
IS	40 ± 10.9 µm	21.8 ± 6 µm	10.5 ± 3.6 µm	$p < 0.001$	$p < 0.001$	$p < 0.001$	41 ± 6.4 µm	22.5 ± 9 µm	9 ± 4.6 µm	$p < 0.001$	$p < 0.001$	$p < 0.001$
200 µm CFI	39 ± 9.8 µm	25.8 ± 9 µm	13.7 ± 6.5 µm	$p < 0.001$	$p < 0.001$	$p < 0.001$	43 ± 2.6 µm	29 ± 8 µm	14 ± 4.2 µm	$p < 0.001$	$p < 0.001$	$p < 0.001$

INT, intact; IWOT, injured without tamoxifen; IWT, injured with tamoxifen; RFI, rostral from injury; IS, injury site; CFI, caudal from injury.

Axonal myelin and cytoskeletal proteins degenerate after a SCI [20]. Our results reveal a myelin loss in IWOT cats. In IWT animals, partial myelin preservation occurred. However, it is unknown whether myelin preservation was due to remyelination. Previous works indicate that tamoxifen promotes NG2 multipotent progenitor cell differentiation changing into oligodendrocytes and could favor remyelination after rat brain penetrating injury [7, 21]. Tamoxifen also spared mature oligodendrocytes after rat SCI favoring remyelination [2].

Rat spinal cord contusion produces deleterious effects in neurons at 24 hours [22, 23]. After one month, they were attributed to an inflammatory process. In IWOT cats, at 30 DAI, after the spinal cord injury, the number of positive FOX-3 cells was reduced on both ipsilateral and contralateral sides. In IWT cats, the number of neurons in VH and DH is similar to the number in INT cats. This result could be related to the morphological ER distribution in the thoracolumbar spinal cord, as reported in other animal species [24–26]. The number of neurons in the PAZ did not recover after treatment. This effect could be attributed to a minor amount of ER of the PAZ neurons. It has been demonstrated that estrogen receptors are poorly expressed in periaqueductal neurons and are present mostly in the ventral horn in the female cat's lumbosacral spinal cord [27]. Further experiments must be performed for evaluating the spinal cord ER distribution in male cats.

PAZ neurons are involved in locomotion alternation [28]. Therefore, important contralateral plastic changes could be contributing to a rapid locomotion recovery but not through the PAZ neurons pathway.

In this study we analyzed overground locomotion. At 16 DAI, tamoxifen recovered the hindlimbs AD in walking cats. In adult cats, spinal cord injury models had been previously described [29–31]. In these models, the locomotion recovery was related to the severity of the SCI. In the present experiments, all cats suffered a similar damage at the T13-L1 level (Figure 2). Therefore, the locomotion recovery by tamoxifen treatment was consistent because the damage of the spinal cord extension was similar in all cats. In the present experiments, the locomotion onset might depend more on the undamaged contralateral spinal cord than a step training plasticity process, given that the cats were not trained for walking.

The kinematic parameters were altered during the first 16 DAI in both hindlimbs but were partially or fully restored after 30 DAI. It is of interest that, in IWT cats, recovery to nearly normal values already occurred at 16 days; therefore tamoxifen shortened the recovery time. To the best of our knowledge, hemisected cats treated with tamoxifen and walking overground were studied for the first time. Locomotion recovery results observed in this study highlight the importance of preserving contralateral descending pathways for locomotion initiation and kinematic recuperation [32]. It would be of interest to study the effects of tamoxifen in relation to avoiding obstacles during a cat's normal walking task. A previous study sheds light on this question, in which

they assessed hemisected spinal cord cats during overground walking while avoiding obstacles in their way [33].

In addition to what was previously stated, a contusion model in rats has been used for studying tamoxifen anti-inflammatory effects, but the kinematics in injured rats under tamoxifen treatment remain to be established [5, 34].

At present time, we consider that a study must be made in which the combined treatment with tamoxifen and treadmill training to improve the outcome of hemisected animals should be carried out.

5. Conclusions

The current study demonstrates that hemisected spinal cord produces important locomotion alterations in both hindlimbs. Tamoxifen has important effects on axonal and myelin preservation, favoring cat locomotion recovery. The drug has been previously tested in the murine species with positive neuroprotective effects. This study shows beneficial outcomes in a repertory of motor patterns. Tamoxifen may be useful in several animal species as therapeutic treatment in spinal cord injury.

Conflict of Interests

The authors declare that there is no conflict of interests regarding the publication of this paper.

Acknowledgments

This work was funded by Universidad de Guadalajara; the authors thank Dr. Hugo Guerrero-Cazares for reviewing the paper and assessing them in the writing process. They would also deeply like to thank Dr. Eduardo Gerardo Mendizabal Ruiz from CUCEI, Universidad de Guadalajara, for his statistical analysis and his great cooperation towards their research group.

References

[1] R. R. Jacobs, M. A. Asher, and R. K. Snider, "Thoracolumbar spinal injuries. A comparative study of recumbent and operative treatment in 100 patients," Spine, vol. 5, no. 5, pp. 463–477, 1980.

[2] J. Guptarak, J. E. Wiktorowicz, R. G. Sadygov et al., "The cancer drug tamoxifen: a potential therapeutic treatment for spinal cord injury," Journal of Neurotrauma, vol. 31, no. 3, pp. 268–283, 2014.

[3] N. J. Tester and D. R. Howland, "Chondroitinase ABC improves basic and skilled locomotion in spinal cord injured cats," Experimental Neurology, vol. 209, no. 2, pp. 483–496, 2008.

[4] S. Rossignol, N. Giroux, C. Chau, J. Marcoux, E. Brustein, and T. A. Reader, "Pharmacological aids to locomotor training after spinal injury in the cat," Journal of Physiology, vol. 533, no. 1, pp. 65–74, 2001.

[5] V. Pertici, C. Pin-Barre, M.-S. Felix, J. Laurin, J. Brisswalter, and P. Decherchi, "A new method to assess weight-bearing distribution after central nervous system lesions in rats," Behavioural Brain Research, vol. 259, pp. 78–84, 2014.

[6] M. Martinez, H. Delivet-Mongrain, H. Leblond, and S. Rossignol, "Recovery of hindlimb locomotion after incomplete spinal

cord injury in the cat involves spontaneous compensatory changes within the spinal locomotor circuitry," *Journal of Neurophysiology*, vol. 106, no. 4, pp. 1969–1984, 2011.

[7] N. Franco Rodríguez, J. Dueñas Jiménez, B. De la Torre Valdovinos, J. López Ruiz, L. Hernández Hernández, and S. Dueñas Jiménez, "Tamoxifen favoured the rat sensorial cortex regeneration after a penetrating brain injury," *Brain Research Bulletin*, vol. 98, pp. 64–75, 2013.

[8] D.-S. Tian, J.-L. Liu, M.-J. Xie et al., "Tamoxifen attenuates inflammatory-mediated damage and improves functional outcome after spinal cord injury in rats," *Journal of Neurochemistry*, vol. 109, no. 6, pp. 1658–1667, 2009.

[9] Ö. İsmailoğlu, B. Oral, A. Görgülü, R. Sütçü, and N. Demir, "Neuroprotective effects of tamoxifen on experimental spinal cord injury in rats," *Journal of Clinical Neuroscience*, vol. 17, no. 10, pp. 1306–1310, 2010.

[10] D. Luque Contreras, I. Jiménez Estrada, D. Martínez Fong et al., "Hindlimb claudication reflects impaired nitric oxide-dependent revascularization after ischemia," *Vascular Pharmacology*, vol. 46, no. 1, pp. 10–15, 2007.

[11] K. K. Kim, R. S. Adelstein, and S. Kawamoto, "Identification of neuronal nuclei (NeuN) as Fox-3, a new member of the Fox-1 gene family of splicing factors," *The Journal of Biological Chemistry*, vol. 284, no. 45, pp. 31052–31061, 2009.

[12] J. Cohen-Adad, H. Leblond, H. Delivet-Mongrain, M. Martinez, H. Benali, and S. Rossignol, "Wallerian degeneration after spinal cord lesions in cats detected with diffusion tensor imaging," *NeuroImage*, vol. 57, no. 3, pp. 1068–1076, 2011.

[13] B. Beirowski, A. Nógrádi, E. Babetto, G. Garcia-Alias, and M. P. Coleman, "Mechanisms of axonal spheroid formation in central nervous system Wallerian degeneration," *Journal of Neuropathology & Experimental Neurology*, vol. 69, no. 5, pp. 455–472, 2010.

[14] D. F. C. Gibson, M. M. Gottardis, and V. C. Jordan, "Sensitivity and insensitivity of breast cancer to tamoxifen," *The Journal of Steroid Biochemistry and Molecular Biology*, vol. 37, no. 6, pp. 765–770, 1990.

[15] D. Lymperatou, E. Giannopoulou, A. K. Koutras, and H. P. Kalofonos, "The exposure of breast cancer cells to fulvestrant and tamoxifen modulates cell migration differently," *BioMed Research International*, vol. 2013, Article ID 147514, 14 pages, 2013.

[16] K. M. Dhandapani and D. W. Brann, "Protective effects of estrogen and selective estrogen receptor modulators in the brain," *Biology of Reproduction*, vol. 67, no. 5, pp. 1379–1385, 2002.

[17] S. Tapia-Gonzalez, P. Carrero, O. Pernia, L. M. Garcia-Segura, and Y. Diz-Chaves, "Selective oestrogen receptor (ER) modulators reduce microglia reactivity in vivo after peripheral inflammation: potential role of microglial ERs," *Journal of Endocrinology*, vol. 198, no. 1, pp. 219–230, 2008.

[18] A. R. Blight and V. Decrescito, "Morphometric analysis of experimental spinal cord injury in the cat: the relation of injury intensity to survival of myelinated axons," *Neuroscience*, vol. 19, no. 1, pp. 321–341, 1986.

[19] J.-R. Kuo, C.-C. Wang, S.-K. Huang, and S.-J. Wang, "Tamoxifen depresses glutamate release through inhibition of voltage-dependent Ca^{2+} entry and protein kinase $C\alpha$ in rat cerebral cortex nerve terminals," *Neurochemistry International*, vol. 60, no. 2, pp. 105–114, 2012.

[20] R. E. Ward, W. Huang, M. Kostusiak, P. N. Pallier, A. T. Michael-Titus, and J. V. Priestley, "A characterization of white matter pathology following spinal cord compression injury in the rat," *Neuroscience*, vol. 260, pp. 227–239, 2014.

[21] R. Nadella, M. H. Voutilainen, M. Saarma et al., "Transient transfection of human CDNF gene reduces the 6-hydroxydopamine-induced neuroinflammation in the rat substantia nigra," *Journal of Neuroinflammation*, vol. 11, no. 1, article 209, 2014.

[22] S. D. Grossman, L. J. Rosenberg, and J. R. Wrathall, "Temporal-spatial pattern of acute neuronal and glial loss after spinal cord contusion," *Experimental Neurology*, vol. 168, no. 2, pp. 273–282, 2001.

[23] S. D. Grossman, B. B. Wolfe, R. P. Yasuda, and J. R. Wrathall, "Changes in NMDA receptor subunit expression in response to contusive spinal cord injury," *Journal of Neurochemistry*, vol. 75, no. 1, pp. 174–184, 2000.

[24] H. C. Evrard and J. Balthazart, "Localization of oestrogen receptors in the sensory and motor areas of the spinal cord in Japanese quail (*Coturnix japonica*)," *Journal of Neuroendocrinology*, vol. 14, no. 11, pp. 894–903, 2002.

[25] E. Hösli and L. Hösli, "Cellular localization of estrogen receptors on neurones in various regions of cultured rat CNS: Coexistence with cholinergic and galanin receptors," *International Journal of Developmental Neuroscience*, vol. 17, no. 4, pp. 317–330, 1999.

[26] R. E. Papka, M. Storey-Workley, P. J. Shughrue et al., "Estrogen receptor-α and -β immunoreactivity and mRNA in neurons of sensory and autonomic ganglia and spinal cord," *Cell and Tissue Research*, vol. 304, no. 2, pp. 193–214, 2001.

[27] V. G. J. M. VanderHorst, E. Meijer, F. C. Schasfoort, F. W. Van Leeuwen, and G. Holstege, "Estrogen receptor-immunoreactive neurons in the lumbosacral cord projecting to the periaqueductal gray in the ovariectomized female cat," *Neuroscience Letters*, vol. 236, no. 1, pp. 25–28, 1997.

[28] S. A. Crone, K. A. Quinlan, L. Zagoraiou et al., "Genetic ablation of V2a ipsilateral interneurons disrupts left-right locomotor coordination in mammalian spinal cord," *Neuron*, vol. 60, no. 1, pp. 70–83, 2008.

[29] J. B. Campbell, V. DeCrescito, J. J. Tomasula, H. B. Demopoulos, E. S. Flamm, and J. Ransohoff, "Experimental treatment of spinal cord contusion in the cat," *Surgical Neurology*, vol. 1, no. 2, pp. 102–106, 1973.

[30] E. Brustein and S. Rossignol, "Recovery of locomotion after ventral and ventrolateral spinal lesions in the cat. I. Deficits and adaptive mechanisms," *Journal of Neurophysiology*, vol. 80, no. 3, pp. 1245–1267, 1998.

[31] E. Brustein and S. Rossignol, "Recovery of locomotion after ventral and ventrolateral spinal lesions in the cat. II. Effects of noradrenergic and serotoninergic drugs," *Journal of Neurophysiology*, vol. 81, no. 4, pp. 1513–1530, 1999.

[32] L. M. Jordan, J. Liu, P. B. Hedlund, T. Akay, and K. G. Pearson, "Descending command systems for the initiation of locomotion in mammals," *Brain Research Reviews*, vol. 57, no. 1, pp. 183–191, 2008.

[33] A. E. Doperalski, N. J. Tester, S. C. Jefferson, and D. R. Howland, "Altered obstacle negotiation after low thoracic hemisection in the cat," *Journal of Neurotrauma*, vol. 28, no. 9, pp. 1983–1993, 2011.

[34] C. Hurd, N. Weishaupt, and K. Fouad, "Anatomical correlates of recovery in single pellet reaching in spinal cord injured rats," *Experimental Neurology*, vol. 247, pp. 605–614, 2013.

22

Prevalence of Subclinical Mastitis and Distribution of Pathogens in Dairy Farms of Rubavu and Nyabihu Districts, Rwanda

J. P. Mpatswenumugabo,[1,2] L. C. Bebora,[2] G. C. Gitao,[2] V. A. Mobegi,[3] B. Iraguha,[4]
O. Kamana,[5] and B. Shumbusho[1]

[1]*Department of Veterinary Medicine, University of Rwanda, P.O. Box 210, Musanze, Rwanda*
[2]*Department of Veterinary Pathology, Microbiology and Parasitology, University of Nairobi, P.O. Box 29053-00625, Kangemi, Kenya*
[3]*Department of Biochemistry, University of Nairobi, P.O. Box 30197, Nairobi, Kenya*
[4]*Rwanda Dairy Competitiveness Program II, P.O. Box 569, Kigali, Rwanda*
[5]*Department of Food Safety and Food Quality Management, University of Rwanda, P.O. Box 210, Musanze, Rwanda*

Correspondence should be addressed to J. P. Mpatswenumugabo; mugajpierre@yahoo.fr

Academic Editor: Nora Mestorino

A cross-sectional study was conducted from May 2016 to January 2017 in Rubavu and Nyabihu districts, Western Rwanda, aiming at estimating the prevalence of subclinical mastitis (SCM) and identifying its causative bacteria. Management practices and milking procedures were recorded through a questionnaire. 123 crossbreed milking cows from 13 dairy farms were randomly selected and screened for SCM using California Mastitis Test (CMT). Composite CMT positive milk samples were processed for bacterial isolation and identification. The overall SCM prevalence at cow level was 50.4%. 68 bacterial isolates were identified by morphological and biochemical characteristics. They included, Coagulase Negative Staphylococci (51.5%), *Staphylococcus aureus* (20.6%), *Streptococcus* species (10.3%), *Bacillus* species (10.3%), *Streptococcus agalactiae* (5.8%), and *Escherichia coli* (1.5%). About 67.1% of the farmers checked for mastitis; of these, 58.9% relied on clinical signs and only 6.8% screened with CMT. Only 5.5% and 2.7% of the farmers tried to control mastitis using dry cow therapy and teat dips, respectively. Thus, to reduce the prevalence of SCM, farmers in the study area need to be trained on good milking practices, including regular use of teat dips, application of dry cow therapy, and SCM screening. This will improve their sales and their financial status.

1. Introduction

Mastitis is defined as inflammation of mammary gland. It is divided into two types: clinical and subclinical. Clinical mastitis (CM) is characterized by visible changes in milk (e.g., clots, color changes or consistence, and decreased production) that may be associated with inflammation signs of the udder (e.g., redness, swelling, heat, or pain) or the cow (e.g., dehydration, hyperthermia, and lethargy) [1]. SCM is asymptomatic; therefore, produced milk appears to be normal. On the other hand, according to the course of the disease and the severity of the inflammatory response, mastitis may be classified as peracute, acute, subacute, and chronic [2].

According to [3], mastitis is the major disease that affects the dairy subsector. Different studies have shown mastitis to be one of the most costly diseases of the dairy industry worldwide [4, 5]. Several economic losses result due to mastitis such as reduction of milk yields, milk discards due to bacterial or antibiotic contamination, veterinary intervention costs, and occasionally deaths [6].

While it is easy to detect CM (seeing clotted milk), SCM can only be demonstrated using various tests such as California Mastitis Test (CMT), Whiteside test (WST), Surf field mastitis test (SFMT), sodium lauryl sulphate test (SLST), Microscopic Somatic Cell Count (MSCC) [7, 8], and Electrical Conductivity (EC) [9]. Enzymatic analyses such as colourimetric and fluorometric assays have also been developed [10]. New advanced techniques such proteomics have been recently developed and used in detection of proteins involved in mastitis [11–13]. Most of these tests are preferred as screening tests indicating SCM since they are easy to use and yield rapid as well as satisfactory results. However, CMT has been recognized as a highly sensitive test to detect bovine subclinical mastitis [14, 15]. It has been reported by [8] that the sensitivity of the CMT was 86.1 while specificity was 59.7% with percentage accuracy of 75.5%. In a similar study, [14] found that sensitivity for the Modified California Mastitis Test (MCMT) was 95.2% while its specificity was 98.0%. In order to identify mastitis causing microorganisms, the microbiological culture procedures still are the gold standard [10].

Different studies have shown that SCM is mainly caused by Coagulase Negative Staphylococci (CNS), *Staphylococcus aureus (S. aureus)*, *Streptococcus agalactiae (Str. agalactiae)*, other *Streptococcus* species, and coliforms [9, 16].

So far, the prevalence of SCM and causative bacteria in lactating cows of Rubavu and Nyabihu district in Rwanda is not known. Therefore, this study was conducted to determine the prevalence of subclinical mastitis as well as isolate and identify the bacterial agents associated with SCM in lactating cows in these two districts and to assess possible association with SCM within the two production systems (extensive and intensive). Milking procedures and management practices that influence the prevalence of mastitis in the study area were also evaluated.

2. Materials and Methods

2.1. Study Area. The current study was carried out in Rubavu and Nyabihu districts which are located in the Western Province of Rwanda (−1°40′52.54″S, 29°19′45.55″E and −1°39′9.90″S, 29°30′24.62″E, resp.). They are 152 km far from Kigali, the capital city of Rwanda, and are boarded by Democratic Republic of Congo (DRC) through Virunga National Park (VNP) and Lake Kivu. The altitude varies from 1830 to 2437 m in Rubavu and Nyabihu, respectively.

Rubavu district has an average annual temperature of 18.1°C with an average annual rainfall of 1,377 mm whereas Nyabihu district has average annual temperature of 15°C and rainfall reaching 1,400 mm per year. Their main types of soils can be grouped into three categories: volcanic soils, lateritic and humus-bearing soils, and clayey soils.

Rubavu and Nyabihu districts are characterised by two dry seasons as well as two rainy seasons: the long dry one stretches from June to mid-September and the short one from January to mid-March; the long rainy season stretches from March till the end of May and the short rainy season from September to December. Heaviest rains fall in April and May, whereas moderate rains fall in October and November.

2.2. Sample Size and Sampling Method. The study was carried out on 123 lactating crossbreed (Friesian versus Ankole and Jersey versus Ankole) cows, 61 from intensive system and 62 from extensive system randomly selected from 13 smallholder dairy farmers, 6 in Rubavu and 7 in Nyabihu. The sample size was determined by using the formula stated by [17]. The basis for sampling was the production system (extensive or intensive) practiced by dairy farmers in the study area. Extensive system was defined as production system where livestock are left to wander and graze during the day and are enclosed during the night whereas intensive system was defined as a production system where cows are kept in zero grazing, being served with grass, supplements, and water, and spend the night in kraal. During farm visits, a structured questionnaire was used to collect information at herd and animal levels regarding herd size, milk production, record keeping, milking practices, mastitis screening, and control measures. Observational assessment was also made on the hygiene of animals as well as cow sheds.

2.3. California Mastitis Test and Detection of SCM. Prior to milk collection for mastitis screening, clinical examination was performed on the every lactating cow. Thorough palpation of the udder to detect any fibrosis, swelling, and other clinical signs was performed. Watery milk, milk with pus or clots, and blind quarters were also examined. Identification of at least one of these signs was enough to consider the mammary quarter as positive to CM and was excluded from the study [16].

Subclinical mastitis prevalence was obtained by the use of California Mastitis Test (CMT) which was conducted using scores from 0 to 4 from the modified Scandinavian scoring system, where 0 is negative result (no gel formation), 1 is traceable (possible infection), and 2 or 3 indicates a positive result and 4 has the thickest gel formation. A sample was defined as positive to SCM when one or more quarters with CMT ≥ 2+ were detected [18].

Milk samples were collected from all four quarters and individually analysed with CMT to detect SCM, as previously described [16]. After confirming SCM by CMT, the udder and teats were cleaned with water and wiped using sterile towels. The teat orifice and the skin around the teat were sprayed with 70% alcohol and dried off with sterile towels.

2.4. Processing of Milk Samples and Bacteriological Assays. The samples were taken shortly prior to milking and only cows expressing no clinical signs of mastitis were sampled. Composite milk samples from CMT positive cows (all cows whose composite milk tested positive to CMT) were aseptically collected directly from quarters into aseptic tubes and taken to the laboratory for bacteriological analysis to identify SCM causative microorganisms [19].

Milk samples were bacteriologically examined according to the procedure previously described [20]. After reaching the laboratory (1-2 hours), milk samples were aseptically removed from the cooler box for examination. Composite CMT positive milk samples were inoculated separately onto MacConkey agar and Blood agar plates by streaking method. Inoculated plates were then incubated aerobically at 37°C for 24–48 hours. After 24 hours, primary bacteriological identification was made based on colony morphology, color, and haemolytic characteristics; these were considered as pure or individual cultures. After primary culture readings, pure cultures were prepared through subculturing and incubation. The purified isolates were then subjected to Gram staining and further biochemical testing. Staphylococci were identified based on catalase test and tube coagulase test. Streptococci were identified based on catalase and Christie, Atkins, and Munch-Peterson (CAMP) test. Gram negative

TABLE 1: Characterization of respondents and herds per production system in the study area.

Parameter	Intensive ($n = 10$)		Extensive ($n = 63$)		Total percentage
	Number of responses	Percentage	Number of responses	Percentage	
Sex					
Male	10	13.7%	60	82.2%	**95.9%**
Female	0	0.0%	3	4.1%	**4.1%**
Age					
[21–30]	0	0.0%	1	1.4%	**1.4%**
[31–40]	3	4.1%	6	8.2%	**12.3%**
[41–50]	2	2.7%	23	31.5%	**34.2%**
>50	5	6.8%	33	45.2%	**52.1%**
Education level					
Informal	1	1.4%	10	13.7%	**15.1%**
Primary	5	6.8%	46	63.0%	**69.9%**
Secondary	1	1.4%	4	5.5%	**6.8%**
University	3	4.1%	3	4.1%	**8.2%**
Cattle breed					
Cross breeds	10	13.7%	63	86.3%	**100.0%**
Herd size (mean)	30	—	21	—	—
Lactating cows (mean)	14	—	10	—	—
Milk production (mean L/day)	110	—	53	—	—
Milking frequency/day					
Once	0	0.0%	0	0.0%	**0.0%**
Twice	10	13.7%	63	86.3%	**100.0%**

isolates were identified based on growth characteristics on MacConkey agar and reactions to strip oxidase test, catalase test, Triple Sugar Iron (TSI) agar, and the "IMViC" tests (Indole, Methyl-Red, Vogas Proskaur and Citrate utilisation) [16]. Composite CMT results, culture, Gram stain, and readings of biochemical tests were encoded in excel spreadsheet to determine the prevalence of SCM and related causative bacteria. Milk samples were collected during the rainy season.

2.5. Descriptive Statistics. Information regarding respondents' particulars (age, sex, and level of education), herd characteristics, management practices, and milking procedures were encoded into excel spreadsheet for descriptive analysis. Correlations between production systems and prevalence of SCM were computed by Statistical Package for Social Sciences (SPSS).

3. Results

Respondent's identification and herds characteristics were presented (Table 1). 100% of the studied animals were crossbreed of Friesian and Ankole (local cattle) while milk production per day doubled in intensive system compared to extensive system. On the other hand, following our field observations, it was noticed that milking practices and procedures are inadequate in the study area (Table 2). Management practices employed by farmers in the study area were reported (Table 2). Among 67.1% of dairy farmers who screen for

mastitis only 6.8% use CMT while 58.9% observe appearance of clinical signs. Out of 84.9% who control mastitis and 2.7% use teat dips, 65.8% treat clinical mastitis cases while 5.5% apply dry cow therapy. 100% of all farmers in the study area milk their cows by hands (Table 2) while 89% of dairy farmers milk their cows in open space.

The overall SCM prevalence at cow level was 50.4% (62/123) (Table 3), prevalence being higher in Rubavu district (intensive system) 61.3% (38/61) than in Nyabihu district (extensive system) 38.7% (24/62). However, the differences between these two farming systems were not statistically significant ($P = 0.087$, CI = 95%) (Table 3).

From a total of 62 composite SCM positive samples cultured, 68 bacterial isolates were identified (Table 4); 6 samples contained more than one organism which were *S. aureus* and CNS while the other 56 samples were associated with single infection. In this study, the most predominant bacteria were CNS at 51.5% (35/68) followed by *S. aureus* at 20.6% (14/68), other *Streptococcus* species at 10.3% (7/68), Bacillus spp. at 10.3% (7/68), and *Str. agalactiae* at 5.8% (4/68) and the least was *Escherichia coli* (*E. coli*) at 1.5% (1/68) (Table 4).

4. Discussion

The results from this study show a high prevalence of SCM. A possible explanation for this finding could be that most farmers in the study area do not practice proper farming management and screen for mastitis at earlier stage. Results

TABLE 2: Management practices routines employed by dairy farmers in the study area.

Management practice	Intensive ($n = 10$)		Extensive ($n = 63$)		Total percentage
	Number of responses	Percentage	Number of responses	Percentage	
Mastitis screening					
Yes	6	8.2%	43	58.9%	67.1%
No	4	5.5%	20	27.4%	32.9%
If yes, how?					
CMT	3	4.1%	2	2.7%	6.8%
Strip cup	0	0.0%	1	1.4%	1.4%
Clinical signs	3	4.1%	40	54.8%	58.9%
If no, why?					
Lack of knowledge	3	4.1%	17	23.3%	27.4%
Lack of screening materials	1	1.4%	1	1.4%	2.7%
No mastitis cases	0	0.0%	2	2.7%	2.7%
Mastitis control					
Yes	10	13.7%	52	71.2%	84.9%
No	0	0.0%	11	15.1%	15.1%
If yes, how?					
Cow hygiene	1	1.4%	7	9.6%	11.0%
Dry cow therapy	0	0.0%	4	5.5%	5.5%
Use of teat dips	2	2.7%	0	0.0%	2.7%
Treatment of clinical cases	7	9.6%	41	56.2%	65.8%
If no, why?					
Lack of knowledge	0	0.0%	11	15.1%	15.1%
Milking technique					
Hand milking	10	13.7%	63	86.3%	100.0%
Milking machine	0	0.0%	0	0.0%	0.0%
Milking place					
Open space	2	2.7%	63	86.3%	89.0%
Milking from stanchion/tie stalls	8	11.0%	0	0.0%	11.0%

TABLE 3: Subclinical mastitis prevalence in relation to production system.

Area (district)	Production system	Number of tested cows	Number of CMT mastitis positive	Number of CMT mastitis negative	% mastitis positive	Pvalue
Rubavu	Intensive	61	38	23	61.3	0.087
Nyabihu	Extensive	62	24	38	38.7	
Total		**123**	**62**	**61**		
Overall prevalence					**50.4%**	

from the survey have revealed that only 6.8% screen for SCM using CMT, 58.9% only observe appearance of clinical signs which is difficult in SCM, and 32.9% do not screen for mastitis. This could also be supported by the fact that 97.3% of farmers in the study area do not practice teat dipping.

The current findings corroborate with those reported in recent studies and in the same country (51.8%) [21] using electrical conductivity and in Tanzania (51.6%) [22, 23], in Ethiopia, all have used CMT to screen for SCM at cow level. It was also similar to those reported from other countries: 49.5%, 51.8%, and 52.4% in South Wales in Australia [24], in Bangladesh [25], and in Uruguay [26], respectively, all

using CMT. However, this reported that SCM prevalence was lower than those reported in recent studies in East Africa; 86.2%, 64% and 59.2% in Uganda [27], in Kenya [28], and [23] in Ethiopia, respectively, and elsewhere, 88.6%, by [29] in Vietnam all have used CMT to screen for SCM at cow level. These differences should be due to different screening methods used. For instance, [29] used SCC determinations with or without positive isolation of pathogens to determine SCM while CMT was used in the current study. It has also been noted that the high prevalence recorded in Kenya [28] was attributed to the breed; 62.8% of the studied animals were Friesian and Jersey. However, in the current study, all

TABLE 4: Prevalence of bacterial agents isolated from CMT subclinical mastitis positive.

Number of samples for bacteriological culture	Bacterial isolates	Number of isolates	Prevalence
62	*S. aureus*	14	20.6%
	CNS	35	51.5%
	Bacillus spp.	7	10.3%
	Str. agalactiae	4	5.8%
	Other streptococci	7	10.3%
	E. coli	1	1.5%

cows were crossbreeds which are less prone to mastitis than exotic breeds [30]. In contrast, the prevalence reported in the current study was higher than 34.1% reported by [31] in Njoro District of Kenya, 41.0% by [32] in Ethiopia, 42.5% by [33] in Iran, 28.5% by [34] in Bangladesh, all of which used CMT test. These difference should be supported by farming systems and management practices and cow breeds. The authors of [31] in Kenya has screened for SCM on cows reared in paddocks where animals are grazed on the green pasture. This is also supported by [35] in UK who found that grass-based herds were less exposed to environmental bacteria, hence less prevalence of subclinical mastitis. On the other hand, the authors of [34], using CMT, have found a low SCM prevalence because 74% of their study animals were local breeds (zebu) which are less prone to mastitis [30].

According to [36], mastitis prevalence of 40 % or higher in a farm must sound alarming to the producer; hence, this study reveals how serious mastitis is the problem in the dairy industry sector of Rwanda; it requires attention. Pre- and postmilking teat disinfection have been recommended as important procedures to prevent prevalence and incidence of mastitis [37]; however, it is not practised in any of the farms in the current study.

The distribution of CNS as the most predominant bacteria isolated from the CMT positive samples, followed by S. aureus and Streptococcus species in this study, is confirmed by [38]. In a similar way, [39] found the CNS, coagulase positive staphylococci (CPS; S. aureus), the environmental streptococci, and coliforms as the prevalent mastitis pathogens associated with SCM in lactating cows. The predominance of CNS in SCM in this study is also in line with the findings of [40] in Czech Republic, [27, 41] in Uganda, and [42] in Canada. The high predominance of CNS in the current study areas can be explained by poor milking hygienic practices in the farms, coupled by nonuse of teat dips and lack of routine mastitis screening tests; these provide an opportunity for the CNS to invade the udder and develop into an intramammary infection. It is also stated that staphylococcal mastitis is the most common form of contagious mastitis and these organisms are spread from infected to clean cows on hands or equipment from one udder to another [43].

CNS are considered to be teat skin opportunists that normally reside on the teat skin and cause mastitis via ascending infection through the teat canal [44]. However, recent reports suggest that CNS have become the most common bovine mastitis isolates in many countries and could therefore be described as emerging mastitis pathogens [45–47].

The prevalence rate of S. aureus (20.6%) in the current study agrees with previous findings by authors of [30, 38, 39] who reported S. aureus to be the most predominant bacterial isolate in their studies. Being a contagious pathogen [48], S. aureus prevalence rate could be associated with poor milking hygiene and lack of teat dipping in the current study. It has been reported that S. aureus has adaptive mechanisms that allow it to be shed on the udder and cause intramammary infections during milking processes [49]. In some studies, S. aureus are the second most prevalent pathogens, while in other studies the environmental mastitis pathogens are more prevalent [1]. As reported by [21] in Eastern Rwanda, coliform bacteria were mostly isolated from SCM positive milk samples. It should, however, be noted that Iraguha's study was carried out during dry season (where there was contamination by soil and fecal matter) whereas the current study was conducted during the short rainy season.

Although environmental streptococci (10.3%) were ranked third followed by Str. agalactiae (5.8%) in the current study, [29] in Vietnam reported S. agalactiae as the most predominantly (21%) isolated bacteria. Similar findings have been reported by [9] who found that Streptococci spp. ranked the second among all isolates from subclinical mastitis with a rate of 26.3%. These findings are also in line with these reported by [50] in Uganda, who found S. agalactiae at 8.4% in SCM. S. agalactiae has been associated with SCM and it can also cause CM [9].

Although Bacillus spp. have been reported to be an uncommon cause of mastitis in cattle [51] and affected animals express acute to gangrenous form of mastitis [52], this species has been reported in the current study at a slightly high rate. This could be explained by the poor hygienic conditions of milkers in the study area. It has been found that Bacillus spp. are widely distributed in nature and most species exist in soil, in water, in dust, in air, in feces, and on vegetation [53]. Therefore, Bacillus spp. should be considered as a cause of intramammary infection in a cow with high SCC or clinical signs of udder disease; otherwise, the presence of few Bacillus spp. colonies on blood agar would be expressed as contamination [53].

The findings of the current study have shown a low prevalence of E. coli, though the study was conducted during the rainy season, case which should depict the opposite findings as coliforms being environmental bacteria associated with wet and muddy conditions [54]. However, the same authors have reported coliform bacteria to be of more importance in CM than subclinical mastitis, despite the environmental factors. This confirms that the prevalence of coliform bacteria in this study would be low, as the selection criteria identified cows with SCM as opposed to CM. On the other hand, coliforms have been confirmed to commonly be involved in CM characterized by a rapid onset associated with acute and peracute forms [16], of short duration [55], and rarely cause SCM [50]. These findings corroborate with those reported in Tanzania, whereby [56] found that SCM was associated with coliforms at 4.1%. However, it has been found that chronic and subclinical infections occur and recurring infections with *E. coli* may be more common than previously thought [57] and could also be associated with immune-depressed animals [58].

The poor management and udder health practices, inadequate milking procedures observed by the farmers and milkers, would expose the cows to SCM caused by environmental and contagious bacteria during milking by miller's hands, as was mostly found in this study. On the other hand, nonuse of teat dips and other mastitis control techniques due to lack of knowledge should have greatly contributed to the high prevalence of SCM in the study area. Farmers in the study area, therefore, need to be educated and encouraged to practice good farming, animal health management practices, and milking practices at all times; this will reduce udder contamination and subsequent SCM or CM. Adequate proper housing with sanitation, regular screening for early detection, and appropriate treatment of subclinical cases, dry cow therapy, and application of pre- and postdipping practices are also highly recommended.

Conflicts of Interest

The authors declare that they have no financial or personal relationships which may have inappropriately influenced them in writing this article.

Authors' Contributions

J. P. Mpatswenumugabo (University of Rwanda and University of Nairobi) contributed to the conceptualization of the work, data collection, laboratory analysis to identify SCM causative bacteria, and article writing. L. C. Bebora (University of Nairobi) contributed to data analysis and critically revised the manuscript. G. C. Gitao (University of Nairobi), O. Kamana (University of Rwanda), and V. A. Mobegi (University of Nairobi) contributed to manuscript review. B. Iraguha (Rwanda Dairy Competitiveness Program II) contributed to article drafting and review. B. Shumbusho (University of Rwanda) contributed to data collection and laboratory analysis.

Acknowledgments

This material is based upon work supported by the United States Agency for International Development, as part of the Feed the Future initiative, under the CGIAR Fund, Award no. BFS-G-11-00002, and the predecessor fund of the Food Security and Crisis Mitigation II grant, Award no. EEM-G-00-04-00013. The authors thank the University of Rwanda for laboratory provision and host institution, University of Nairobi. They also sincerely thank the Rubavu and Nyabihu district farmers who offered their time to work with them in conducting this research.

References

[1] L. K. Fox, "Prevalence, incidence and risk factors of heifer mastitis," *Veterinary Microbiology*, vol. 134, no. 1-2, pp. 82–88, 2009.

[2] Mastitis Clinical Syndromes, http://ansci.illinois.edu/static/ansc438/Mastitis/syndromes.html.

[3] P. Chatikobo, "Mastitis control for quality milk," *Dairy Mail Africa*, vol. 5, no. 1, pp. 1–8, 2010.

[4] D. Biffa, E. Debela, and F. Beyene, "Prevalence and risk factors of mastitis in lactating dairy cows in Southern Ethiopia," *International Journal of Applied Research and Veterinary Medicine*, vol. 3, no. 3, pp. 189–198, 2005.

[5] M. A. Kossaibati and R. J. Esslemont, "The costs of production diseases in dairy herds in England," *The Veterinary Journal*, vol. 154, no. 1, pp. 41–51, 1997.

[6] M. Vaarst and C. Enevoldsen, "Patterns of clinical mastitis manifestations in Danish organic dairy herds," *Journal of Dairy Research*, vol. 64, no. 1, pp. 23–37, 1997.

[7] M. N. Hoque, Z. C. Das, A. K. Talukder, M. S. Alam, and A. N. M. A. Rahman, "Different screening tests and milk somatic cell count for the prevalence of subclinical bovine mastitis in Bangladesh," *Tropical Animal Health and Production*, vol. 47, no. 1, pp. 79–86, 2014.

[8] N. Sharma, V. Pandey, and N. A. Sudhan, "Comparison of some indirect screening tests for detection of subclinical mastitis in dairy cows," *Bulgarian Journal of Veterinary Medicine*, vol. 13, no. 2, pp. 98–103, 2010.

[9] R. Hegde, S. Isloor, K. N. Prabhu et al., "Incidence of subclinical mastitis and prevalence of major mastitis pathogens in organized farms and unorganized sectors," *Indian Journal of Microbiology*, vol. 53, no. 3, pp. 315–320, 2013.

[10] C. Viguier, S. Arora, N. Gilmartin, K. Welbeck, and R. O'Kennedy, "Mastitis detection: current trends and future perspectives," *Trends in Biotechnology*, vol. 27, no. 8, pp. 486–493, 2009.

[11] J. D. Lippolis and T. A. Reinhardt, "Proteomic survey of bovine neutrophils," *Veterinary Immunology and Immunopathology*, vol. 103, no. 1-2, pp. 53–65, 2005.

[12] W. B. Van Leeuwen, D. C. Melles, A. Alaidan et al., "Host- and tissue-specific pathogenic traits of Staphylococcus aureus," *Journal of Bacteriology*, vol. 187, no. 13, pp. 4584–4591, 2005.

[13] G. Smolenski, S. Haines, F. Y.-S. Kwan et al., "Characterisation of host defence proteins in milk using a proteomic approach," *Journal of Proteome Research*, vol. 6, no. 1, pp. 207–215, 2007.

[14] S. Joshi and S. Gokhale, "Status of mastitis as an emerging disease in improved and periurban dairy farms in India," *Annals of the New York Academy of Sciences*, vol. 1081, pp. 74–83, 2006.

[15] N. A. Madut, A. Elamin, A. Gadir, I. Mohamed, and E. Jalii, "Host determinants of bovine mastitis in semi-intensive production system of Khartoum state, Sudan," *Journal of Cell and Animal Biology*, vol. 3, no. 5, 2009.

[16] P. J. Quinn, B. K. Markey, F. C. Leonard, E. S. Fitzpatrick, S. Fanning, and P. J. Hartigan, *Veterinary Microbiology and Microbial Disease*, Blackwell Science Ltd, 2011.

[17] I. Dohoo, W. Martin, and H. Stryhn, *Veterinary Epidemilogic Research*, Atlantic Veterinary College, University of Prince Edward Island, Charlottetown, Canada, 2003.

[18] Y. H. Schukken, D. J. Wilson, F. Welcome, L. Garrison-Tikofsky, and R. N. Gonzalez, "Monitoring udder health and milk quality using somatic cell counts," *Veterinary Research*, vol. 34, no. 5, pp. 579–596, 2003.

[19] O. Klastrup, "Scandinavian recommendations on examination of quarter milk samples," in *Proceedings of the IDF Seminar on Mastitis Control*, F. H. Dodd, Ed., vol. 85, pp. 49–52, International Dairy Federation, 1975.

[20] B. Markey, F. C. Leonard, M. Archambault, A. Cullinane, and D. Maguire, *Clinical Veterinary Microbiology*, 2nd edition, 2013.

[21] B. Iraguha, H. Hamudikuwanda, and B. Mushonga, "Bovine mastitis prevalence and associated risk factors in dairy cows in Nyagatare District, Rwanda," *Journal of the South African Veterinary Association*, vol. 86, no. 1, 6 pages, 2015.

[22] R. H. Mdegela, R. Ryoba, E. D. Karimuribo et al., "Prevalence of clinical and subclinical mastitis and quality of milk on smallholder dairy farms in Tanzania," *Journal of the South African Veterinary Association*, vol. 80, no. 3, pp. 163–168, 2009.

[23] R. Abebe, H. Hatiya, M. Abera, B. Megersa, and K. Asmare, "Bovine mastitis: prevalence, risk factors and isolation of Staphylococcus aureus in dairy herds at Hawassa milk shed, South Ethiopia," *BMC Veterinary Research*, vol. 12, no. 1, article 270, 11 pages, 2016.

[24] K. Plozza, J. J. Lievaart, G. Potts, and H. W. Barkema, "Subclinical mastitis and associated risk factors on dairy farms in New South Wales," *Australian Veterinary Journal*, vol. 89, no. 1-2, pp. 41–46, 2011.

[25] T. K. Tripura, S. C. Sarker, S. K. Roy et al., "Prevalence of subclinical mastitis in lactating cows and efficacy of intramammary infusion therapy," *Bangladesh Journal of Veterinary Medicine*, vol. 12, no. 1, pp. 55–61, 2014.

[26] R. Gianneechini, C. Concha, R. Rivero, and I. Delucci, "Occurrence of clinical and sub-clinical mastitis in dairy herds in the west littoral region in Uruguay," *Acta Veterinaria Scandinavica*, vol. 43, no. 4, pp. 221–230, 2002.

[27] M. Abrahmsén, Y. Persson, B. M. Kanyima, and R. Båge, "Prevalence of subclinical mastitis in dairy farms in urban and peri-urban areas of Kampala, Uganda," *Tropical Animal Health and Production*, vol. 46, no. 1, pp. 99–105, 2014.

[28] D. K. Mureithi and M. N. Njuguna, "Prevalence of subclinical mastitis and associated risk factors in dairy farms in urban and peri-urban areas of Thika Sub County, Kenya," *Livestock Research for Rural Development*, vol. 28, no. 2, 2016.

[29] K. Östensson, V. Lam, N. Sjögren, and E. Wredle, "Prevalence of subclinical mastitis and isolated udder pathogens in dairy cows in Southern Vietnam," *Tropical Animal Health and Production*, vol. 45, no. 4, pp. 979–986, 2013.

[30] M. M. Kurjogi and B. B. Kaliwal, "Epidemiology of bovine mastitis in cows of Dharwad district," *International Scholarly Research Notices*, vol. 2014, Article ID 968076, 9 pages, 2014.

[31] J. O. Ondiek, P. S. Ogore, E. K. Shakala, and G. M. Kaburu, "Prevalence of bovine mastitis, its therapeutics and control in Tatton Agriculture Park, Egerton University, Njoro District of Kenya," *Basic Research Journals of Agricultural Science and Review*, vol. 2, no. 1, pp. 15–20, 2013.

[32] A. A. Ayano, F. Hiriko, A. M. Simyalew, and A. Yohannes, "Prevalence of subclinical mastitis in lactating cows in selected commercial dairy farms of Holeta district," *J. Vet. Med. Anim. Heal*, vol. 5, no. 3, pp. 67–72, 2013.

[33] M. Hashemi, M. Kafi, and M. Safdarian, "The prevalence of clinical and subclinical mastitis in dairy cows in the central region of Fars province, south of Iran," *Iranian Journal of Veterinary Research*, vol. 12, no. 3, pp. 236–241, 2011.

[34] M. Kayesh, M. Talukder, and A. Anower, "Prevalence of subclinical mastitis and its association with bacteria and risk factors in lactating cows of Barisal district in Bangladesh," *International Journal of Biological Research*, vol. 2, no. 2, pp. 35–38, 2014.

[35] D. J. Barrett, A. M. Healy, F. C. Leonard, and M. L. Doherty, "Prevalence of pathogens causing subclinical mastitis in 15 dairy

herds in the Republic of Ireland," *Irish Veterinary Journal*, vol. 58, no. 6, pp. 333–337, 2005.

[36] P. Lévesque, *Moins de Mammite, Meilleur Lait*, Institut de Technologie Agroalimentaire, Campus de la Pocatière, Québec, Canada, 2004.

[37] O. C. Sampimon, O. Riekerink, and T. J. G. M. Lam, "Prevalence of subclinical mastitis pathogens and adoption of udder health management practices on Dutch dairy farms: preliminary results," in *Mastitis Control: From Science to Practice*, pp. 39–46, 2008.

[38] B.-M. Thorberg, *Coagulase-Negative Staphylococci in Bovine Sub-Clinical Mastitis*, Sveriges lantbruksuniv, Uppsala, Sweden, 2008.

[39] J. S. Hogan and K. L. Smith, "Occurrence of clinical and subclinical environmental streptococcal mastitis," in *Proceedings of the Symposium on Udder Health Management for Environmental Streptococci*, pp. 36–41, 1997.

[40] D. Cervinkova, H. Vlkova, I. Borodacova et al., "Prevalence of mastitis pathogens in milk from clinically healthy cows," *Veterinarni Medicina*, vol. 58, no. 11, pp. 567–575, 2013.

[41] S. Björk, R. Båge, B. M. Kanyima et al., "Characterization of coagulase negative staphylococci from cases of subclinical mastitis in dairy cattle in Kampala, Uganda," *Irish Veterinary Journal*, vol. 67, no. 1, article 12, 3 pages, 2014.

[42] G. H. Lim, K. E. Leslie, D. F. Kelton, T. F. Duffield, L. L. Timms, and R. T. Dingwell, "Adherence and efficacy of an external teat sealant to prevent new intramammary infections in the dry period," *Journal of Dairy Science*, vol. 90, no. 3, pp. 1289–1300, 2007.

[43] C. V. Bagley, "Staphylococcus mastitis: Herd control program," Logan UT 84322-5600, 1997.

[44] O. M. Radostits, C. C. Gay, K. W. Hinchcliff, and P. D. Constable, *Veterinary Medicine: A Textbook of the Diseases of Cattle, Horses, Sheep, Pigs and Goats*, Saunders, Elsevier, Barcelona, Spain, 10th edition, 2007.

[45] D. J. Wilson, R. N. Gonzalez, and H. H. Das, "Bovine mastitis pathogens in New York and Pennsylvania: prevalence and effects on somatic cell count and milk production," *Journal of Dairy Science*, vol. 80, no. 10, pp. 2592–2598, 1997.

[46] S. Pyörälä and S. Taponen, "Coagulase-negative staphylococci—emerging mastitis pathogens," *Veterinary Microbiology*, vol. 134, no. 1-2, pp. 3–8, 2009.

[47] S. Taponen, *Bovine Mastitis Caused by Coagulase-Negative Staphylococci*, University of Helsinki, 2008.

[48] G. M. Jones, T. L. Bailey, and J. R. Roberson, *Staphylococcus aureus Mastitis: Cause, Detection, and Control*, Virginia State University, 1998.

[49] O. M. Radostits, K. E. Leslie, W. B. Saunders, K. E. Leslie, and J. Fetrow, *Herd Health: Food Animal Production Medicine*, W.B Saunders, Philadelphia, Pa, USA, 2nd edition, 1994.

[50] S. Björk, *Clinical and Subclinical Mastitis in Dairy Cattle in Kampala, Uganda*, Swedish University of Agricultural Sciences, 2013.

[51] T. Parkinson, M. Merrall, and S. Fenwick, "A case of bovine mastitis caused by Bacillus cereus Continued next page," *New Zealand Veterinary Journal*, vol. 47, no. 4, pp. 151-152, 1999.

[52] N. A. Logan, "Bacillus species of medical and veterinary importance," *Journal of Medical Microbiology*, vol. 25, no. 3, pp. 157–165, 1988.

[53] R. N. Gonzalez, "Prototheca, yeast, and bacillus as a cause of mastitis," in *Proceedings of the National Mastitis Council Annual Meeting*, no. 8, pp. 82–90, 1996.

[54] J. Hogan and K. L. Smith, "Coliform mastitis," *Veterinary Research*, vol. 34, no. 5, pp. 507–519, 2003.

[55] NMC, *A Practical Look at Environmental Audits*, National Mastitis Council, 2010.

[56] F. M. Kivaria, J. P. T. M. Noordhuizen, and M. Nielen, "Interpretation of California mastitis test scores using Staphylococcus aureus culture results for screening of subclinical mastitis in low yielding smallholder dairy cows in the Dar es Salaam region of Tanzania," *Preventive Veterinary Medicine*, vol. 78, no. 3-4, pp. 274–285, 2007.

[57] A. J. Bradley and M. J. Green, "Aetiology of clinical mastitis in six Somerset dairy herds," *Veterinary Record*, vol. 148, no. 22, pp. 683–686, 2001.

[58] W. D. Kremer, E. N. Noordhuizen-Stassen, and J. A. Lohuis, "Host defence and bovine coliform mastitis. Host defence mechanisms and characteristics of coliform bacteria in coliform mastitis in bovine: a review," *Veterinary Quarterly*, vol. 12, no. 2, pp. 103–113, 1990.

23

Cloacael Carriage and Multidrug Resistance *Escherichia coli* O157:H7 from Poultry Farms, Eastern Ethiopia

Mude Shecho,[1] **Naod Thomas,**[1] **Jelalu Kemal,**[2] **and Yimer Muktar**[2]

[1]*School of Veterinary Medicine, Wolaita Sodo University, Wolaita Sodo, Ethiopia*
[2]*College of Veterinary Medicine, Haramaya University, P.O. Box 138, Dire Dawa, Ethiopia*

Correspondence should be addressed to Jelalu Kemal; jelaluk@gmail.com

Academic Editor: Antonio Ortega-Pacheco

A cross-sectional study was carried out to determine antimicrobial drug resistance patterns of *E. coli* O157:H7 isolates and estimate the level of the pathogen. A total of 194 cloacae swab samples were collected randomly in two poultry farms. Standard cultural, biochemical, and serological (latex agglutination) methods were used to isolate *E. coli* O157:H7. The isolates were subjected to antimicrobial susceptibility testing using disc diffusion method. Out of 194 cloacae samples examined, 13.4% ($n = 26$) were found to be positive for *E. coli* O157:H7. The finding indicated differences in *E. coli* O157:H7 infection among the different risk factors. Chicken from Adele Poultry Farm showed higher *E. coli* O157:H7 infection (OR = 3.89) than Haramaya University poultry farm and young birds had more infection (OR = 4.62) than adult birds. Of the total 14 antimicrobials included in the panel of study, the susceptibility results were varied with 96.15% and 0% *E. coli* O157:H7 isolates expressing resistance to erythromycin, clindamycin, spectinomycin, and ciprofloxacin, respectively. Multidrug resistance to more than two antimicrobial agents was detected in 24 (92.30%) of the isolates. The study showed high presence of antimicrobial resistant isolates of *E. coli* O157:H7. Further study is required to better understand the ecology and evolution of bacterial resistance to antimicrobial agents.

1. Introduction

Poultry is a major fast growing source of food in the world today [1]. However, it is one of the commodities most commonly associated with food-borne disease outbreaks. Pathogens can be transmitted to humans directly through contact with poultry litter or indirectly through contaminated poultry products [2]. The avian intestines have been considered as a reservoir of potential *E. coli* with zoonotic potential that could be transferred directly from birds to humans.

E. coli is a commensal bacterium in humans and animals and has a wide range of hosts. It is commonly present in the environment and considered an indicator of fecal contamination in food and water. It can acquire, maintain, and transmit resistance genes from other organisms in the environment. *E. coli* serotype O157:H7 is an enterohaemorrhagic strain, which was initially recognized in the United States of America, as a cause of food-borne illness, and has now emerged as an important enteric pathogen of considerable public health significance [3].

In animal production antimicrobials are widely used as growth promoter and in treatment of infectious diseases. The use of antimicrobials in poultry production industries for promotion of growth largely contributes to the high resistance to antimicrobial agents in normal flora of poultry and pathogenic microorganism [4]. The practice of using antimicrobials in feed may modify the intestinal flora by creating a selective pressure in favor of resistant bacteria populations (such as resistant *E. coli*) that could find their way into the environment and food chain [5]. Due to its ubiquity in humans and animals and its role as a pathogenic and commensal organism, *E. coli* has become one of the microorganisms that are commonly resistant to antimicrobials [6]. With the constant use of antimicrobials over a period of time, bacteria resist not only single but also multiple antimicrobials making some diseases troublesome to treat [7].

In recent years, antimicrobial resistance especially multidrug resistance has become very common in clinical isolates, including *E. coli* isolates of animal origin [8]. Antimicrobial resistance among *E. coli* in food animals such as

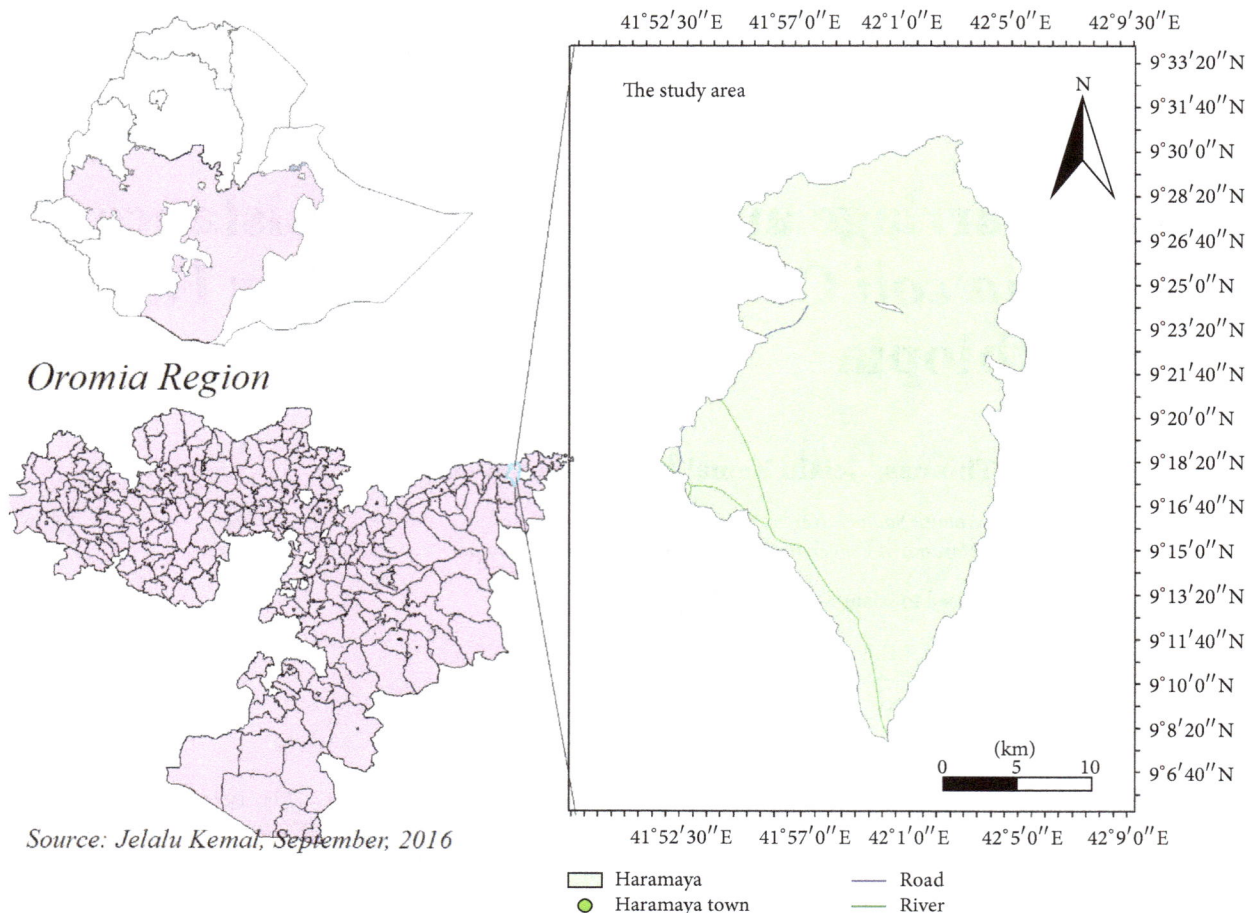

FIGURE 1: Map showing the study area.

chicken is of increasing concern due to the potential for transfer of these resistant pathogens to the human population [9]. Antimicrobial resistance is a global problem, and emerging antimicrobial resistance has become a public health fact worldwide [10]. The use of antimicrobials in food animals, as well as their role in promoting resistance in food-borne bacteria, is an important public health issue. To measure the baseline resistance rates and the impact of different targeted interventions, an ongoing monitoring system is necessary [6]. Even though there have been few studies about the level and antimicrobial resistance pattern of *E. coli* O157:H7 in poultry in Ethiopia, information is lacking. Thus, objectives of the study were to determine the antimicrobial resistance patterns of *E. coli* O157:H7 isolates and estimate the level of the pathogen in apparently healthy birds.

2. Materials and Methods

2.1. Study Site Description and Study Population. The study was conducted at Haramaya district Adele Poultry Farm and poultry farm in Haramaya University. Haramaya district is located in eastern Hararge Zone of Oromia Regional State, along the high way from Addis Ababa to Harar 508 km from Addis Ababa and 19 km ahead to reach Harar at an altitude

of 1980 meters above sea level (m.a.s.l.), 9°26'N latitude and 42°3'E longitude (Figure 1). The mean annual rainfall is 780 mm. The mean annual minimum and maximum temperatures are 8.5 and 24.4°C, respectively. Haramaya University poultry farm is located at 42°3'E longitude, 9°26'N latitude, and an elevation of 1980 m.a.s.l. and 513 km away from Addis Ababa. The annual mean rain fall of the area amounts to 780 mm and the average minimum and maximum temperature are 8°C and 24°C, respectively. The total poultry population of the country is estimated to be 56.87 million and it comprises 95.86% indigenous breeds, 2.79% crossbreeds, and 1.35% exotic breeds [12].

This study was conducted on exotic breed chicken under intensive management system. The target population was apparently healthy exotic breed of white leg horn and Feyumi (Egyptian breed) breed chickens. Both farms comprise the aforementioned breeds. Most of these breeds have been from Debre Zeit farms and the fertilized egg was imported from Egypt, Holland, and other countries. Poultry were selected according to their age groups and breeds. The age was conveniently subdivided into young growers up to six months of age and adult chicken. The main purpose of these poultry farms is to supply egg, live chicken for meat, and 3-month-old chick to the surrounding farmers and backyard and private producers. Furthermore, Haramaya University satisfies its egg demand for its cafeteria of all campuses and the community residing within the university from own farm production. The farms use formulated feed either buying from Debre Zeit or formulating feed on their farm by mixing with local available cereals, pulses, university cafeteria and staff lounge leftovers, and carcass from abattoirs in order to reduce the cost of input.

2.2. Study Design. A cross-sectional purposive type of study was conducted from October 2015 to May 2016 aimed to isolate, identify, and determine the antimicrobial susceptibility profiles *E. coli* O157:H7 in the area. A total of 194 samples of cloacae swabs were collected randomly from healthy chickens from two poultry farms located in Haramaya University ($n =$ 106) and Haramaya district Adele Poultry Farm ($n = 88$), eastern Ethiopia. During the study hypothesized risk factors such as the age, breed, and farm location of the birds were taken into account and recorded.

2.3. Sample Collection. All samples were taken using sterile swabs which were moistened with sterile buffered peptone water (Oxoid Ltd., Cambridge, UK), placed in sterile vial tubes containing 8 mL buffered peptone water which is used to avoid drying out of the swabs. Samples were kept in ice box containing ice pack for transporting to Haramaya University, College of Veterinary Medicine, Microbiology Laboratory, immediately for further analysis.

2.4. Isolation and Identification of E. coli O157:H7. Isolation and identification of *E. coli* O157:H7 were performed by standard bacteriological methods. The samples were incubated at 37°C for 24 hrs on the same day upon arrival at the laboratory on MacConkey agar (Oxoid Ltd., Cambridge, UK) which is selective and differential medium for *E. coli* [13]. A pink colony was picked and subcultured on Eosin Methylene Blue (EMB) agar (Oxoid Ltd., Cambridge, UK) to obtain pure colony. Colonies with metallic green sheen on EMB (characteristic of *E. coli*) were later characterized microscopically using Gram's stain according to the method described by Merchant and Packer [14]. After isolation of the organism on the selective media, differential screening media, triple sugar iron (TSI) agar (Difco, MI, USA) was used for further characterization. Yellow slant, yellow butt, presence of gas bubbles, and absence of black precipitate in the butt was observed which indicates *E. coli* [15]. Then the isolates were subjected to different biochemical tests according to Quinn et al. [16] such as sugar fermentation test and indole production test, methyl-red, Voges-Proskauer, and citrate utilization (IMViC) test. Then the bacterium that was confirmed as *E. coli* was subcultured onto Sorbitol MacConkey agar (Oxoid Ltd., Cambridge, UK) from nutrient agar and colorless colonies (nonsorbitol fermenter) were again subcultured onto nutrient agar and latex *E. coli* O157:H7 agglutination test was performed to determine strains using polyvalent antisera (DENKA SEIKEN Co. Ltd., Tokyo, Japan).

2.5. Antimicrobial Susceptibility Testing for E. coli O157:H7 Isolates. The antimicrobial susceptibility testing *E. coli* O157:H7 isolates was conducted using disc diffusion method (Kirby-Bauer method) on Mueller-Hinton agar (Oxoid Ltd., Cambridge, UK) according to the guidelines of the Clinical and Laboratory Standards Institute [11]. All *E. coli* O157:H7 isolates were evaluated for antimicrobial susceptibility to 14 antimicrobial agents. A McFarland 0.5 (the turbidity of the test broth was adjusted with saline until the turbidity of the test suspension equated that of the standard) standardized suspension of the bacteria in tryptone soya broth (Oxoid Ltd., Cambridge, UK) was prepared. A bacterial suspension incubated for 6–8 hours was swabbed over the entire surface of Mueller-Hinton agar (Oxoid Ltd., Cambridge, UK) with a sterile cotton swab. The inoculated pates were allowed to stand for 3–5 minutes to observe any excess moisture from the medium before the antimicrobial discs were applied. A ring of discs containing single concentrations of each antimicrobial agent was then placed onto the inoculated surface using disc dispenser, gently pressed with the point of the forceps for ensuring complete contact with the agar surface, and then inverted. After 16–18 hours of incubation at 35°C ± 2°C, aerobically, clear zones produced by antimicrobial inhibition of bacterial growth were measured in mm using a measuring caliper. For the susceptibility testing, the following 14 antimicrobial drugs and concentrations were used: ampicillin (10 μg), amoxicillin (20 μg), cefoxitin (30 μg), chloramphenicol (30 μg), ciprofloxacin (5 μg), clindamycin (30 μg), erythromycin (15 μg), gentamycin (10 μg), kanamycin (30 μg), nalidixic acid (30 μg), spectinomycin (30 μg), streptomycin (10 μg), tetracycline (30 μg), and trimethoprim (5 μg) (Oxoid Ltd., Cambridge, UK). The antimicrobials used were selected from the currently available and commonly used chemotherapeutic agents for the treatment of *E. coli* infection in humans and animals. *E. coli* ATCC25922 and *E. coli* ATCC35218 were used as quality control during the test. Finally, the findings of antimicrobial resistance testing were recorded as susceptible, intermediate, and resistant according to Clinical and Laboratory Standards Institute break points [11] (Table 1).

2.6. Data Analysis. All the data were coded and entered into Microsoft Excel® 2007. The data were then exported to SPSS windows version 20.0 (SPSS) (IBM, Armonk, USA) for appropriate statistical analysis. The occurrence of the pathogen was determined by using descriptive statistics. Chi square (χ^2) and odds ratio were used to measure the association between the different risk factors and occurrence of *E. coli* O157:H7 in chicken cloacae. Effects were reported as statistically significant if *P* value is less than 5% ($P < 0.05$).

3. Results

3.1. Level of E. coli O157:H7 from Cloacal Fecal Sample. Based on colonial morphology and biochemical and latex agglutination tests, *E. coli* O157:H7 were isolated from cloacal swab sample of chickens (Table 2). Out of the 194 cloacae samples examined, 26 (13.4%) were found positive for *E. coli* O157:H7. The results indicated different level of *E. coli* O157:H7 among the different selected risk factors (source, age, and breed) of examined poultry; Haramaya University

TABLE 1: Zone diameter interpretive standard chart for *Enterobacteriaceae* [11].

Antimicrobial agents and symbols	Disc potency (μg)	Zone diameter, nearest whole mm		
		Resistance	Intermediate	Susceptible
Amoxicillin (AML)	20	≤13	14–16	≥17
Ampicillin (AMP)	10	≤13	14–16	≥17
Cefoxitin (FOX)	30	≤14	15–17	≥18
Chloramphenicol (C)	30	≤12	13–17	≥18
Ciprofloxacin (CIP)	5	≤14	15–17	≥21
Clindamycin (CLI)	30	≤16	—	≥17
Erythromycin (E)	15	≤13	14–22	≥18
Gentamycin (CN)	10	≤12	13-14	≥15
Kanamycin (K)	30	≤13	14–17	≥18
Nalidixic acid (NAL)	30	≤17	—	≥18
Spectinomycin (SPT)	30	≤11	12–14	≥15
Streptomycin (S)	10	≤11	12–14	≥15
Tetracycline (TE)	30	≤11	12–14	≥15
Trimethoprim (TRI)	5	≤13	14–17	≥17

TABLE 2: Level of *E. coli* O157:H7 isolates with different hypothesized risk factors from Haramaya University and Adele Poultry Farms.

Risk factors	Risk categories	Number examined	Number positive	Proportion (%)	OR (95% CI)	*P* value
Source	HUPF[a]	106	7	6.6	1	
	APF[b]	88	19	21.6	3.89 (1.5–11.5)	0.002
Age	Adult	93	5	7.5	1	
	Young	101	21	18.8	4.62 (1.6–16.3)	0.021
Breed	Feyumi	85	7	10.6	1	
	White Leghorn	109	19	15.6	2.35 (0.9–6.9)	0.310
Total		*194*	*26*	*13.4*		

[a]Haramaya University Poultry Farm.
[b]Adele Poultry Farm.

poultry farm (7; 6.6%), Adele Poultry Farm (19; 21.6%), young (21; 18.8%), adult chicken (5; 7.5%), White Leghorn (19; 15.6%), and Feyumi (7; 10.6%) showed level of *E. coli* O157:H7, respectively. There was a significant difference in *E. coli* O157:H7 among the farms and age groups ($P < 0.05$). Chicken from Adele Poultry Farm showed *E. coli* O157:H7 infection four times higher than Haramaya University poultry farm and young birds had more infection than adult birds. However there was an equal chance of *E. coli* O157:H7 infection among different breeds of chicken.

A total of 26 isolates of *E. coli* O157:H7 were analyzed, 7 from Haramaya University poultry farm and 19 from Adele Poultry Farm for antimicrobial resistance test. The percentage of isolates susceptible, intermediate, and resistant to each antimicrobial agent is outlined in Table 3. Of the total 14 antimicrobials included in the panel of study, the susceptibility results were varied with 96.15% and 0% *E. coli* O157:H7 isolates expressing resistance to erythromycin, clindamycin, spectinomycin, and ciprofloxacin, respectively. The isolates expressed resistance to ampicillin and amoxicillin at frequencies of 92.30% and 34.61%, respectively. Cefoxitin and tetracycline resistance occurred at a frequency of 84.61% and 76.92%, respectively. Relatively similar resistance was observed among kanamycin (15.38), nalidixic acid (23.07),

and streptomycin (34.61) while lower resistance was recorded between chloramphenicol (3.84) and gentamycin (7.69). Ciprofloxacin, chloramphenicol, trimethoprim, gentamicin, and streptomycin were the most sensitive antibiotics in the study. Intermediate resistance/susceptibility to various antibiotics were observed for 0–46.15% *E. coli* O175:H7 strains.

The level of multiple resistance patterns in *E. coli* O157:H7 isolates is given in Table 4. Single and multiple resistance to most of the antimicrobials tested were observed. Multidrug resistance was recorded in case of 2–9 antimicrobials for the tested strains. Multidrug resistance to more than two antimicrobial agents was detected in 24 (92.30%) of the isolates. One isolate was resistant to up to nine antimicrobials tested. The resistance pattern most frequently observed in the isolates was resistance to erythromycin in combination with clindamycin, ampicillin, and cefoxitin 3 (12.5%). The next most frequent resistance isolates were resistance to erythromycin, cefoxitin, clindamycin, ampicillin, amoxicillin, tetracycline, and kanamycin 2 (8.33%). Multidrug resistance was defined as resistance exhibited to two or more antimicrobials.

Among the *E. coli* O157:H7 isolates, 37.5%, 33.33%, and 4.16% expressed resistance to two, four, and nine antimicrobials, respectively (Table 4; Figure 2), and resistance to three and eight antimicrobials occurred at a frequency of

TABLE 3: Antimicrobial resistance profiles of isolated *E. coli* O157:H7 from Haramaya University and Adele Poultry Farms.

Antimicrobial agents	Disc potency (μg)	Number of isolates	Susceptible N (%)	Intermediate N (%)	Resistant N (%)
Amoxicillin	20	26	7 (26.92)	10 (38.46)	9 (34.61)
Ampicillin	10	26	0 (0.0)	2 (7.69)	24 (92.30)
Cefoxitin	30	26	2 (7.69)	2 (7.69)	22 (84.61)
Chloramphenicol	30	26	25 (96.15)	0 (0.0)	1 (3.84)
Ciprofloxacin	5	26	27 (100)	0 (0.0)	0 (0.0)
Clindamycin	30	26	0 (0.0)	1 (3.84)	25 (96.15)
Erythromycin	15	26	1 (3.84)	0 (0.0)	25 (96.15)
Gentamycin	10	26	23 (88.46)	1 (3.84)	2 (7.69)
Kanamycin	30	26	10 (38.46)	12 (46.15)	4 (15.38)
Nalidixic acid	30	26	16 (61.53)	3 (11.53)	6 (23.07)
Spectinomycin	30	26	18 (69.23)	8 (30.76)	0 (0.0)
Streptomycin	10	26	17 (65.38)	0 (0.0)	9 (34.61)
Tetracycline	30	26	2 (7.69)	4 (15.38)	20 (76.92)
Trimethoprim	5	26	24 (92.30)	0 (0.0)	2 (7.69)

TABLE 4: Resistance patterns of *E. coli* O157:H7 isolates form Haramaya University and Adele Poultry Farms against 14 antimicrobial agents.

Antimicrobials	*E. coli* O157:H7	
	Frequency	%
E, K	1	4.16
E, TE	2	8.33
E, C	1	4.16
E, CLI	1	4.16
E, SPT	1	4.16
E, AMP	2	8.33
E, FOX	1	4.16
E, CLI, TE	1	4.16
E, K, TE	1	4.16
CN, E, TE	1	4.16
E, C, CLI, AMP	3	12.5
E, FOX, C, AML	1	4.16
E, CLI, C, AMP	1	4.16
E, S, C, AML	1	4.16
E, AMP, TE, AML	1	4.16
CN, E, S, AMP	1	4.16
E, CLI, K, AMP, FOX, C, TE, AML	2	8.33
E, CLI, K, AMP, C, TE, TRI, AML	1	4.16
E, S, K, NAL, CLI, C, TE, TRI, AML	1	4.16
Total	24	92.30

E: erythromycin, S: streptomycin, Nal = nalidixic acid, K: kanamycin, AMP: ampicillin, TE: tetracycline, RIT: trimethoprim, AML: amoxicillin, CIP: ciprofloxacin, CN: gentamycin, FOX: cefoxitin, C: chloramphenicol, and SPT: spectinomycin.

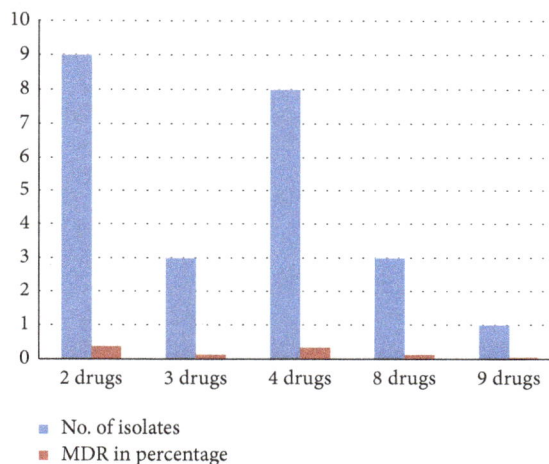

FIGURE 2: Multidrug resistant profiles of *E. coli* O157:H7 isolates of the farms.

4. Discussion

The occurrence of *E. coli* O157:H7 among poultry farms varies considerably [17]. Several studies showed 0.0% to 27.8% level of *E. coli* O157:H7 on poultry farms in different countries [18–20]. In the current study, 13.4% ($n = 26$) of *E. coli* O157:H7 was isolated from cloacal samples taken from poultry farms which agrees with the findings of Olatoye et al. [21] who reported 13 and 14% level of *E. coli* O157:H7 from Lagos and Ibadan poultry farms, respectively. In another study, Ojo et al. [22] confirmed *E. coli* O157:H7 strains in the faeces of poultry sampled from different farms in Nigeria and Aibinu et al. [23] also isolated *E. coli* O157:H7 from chicken in Lagos and Ogun State in Nigeria who found 14.5%.

Moderately comparable levels of *E. coli* O157:H7 were reported from different countries: 8% [24] and 8.1% [25] in Ethiopia, 9% [26] in India, and 6% [27] in Turkey. However, the current finding is higher than the reports of

12.5% each. 8.33% of the isolates showed resistance to a single antimicrobial (kanamycin, tetracycline, ampicillin, and gentamycin).

Baran and Gulmez [28], Dutta et al. [29], and McCluskey et al. [30] who reported 2%, 3.2%, and 2.8% level of *E. coli* O157:H7 in Canada, the United Kingdom, and South Africa, respectively. In addition, 4.4% occurrence was reported in Kenya [31]. These variations might be due to different sampling techniques, areas, and time and lack of strict hygienic measures among the farms and cross contamination with other principal reservoirs [24] and also due to the low isolation rate of culture methods compared to more sensitive immunological and molecular methods [32].

Chicken from Adele Poultry Farm showed *E. coli* O157:H7 infection four times higher than Haramaya University poultry farm and young birds had more infection than adult birds. However there was an equal chance of *E. coli* O157:H7 infection among different breeds of chicken. Zhao et al. [33] described young animals tend to carry *E. coli* O157:H7 more frequently than adults. Moreover, as young chicks are not fully immunocompetent and have also lost protection from maternal antibodies [34]. Regarding *E. coli* O157:H7 infection variation between the two farms might be due to security differences among the farms. However there was no statistically significant association between different breeds; this might be due to equal chance of infection among the breeds.

Antimicrobial resistance has become a global concern [35]. Indiscriminate use of antimicrobial agents in humans, veterinary, and agriculture is considered the most important factor promoting the emergence, selection, and dissemination of antimicrobial resistant microorganisms in both veterinary and human medicine [36]. There were variations in antimicrobial susceptibility of *E. coli* O157:H7 isolates in the present study. A complete (100%) susceptibility was observed against ciprofloxacin and large numbers of isolates were also found to be susceptible against chloramphenicol (96.15%), trimethoprim (92.30), gentamycin (88.46%), spectinomycin (69.23%), streptomycin (65.38%), and nalidixic acid (61.53%). Zinnah et al. [37] reported high susceptible *E. coli* isolates against ciprofloxacin. Similar to the current finding Hailu and Tefera [38] had reported susceptible *E. coli* O157:H7 isolates to chloramphenicol (100%), spectinomycin (62.61%), and nalidixic acid (61.76%). Taye et al. [39] also reported most isolated strains were found susceptible to chloramphenicol and spectinomycin. Closely related chloramphenicol susceptibility to our finding was also reported by Hamisi et al. [13] and Talebiyan et al. [40] from Tanzania and Iran, respectively. The current study finding is distantly related to the finding of Moniri and Dastehgoli [41] who found 36% of healthy broilers susceptibility to chloramphenicol and with the finding of Zakeri and Kashefi [42] who reported 51% from cases of colibacillosis in Iran. 100% chloramphenicol resistance isolates were reported by Islam et al. [43] from poultry in Dhaka, Bangladesh, which is in disagreement with the current study finding.

Comparable susceptible isolates (94.34%) were reported by Talebiyan et al. [40] from chickens in Iran. Muhammad et al. [44] reported 80% susceptible *E. coli* isolate to gentamicin from Bangladesh which is comparable to our finding. Gentamicin was also observed in 71.7% *E. coli* O157:H7 isolates of poultry sample in Saudi Arabia [45]. In another work,

Miles et al. [35] had reported gentamicin susceptibility to all tested *E. coli* isolates. According to the report of Hassan [46] isolates were also 100% susceptible for gentamicin in layer poultry reported from Bangladesh. Susceptibility to gentamicin in the current study is distantly related to finding of Zinnah et al. [37] who reported 40% in Bangladesh. Resistance gentamicin was reported to 46.6% isolates by Abd El Tawab et al. [47] from broiler chickens which is higher than the current study. In contrast to the present finding low susceptible *E. coli* isolates were reported to nalidixic acid (29.7%) [45], spectinomycin, trimethoprim (6%) [48], and streptomycin (30%) [44].

Antimicrobial resistance to clindamycin (96.15%), erythromycin (96.15%), ampicillin (92.30%), cefoxitin (84.61%), and tetracycline (76.92%) was noted in *E. coli* O157:H7 isolates (Table 3). The presence and frequency of drug resistance in *E. coli* O157:H7 from cloacal samples agree with findings of other studies on antimicrobial resistance in *E. coli* [38, 49, 50]. High level of *E. coli* isolates resistant to ampicillin, erythromycin, and amoxicillin were also reported by former study [37]. Similar resistant isolates to tetracycline were reported by different researchers [4, 47, 51, 52]. Resistance patterns of these drugs could be due to the widespread, indiscriminate, and lengthy use of the drugs in the poultry farms [49, 53]. Bacteria can be exposed to these antimicrobial agents in nature and used for disease treatment, for prophylaxis, or for livestock growth promotion which can lead to resistance. Plasmid mediated with a wide variety of genetic determinants also contributes to resistance in these antimicrobials [54]. This makes it more possible for a susceptible bacterium to acquire resistance factors through conjugation or transformation [35]. Furthermore, the problem is probably associated with the widespread use of these antimicrobials in humans and animals for treatment of enteric infections.

In the present study, multidrug resistance to more than two antimicrobial agents was detected in 24 (92.30%) of the isolates. The resistance pattern most frequently observed in the isolates was resistance to erythromycin in combination with clindamycin, ampicillin, and cefoxitin 3 (12.5%). The next most frequent resistance isolates were resistance to erythromycin, cefoxitin, clindamycin, ampicillin, amoxicillin, tetracycline, and kanamycin 2 (8.33%) (Table 4). Among the *E. coli* O157:H7 isolates, 37.5%, 33.33%, and 4.16% expressed resistance to two, four, and nine antimicrobials, respectively (Table 4; Figure 2), and resistance to three and eight antimicrobials occurred at a frequency of 12.5% each. 8.33% of the isolates showed resistance to a single antimicrobial (Figure 2).

Similar findings on multidrug resistance of *E. coli* strains has been reported from Ethiopia [38, 39, 51] and other parts of the world (Khan et al. 2002; [33, 37, 43, 44, 55, 56]). Such high incidence of multidrug resistance may apparently have occurred due to indiscriminate utilization of antimicrobial agents which may ultimately replace the susceptible microorganisms [53, 57]. Feed additives for poultry suggest encountering such resistance emergence with reduced and unsafe application of antimicrobials in animal farming and clinical purposes. The multidrug resistance observed in this study might also be mediated by genetic mobile elements such as plasmids, transposons, and integrons as seen in the case of other studies.

5. Conclusion

The study showed 13.4% of *E. coli* O157:H7 in cloacal swab samples in the study poultry farms. Chickens younger than six months had significantly higher level of *E. coli* O157:H7 compared to older chickens. A significant variation of infection was also recorded in Adele Poultry Farm compared to Haramaya University poultry farm. The study showed the presence of antimicrobial resistant isolates of *E. coli* O157:H7 in the studied poultry farms. *E. coli* O157:H7 isolates showed high level resistance to clindamycin, erythromycin, ampicillin, cefoxitin, and tetracycline which are commonly used antimicrobial agents in veterinary and human practices. The vast majority of *E. coli* O157:H7 isolates showed multiple drugs resistance for two to nine antimicrobials. This could have a significant public health consequence if these microorganisms are transmitted to humans through food chain. Therefore, further study is required to better understand bacterial resistance to antimicrobial agents with emphasis on surveillance of multidrug resistant *E. coli* O157:H7 isolates.

Competing Interests

The authors have not declared any conflict of interests.

Acknowledgments

The authors are very grateful to Haramaya University, College of Veterinary Medicine, for the material support and allowing laboratory facilities. Poultry farm workers were also acknowledged for their overall cooperation.

References

[1] J. T. Hemen, J. T. Johnson, E. E. Ambo, V. S. Ekam, M. O. Odey, and W. A. Fila, "Multi-antibiotic resistance of some gram negative bacterial isolates from poultry litters of selected farms in Benue State," *International Journal of Sciences and Technology*, vol. 2, no. 8, pp. 543–547, 2012.

[2] Z. Chen and X. Jiang, "Microbiological safety of chicken litter or chicken litter-based organic fertilizers: a review," *Agriculture*, vol. 4, no. 1, pp. 1–29, 2014.

[3] H. Karch, P. I. Tarr, and M. Bielaszewska, "Enterohaemorrhagic *Escherichia coli* in human medicine," *International Journal of Medical Microbiology*, vol. 295, no. 6-7, pp. 405–418, 2005.

[4] I. I. Romanus, O. E. Chinyere, N. E. Amobi et al., "Antimicrobial resistance of *Escherichia coli* isolated from animal and human clinical sample," *Global Research Journal of Microbiology*, vol. 2, no. 1, pp. 85–89, 2012.

[5] V. Furtula, E. G. Farrell, F. Diarrassouba, H. Rempel, J. Pritchard, and M. S. Diarra, "Veterinary pharmaceuticals and antibiotic resistance of *Escherichia coli* isolates in poultry litter from commercial farms and controlled feeding trials," *Poultry Science*, vol. 89, no. 1, pp. 180–188, 2010.

[6] S. Zhao, K. Blickenstaff, S. Bodeis-Jones, S. A. Gaines, E. Tong, and P. F. McDermott, "Comparison of the prevalences and antimicrobial resistances of *Escherichia coli* isolates from different retail meats in the United States, 2002 to 2008," *Applied and Environmental Microbiology*, vol. 78, no. 6, pp. 1701–1707, 2012.

[7] S. Moustafa and D. Mourad, "Resistance to 3rd generation cephalosporin of *Escherichia coli* isolated from the feces of healthy broilers chickens in Algeria," *Journal of Veterinary Medicine and Animal Health*, vol. 7, no. 8, pp. 290–295, 2015.

[8] E. T. Elsabet, *Characterization of E. Coli Isolated from Village Chicken and Soil Samples*, 2011.

[9] J. A. Odwar, G. Kikuvi, J. N. Kariuki, and S. Kariuki, "A cross-sectional study on the microbiological quality and safety of raw chicken meats sold in Nairobi, Kenya," *BMC Research*, vol. 7, article 627, 2014.

[10] K. S. Kaye, J. J. Engemann, H. S. Fraimow, and E. Abrutyn, "Pathogens resistant to antimicrobial agents: epidemiology, molecular mechanisms, and clinical management," *Infectious Disease Clinics of North America*, vol. 18, no. 3, pp. 467–511, 2004.

[11] Clinical and Laboratory Standard Institute (CLSI), *Performance Standards for Antimicrobial Susceptibility Testing; Twenty-Third Informational Supplement*, CLSI, Wayne, Pa, USA, 2013.

[12] Central Statistics Authority (CSA), "Agricultural sample survey 2008-2009. Report on livestock and livestock characteristics, vol. II," Statistical Bulletin 446, CSA, Addis Ababa, Ethiopia, 2012.

[13] Z. Hamisi, T. Huruma, and S. Francis, "Antimicrobial resistance phenotypes of *Escherichia coli* isolated from tropical free range chickens," *International Journal of Science and Research*, vol. 3, no. 9, p. 34, 2012.

[14] I. A. Merchant and R. A. Packer, *Veterinary Bacteriology and Virology*, The Iowa State University Press, Ames, Iowa, USA, 7th edition, 1967.

[15] M. N. Islam, M. Sharifuzzaman, and Fakhruzzaman, "Isolation and identification of *E. coli* and *Salmonella* from poultry litter and feed," *International Journal of natural and Social Science*, vol. 1, pp. 1–7, 2014.

[16] P. J. Quinn, B. K. Markey, M. E. Carter, W. J. Donnelly, and F. C. Leonard, *Veterinary Microbiology and Microbial Disease: Pathogenic Bacteria*, Blackwell Scientific Publications, Oxford, London, 2002.

[17] A. O. Onyango, E. U. Kenya, J. J. N. Mbithi, and M. O. Ng'ayo, "Pathogenic *Escherichia coli* and food handlers in luxury hotels in Nairobi, Kenya," *Travel Medicine and Infectious Disease*, vol. 7, no. 6, pp. 359–366, 2009.

[18] P. A. Chapman, A. T. Cerdán Malo, M. Ellin, R. Ashton, and M. A. Harkin, "*Escherichia coli* O157 in cattle and sheep at slaughter, on beef and lamb carcasses and in raw beef and lamb products in South Yorkshire, UK," *International Journal of Food Microbiology*, vol. 64, no. 1-2, pp. 139–150, 2001.

[19] M. P. Doyle and J. L. Schoeni, "Isolation of Escherichia coli O157:H7 from retail fresh meats and poultry," *Applied and Environmental Microbiology*, vol. 53, no. 10, pp. 2394–2396, 1987.

[20] B. O. Abong'o and M. N. B. Momba, "Prevalence and characterization of *Escherichia coli* O157:H7 isolates from meat and meat products sold in Amathole District, Eastern Cape Province of South Africa," *Food Microbiology*, vol. 26, no. 2, pp. 173–176, 2009.

[21] I. O. Olatoye, E. A. Amosun, and G. A. T. Ogundipe, "Multidrug resistant *Escherichia coli* O157 contamination of beef and chicken in municipal abattoirs of Southwest," *Nigeria Natural Sciences*, vol. 10, no. 8, pp. 125–132, 2012.

[22] O. E. Ojo, M. A. Oyekunle, A. O. Ogunleye, and E. B. Otesile, "E. coli O157:H7 in food animals in part of S/Western Nigeria: prevalence and invitro antimicrobial susceptibility," *Tropical Veterinarian*, vol. 26, pp. 23–30, 2009.

[23] I. E. Aibinu, R. F. Peters, K. O. Amisu, S. A. Adesida, M. O. Ojo, and T. Odugbemi, "Multidrug resistance in E. coli O157 strains and the public health implication," *Journal of Animal Science*, vol. 3, no. 3, pp. 22–33, 2007.

[24] A. Hiko, D. Asrat, and G. Zewde, "Occurrence of *Escherichia coli* O157:H7 in retail raw meat products in Ethiopia," *The Journal of Infection in Developing Countries*, vol. 2, no. 5, pp. 389–393, 2008.

[25] G. Mersha, D. Asrat, B. M. Zewde, and M. Kyule, "Occurrence of *Escherichia coli* O157:H7 in faeces, skin and carcasses from sheep and goats in Ethiopia," *Letters in Applied Microbiology*, vol. 50, no. 1, pp. 71–76, 2010.

[26] I. Luga, P. M. Akombo, J. K. P. Kwaga, V. J. Umoh, and I. Ajogi, "Seroprevalence of faecal shedding of *Escherichia coli* O157:H7 from exotic dairy cattle in North-Western Nigeria," *Nigerian Veterinary Journal*, vol. 28, no. 2, pp. 6–11, 2007.

[27] H. K. Trček, "Impact verotoxigenic E. coli O157:H7 in animals on the health of the Slovenian population," *Slovenian Veterinary Research*, vol. 48, pp. 83–92, 2011.

[28] F. Baran and M. Gulmez, "The occurrence of *Escherichia coli* O157:H7 in the ground beef and chicken drumsticks," *Internet Journal of Food Safety*, vol. 2, pp. 13–15, 2010.

[29] S. Dutta, A. Deb, U. K. Chattopadhyay, and T. Tsukamoto, "Isolation of shiga toxin-producing *Escherichia coli* including O157:H7 strains from dairy cattle and beef samples marketed in Calcutta, India," *Journal of Medical Microbiology*, vol. 49, no. 8, pp. 765–767, 2000.

[30] B. J. McCluskey, D. H. Rice, D. D. Hancock et al., "Prevalence of *Escherichia coli* O157 and other Shiga-toxin-producing E. coli in lambs at slaughter," *Journal of Veterinary Diagnostic Investigation*, vol. 11, no. 6, pp. 563–565, 1999.

[31] P. A. Chapman, C. A. Siddons, A. T. Cerdan Malo, and M. A. Harkin, "A one year study of *Escherichia coli* O157 in raw beef and lamb products," *Epidemiology and Infection*, vol. 124, no. 2, pp. 207–213, 2000.

[32] A. Govaris, A. S. Angelidis, K. Katsoulis, and S. Pournaras, "Occurrence, virulence genes and antimicrobial resistance of escherichia coli o157 in bovine, caprine, ovine and porcine carcasses in greece," *Journal of Food Safety*, vol. 31, no. 2, pp. 242–249, 2011.

[33] S. Zhao, J. J. Maurer, S. Hubert et al., "Antimicrobial susceptibility and molecular characterization of avian pathogenic Escherichia coli isolates," *Veterinary Microbiology*, vol. 107, no. 3-4, pp. 215–224, 2005.

[34] J. Pitcovski, D. E. Heller, A. Cahaner, and B. A. Peleg, "Selection for early responsiveness of chicks to *Escherichia coli* and Newcastle disease virus," *Poultry Science*, vol. 66, no. 8, pp. 1276–1282, 1987.

[35] T. D. Miles, W. McLaughlin, and P. D. Brown, "Antimicrobial resistance of *Escherichia coli* isolates from broiler chickens and humans," *BMC Veterinary Research*, vol. 2, article no. 7, 2006.

[36] G. S. Simonsen, J. W. Tapsall, B. Allegranzi, E. A. Talbot, and S. Lazzari, "The antimicrobial resistance containment and surveillance approach—a public health tool," *Bulletin of the World Health Organization*, vol. 82, no. 12, pp. 928–934, 2004.

[37] M. H. Zinnah, M. T. Haque, M. T. Islam et al., "Drug sensitivity pattern of *Escherichia coli* isolated from samples of different

biological and environmental sources," *Bangladesh Journal of Veterinary Medicine*, vol. 6, no. 1, pp. 13–18, 2008.

[38] D. Hailu and G. Tefera, "Isolation and characterization of multidrug resistant *Escherichia coli* isolates from contagion syndrome poultry farm," *International Journal of Current Trends in Pharmacobiology and Medical Sciences*, vol. 1, no. 2, pp. 19–26, 2016.

[39] M. Taye, T. Berhanu, Y. Berhanu, F. Tamiru, and D. Terefe, "Study on carcass contaminating *Escherichia coli* in apparently healthy slaughtered cattle in Haramaya University slaughter house with special emphasis on *Escherichia coli* o157:H7, Ethiopia," *Journal of Veterinary Science and Technology*, vol. 4, no. 1, article no. 132, 2013.

[40] M. K. Talebiyan, K. Faham, and R. F. Mohammad, "Multiple antimicrobial resistance of *Escherichia coli* isolated from chickens in Iran," *Veterinary Medicine International*, vol. 2014, Article ID 491418, 4 pages, 2014.

[41] R. Moniri and K. Dastehgoli, "Fluoroquinolone-resistant *Escherichia coli* isolated from healthy broilers with previous exposure to fluoroquinolones: is there a link?" *Microbial Ecology in Health and Disease*, vol. 17, no. 2, pp. 69–74, 2005.

[42] A. Zakeri and P. Kashefi, "Isolation and drug resistance patterns of *Escherichia coli* from cases of colibacillosis in Tabriz," *Journal of Animal and Veterinary Advances*, vol. 11, no. 19, pp. 3550–3556, 2012.

[43] M. J. Islam, S. Sultana, K. K. Das, N. Sharmin, and M. N. Hasan, "Isolation of plasmid-mediated multidrug resistant *Escherichia coli* from poultry," *International Journal of Sustainable Crop Production*, vol. 3, no. 5, pp. 46–50, 2008.

[44] A. Muhammad, S. Akond, S. M. Alam, R. Hassan, and S. Momena, "Antibiotic resistance of *Escherichia coli* isolated from poultry and poultry environment of Bangladesh," *Internet Journal of Food Safety*, vol. 11, pp. 19–23, 2009.

[45] A. D. Altalhi, Y. A. Gherbawy, and S. A. Hassan, "Antibiotic resistance in *Escherichia coli* isolated from retail raw chicken meat in Taif, Saudi Arabia," *Foodborne Pathogens and Disease*, vol. 7, no. 3, pp. 281–285, 2010.

[46] M. M. Hassan, "Antimicrobial resistance pattern against E. coli and *Salmonella* in layer poultry," *Research Journal for Veterinary Practitioners*, vol. 2, no. 2, pp. 30–35, 2014.

[47] A. A. Abd El Tawab, A. M. Ammar, S. A. Nasef, and R. M. Reda, "Prevalence of E. coli in diseased chickens with its antibiogram pattern," *Benha Veterinary Medical Journal*, vol. 28, no. 2, pp. 224–230, 2015.

[48] J. Isendahl, A. Turlej-Rogacka, C. Manjuba, A. Rodrigues, C. G. Giske, and P. Nauclér, "Fecal carriage of ESBL-producing E. coli and *K. pneumoniae* in children in Guinea-Bissau: a Hospital-Based Cross-Sectional Study," *PLoS ONE*, vol. 7, no. 12, Article ID e51981, 2012.

[49] A. E. van den Bogaard, N. London, C. Driessen, and E. E. Stobberingh, "Antibiotic resistance of faecal *Escherichia coli* in poultry, poultry farmers and poultry slaughterers," *Journal of Antimicrobial Chemotherapy*, vol. 47, no. 6, pp. 763–771, 2001.

[50] R. S. Sayah, J. B. Kaneene, Y. Johnson, and R. Miller, "Patterns of antimicrobial resistance observed in *Escherichia coli* isolates obtained from domestic-and wild-animal fecal samples, human septage, and surface water," *Applied and Environmental Microbiology*, vol. 71, no. 3, pp. 1394–1404, 2005.

[51] T. Zeryehun and B. Bedada, "Antimicrobial resistant pattern of fecal *E. coli* in selected broiler farms of eastern Harare zone, Ethiopia," *International Journal of Applied Biology and Pharmaceutical Technology*, vol. 4, no. 4, pp. 298–304, 2013.

[52] O. O. Adelowo, O. E. Fagade, and Y. Agersø, "Antibiotic resistance and resistance genes in *Escherichia coli* from poultry farms, southwest Nigeria," *Journal of Infection in Developing Countries*, vol. 8, no. 9, pp. 1103–1112, 2014.

[53] A. E. Van Den Bogaard and E. E. Stobberingh, "Antibiotic usage in animals. Impact on bacterial resistance and public health," *Drugs*, vol. 58, no. 4, pp. 589–607, 1999.

[54] J. F. Prescott, J. D. Baggot, and R. D. Walker, *Antimicrobial Therapy in Veterinary Medicine*, Iowa State Press, Ames, Iowa, USA, 3rd edition, 2000.

[55] B. Guerra, E. Junker, A. Schroeter, B. Malorny, S. Lehmann, and R. Helmuth, "Phenotypic and genotypic characterization of antimicrobial resistance in German Escherichia coli isolates from cattle, swine and poultry," *Journal of Antimicrobial Chemotherapy*, vol. 52, no. 3, pp. 489–492, 2003.

[56] E. A. Amosun and I. O. Olatoye, "Molecular characterization and antibiotic resistance profile of *Escherichia coli* from food producing animals from Southwest Nigeria," *American Journal of Science*, vol. 12, no. 8, pp. 51–56, 2016.

[57] J. M. Miranda, B. I. Vázquez, C. A. Fente, J. Barros-Velázquez, A. Cepeda, and C. M. Franco, "Evolution of resistance in poultry intestinal *Escherichia coli* during three commonly used antimicrobial therapeutic treatments in poultry," *Poultry Science*, vol. 87, no. 8, pp. 1643–1648, 2008.

24

The Demographics of Canine Hip Dysplasia in the United States and Canada

Randall T. Loder[1] and Rory J. Todhunter[2]

[1]Department of Orthopaedic Surgery, Indiana University School of Medicine and James Whitcomb Riley Children's Hospital, Indianapolis, IN 46202, USA
[2]Department of Clinical Sciences, College of Veterinary Medicine, Cornell University, Ithaca, NY 14853-6401, USA

Correspondence should be addressed to Randall T. Loder; rloder@iupui.edu

Academic Editor: Antonio Ortega-Pacheco

Canine hip dysplasia (CHD) is a common problem in veterinary medicine. We report the demographics of CHD using the entire hip dysplasia registry from the Orthopedic Foundation for Animals, analyzing differences by breed, sex, laterality, seasonal variation in birth, and latitude. There were 921,046 unique records. Each dog was classified using the American Kennel Club (AKC) and Fédération Cynologique Internationale (FCI) systems. Statistical analysis was performed with bivariate and logistic regression procedures. The overall CHD prevalence was 15.56%. The OR for CHD was higher in females (1.05), those born in spring (1.14) and winter (1.13), and those in more southern latitudes (OR 2.12). Within AKC groups, working dogs had the highest risk of CHD (OR 1.882) with hounds being the reference group. Within FCI groups, the pinscher/molossoid group had the highest risk of CHD (OR 4.168) with sighthounds being the reference group. The similarities between CHD and DDH are striking. Within DDH there are two different types, the typical infantile DDH and the late onset adolescent/adult acetabular dysplasia, with different demographics; the demographics of CHD are more similar to the later onset DDH group. Comparative studies of both disorders should lead to a better understanding of both CHD and DDH.

1. Introduction

Canine hip dysplasia (CHD) is a well-known disorder in veterinary medicine [1–4], especially amongst certain breeds. The human counterpart of CHD, developmental dysplasia of the hip (DDH), is also a well-known problem with differences in prevalence by race/ethnicity [5], analogous to breed differences in CHD. Comprehensive literature reviews of DDH have shown various demographic patterns regarding sex, laterality, latitude, and seasonal variation in birth month [5, 6]. Variation in birth month/season has been described in a few small series of CHD [7–12]. There has been no study of the demographics of CHD using a large data set. The purpose of this study was to investigate the demographics of CHD using a large North American data base and analyze the differences by breed, sex, laterality, seasonal variation in birth, and latitude. Comparison with the demographics of DDH may shed further light on the etiology of both conditions and

specifically support the use of CHD as an animal model for DDH, as well as DDH pointing towards further comparative research areas in CHD.

2. Materials and Methods

2.1. Data Source. The data for this study was the complete hip dysplasia registry (both public and private) collected by the Orthopedic Foundation for Animals (OFA) through April 2015. There were a total of 1,430,979 records. The OFA hip score uses the American Veterinary Medical Association grading system: 1 = excellent, 2 = good, 3 = fair, 4 = borderline CHD, 5 = mild CHD, 6 = moderate CHD, and 7 = severe CHD. These scores were divided into two groups: those with CHD (scores 5–7) and those without CHD (scores 1–3); the borderline score of 4 was excluded. Duplicate records, feline cases, and those with an indeterminate score were deleted. The country of origin was known in 1,130,478 dogs; the vast majority (1,121,961–99.25%) were from the USA (1,046,249) or Canada (75,712). Dogs less than 24 or greater than 60 months of age at the time of the radiograph were next deleted, leaving 921,046 unique records which are the data for this study.

2.2. Data Groups. Each dog was classified into related breed groups using both the American Kennel Club (AKC) (http://www.akc.org) [13] and Fédération Cynologique Internationale (FCI) (http://www.fci.be/en/Nomenclature) [14] systems. Each dog was separately given an AKC and FCI group designation and analyzed separately; the two different systems were not merged. Dogs in each of these groups are relatively similar genetically [15, 16] and thus could be expected to respond to environmental triggers similarly, compared to dogs that do not share a common genetic background. The AKC categories are herding, hound, working, sporting, nonsporting, terrier, toy, native, hybrid, and miscellaneous groups. The FCI categories are (1) sheep and cattle dogs; (2) pinscher, schnauzer, molossoid, and Swiss mountain and Swiss cattle dogs; (3) terriers; (4) dachshunds; (5) spitz and primitive dogs; (6) scent hounds; (7) pointers; (8) retrievers, flushers, and water dogs; (9) companion and toy dogs; and (10) sighthounds.

The variables analyzed were sex, breed, season of birth, hip score, and latitude. Season of birth was arbitrarily defined as follows: winter, December through February, spring, March through May, summer, June through August, and autumn, September through November. Each state and province was grouped by latitude. The latitude where each dog was living at the time of the radiograph was placed into 4 groups defined as (1) <30°N, (2) 30–39°N, (3) 40–49°N, and (4) >50°N. Those <30°N were Florida, Hawaii, Louisiana, Puerto Rico, Virgin Islands, and Guam. Those 30–39°N were Alabama, Arkansas, Arizona, California, Colorado, District of Columbia, Delaware, Georgia, Indiana, Kansas, Kentucky, Maryland, Missouri, Mississippi, North Carolina, New Mexico, Nevada, Oklahoma, South Carolina, Tennessee, Texas, Virginia, and West Virginia. Those 40–49°N were the states of Connecticut, Iowa, Idaho, Illinois, Maryland, Maine, Michigan, Minnesota, Montana, Nebraska, New Hampshire, New Jersey, New York, Ohio, Oregon, Pennsylvania, Rhode Island, South Dakota, Utah, Vermont, Washington, Wisconsin, and Wyoming and the provinces of New Brunswick, Newfoundland, Nova Scotia, Ontario, Prince Edward Island, and Quebec. Those >50°N were the state of Alaska and the provinces of Alberta, British Columbia, Manitoba, Northwest Territories, Saskatchewan, and Yukon Territory. Although a few of the states and provinces straddle these latitude lines, each state/province was placed into the group corresponding to the major population areas.

2.3. Statistical Analysis. Demographic variables were first analyzed using bivariate analyses (Pearson's χ^2 test) to determine differences between those with and without CHD. Next, binary multivariate logistic regression analyses were performed to determine adjusted odds ratios (OR) and 95% [upper, lower] confidence intervals of a dog having CHD. While the American Veterinary Medical Association grading system is a numerical value, it is not a continuous variable such as the Norberg angle, but rather a categorical ordinal variable determined by subjective criteria (http://www.ofa.org/hd_grades.html – hip dysplasia, OFA X-ray procedures). For this reason, CHD grade was considered to be a categorical variable. All statistical analyses were performed with Systat™ 10 software (Chicago, IL, 2000), and $p < 0.05$ was considered statistically significant.

3. Results

3.1. Overall Results. The hip dysplasia scores were 1 in 74,931 dogs; 2 in 601,893; 3 in 95,154; 4 in 6,772; 5 in 86,321; 6 in 47,971; and 7 in 8,004, resulting in an overall CHD prevalence of 15.56%. There was significant variability in the prevalence of CHD by AKC and FCI groups, gender, latitude, and season of birth (Table 1). CHD was overall slightly more common in females, those born in spring and winter (Figure 1(a)), and those born in the more southern latitudes (Figure 1(b)). Within AKC groups, CHD was most prevalent in hybrid breeds (21.5%) and least prevalent in hounds (10.5%) (Figure 1(c)). Within FCI groups, it was most prevalent in group 2 (pinscher, schnauzer, molossoid, and Swiss mountain/Swiss cattle dogs) (20.4%) and least common in group 10 (sighthounds) (5.2%) (Figure 1(d)). Although there was a statistically significant difference in the prevalence of CHD by age at the time of radiography (Figure 1(e)), the variability was less than 2% and considered to not be clinically significant, especially since the oldest group of dogs had a lower prevalence of CHD than the youngest cohort. Age was thus deleted from all further analyses. There was significant variation by individual breeds. The prevalence of CHD by breeds in this study is very similar to that given on the OFA website http://www.ofa.org, even though dogs outside of Canada or the USA were excluded in our study. The complete CHD prevalence data set is given in Supplemental Table 1 in Supplementary Material available online at https://doi.org/10.1155/2017/5723476; the highest prevalence was in the bulldog (77.7%) and the lowest in the Italian greyhound (0.0%).

3.2. Results by Demographic Parameters. The overall OR for CHD was higher in females (1.05 [1.064, 1.039]; $p < 10^{-6}$), those born in spring (1.143 [1.16, 1.13]; $p < 0.004$), and those living in more southern latitudes (<30°N) (OR 2.12; [2.21, 2.04]; $p < 10^{-6}$). These results from the composite data set obviously reflect the proportion of breeds in the OFA database and could likely be different if the breed composition differed. Therefore, analyses for each AKC and FCI group, as well as individual breeds, were performed (Table 2). Due to small numbers in certain groups, those in the native, hybrid, and miscellaneous were excluded when analyzing by AKC groups and the dachshunds when analyzing by FCI groups. Within AKC groups, working dogs had the highest risk of CHD (OR 1.882) with hounds being the reference group. Within FCI groups, group 2 (pinscher, schnauzer, molossoid, and Swiss mountain/Swiss cattle dogs) had the highest risk of CHD (OR 4.168) with sighthounds being the reference group.

TABLE 1: Prevalence of CHD by demographic variables.

Parameter	All	Dogs without CHD	CHD versus no CHD				Bilateral versus unilateral CHD					Right versus left unilateral CHD				
			Dogs with CHD	% CHD	% without CHD	p value	Bilateral CHD	Unilateral CHD	% bilateral	% unilateral	p value	Left CHD	Right CHD	% left	% right	p value
All dogs	914,274	771,978	142,296	15.56	84.44	—	95,376	46,918	67.03	32.97	—	21,657	18,140	54.42	45.58	—
Sex																
Female	582,990	490,884	92,106	15.80	84.20	$<10^{-6}$	62,267	29,839	67.60	32.40	$<10^{-6}$	13,618	11,696	53.80	46.20	0.001
Male	331,281	281,091	50,190	15.15	84.85		33,111	17,079	65.97	34.03		8,039	6,444	55.51	44.49	
AKC group																
Herding	181,497	153,857	27,640	15.23	84.77	$<10^{-6}$	17,870	9,770	64.65	35.35	$<10^{-6}$	4,346	3,922	52.56	47.44	$<10^{-6}$
Hound	24,017	21,490	2,527	10.52	89.48		1,745	782	69.05	30.95		359	307	53.90	46.10	
Working	217,397	178,178	39,219	18.04	81.96		27,004	12,215	68.85	31.15		5,076	4,898	50.89	49.11	
Sporting	404,008	343,284	60,724	15.03	84.97		40,096	20,628	66.03	33.97		10,006	7,694	56.53	43.47	
Nonsporting	51,153	44,226	6,927	13.54	86.46		4,922	2,005	71.06	28.94		1,031	238	81.25	18.75	
Terrier	19,234	16,812	2,422	12.59	87.41		1,789	633	73.86	26.14		341	238	58.89	41.11	
Toy	11,005	9,197	1,808	16.43	83.57		1,311	497	72.51	27.49		277	194	58.81	41.19	
Native	36	32	4	11.11	88.89		2	2	50.00	50.00		1	1	50.00	50.00	
Hybrid	2,514	1,973	541	21.52	78.48		345	196	63.77	36.23		117	66	63.93	36.07	
Miscellaneous	3,413	2,929	484	14.18	85.82		294	190	60.74	39.26		103	77	57.22	42.78	
FCI group																
Sheep and cattle	185,969	157,713	28,256	15.19	84.81	$<10^{-6}$	18,250	10,005	64.59	35.41	$<10^{-6}$	4,465	4,004	52.72	47.28	$<10^{-6}$
Pinscher Schnauzer, molossoid, and	176,144	140,164	35,980	20.43	79.57		24,919	11,061	69.26	30.74		4,571	4,462	50.60	49.40	
Swiss Mtn/cattle dog	14,542	12,374	2,168	14.91	85.09		1,623	545	74.86	25.14		291	209	58.20	41.80	
Terrier	70	63	7	10.00	90.00		7	0	100.00	0.00		0	0	—	—	
Dachshund																
Spitz and primitive	64,683	58,132	6,551	10.13	89.87		4,588	1,963	70.04	29.96		915	740	55.29	44.71	
Scent hounds	16,509	14,782	1,727	10.46	89.54		1,207	520	69.89	30.11		238	200	54.34	45.66	
Pointing dogs	71,170	63,403	7,767	10.91	89.09		5,045	2,721	64.96	35.04		1,293	1,073	54.65	45.35	
Retrievers, flushers, and water dogs	340,551	286,489	54,062	15.87	84.13		35,797	18,265	66.21	33.79		8,912	6,746	56.92	43.08	
Companion and toy dogs	37,085	32,071	5,014	13.52	86.48		3,484	1,530	69.49	30.51		815	586	58.17	41.83	
Sighthounds	5,129	4,860	269	5.24	94.76		148	121	55.02	44.98		48	54	47.06	52.94	
Latitude																
<30°N	43,929	34,779	9,150	20.83	79.17	$<10^{-6}$	6,428	2,721	70.26	29.74	$<10^{-6}$	1,172	1,074	52.18	47.82	0.0037
30–39°N	404,336	343,861	60,475	14.96	85.04		40,594	19,880	67.13	32.87		9,131	7,865	53.72	46.28	
40–49°N	425,790	357,670	68,120	16.00	84.00		45,283	22,837	66.48	33.52		10,650	8,619	55.27	44.73	
≥50°N	37,506	33,364	4,142	11.04	88.96		2,777	1,365	67.04	32.96		655	546	54.54	45.46	

TABLE 1: Continued.

Parameter	All	CHD versus no CHD					Bilateral versus unilateral CHD					Right versus left unilateral CHD				
		Dogs without CHD	Dogs with CHD	% CHD	% without CHD	p value	Bilateral CHD	Unilateral CHD	% bilateral	% unilateral	p value	Left CHD	Right CHD	% left	% right	p value
Season of birth																
Autumn	215,003	182,842	32,161	14.96	85.04		21,362	10,798	66.42	33.58		5,020	4,099	55.05	44.95	
Winter	218,849	183,276	35,573	16.25	83.75	$<10^{-6}$	23,695	11,878	66.61	33.39	0.0016	5,582	4,555	55.07	44.93	0.10
Spring	255,064	213,377	41,687	16.34	83.66		28,146	13,540	67.52	32.48		6,151	5,278	53.82	46.18	
Summer	225,358	192,483	32,875	14.59	85.41		22,173	10,702	67.45	32.55		4,904	4,208	53.82	46.18	

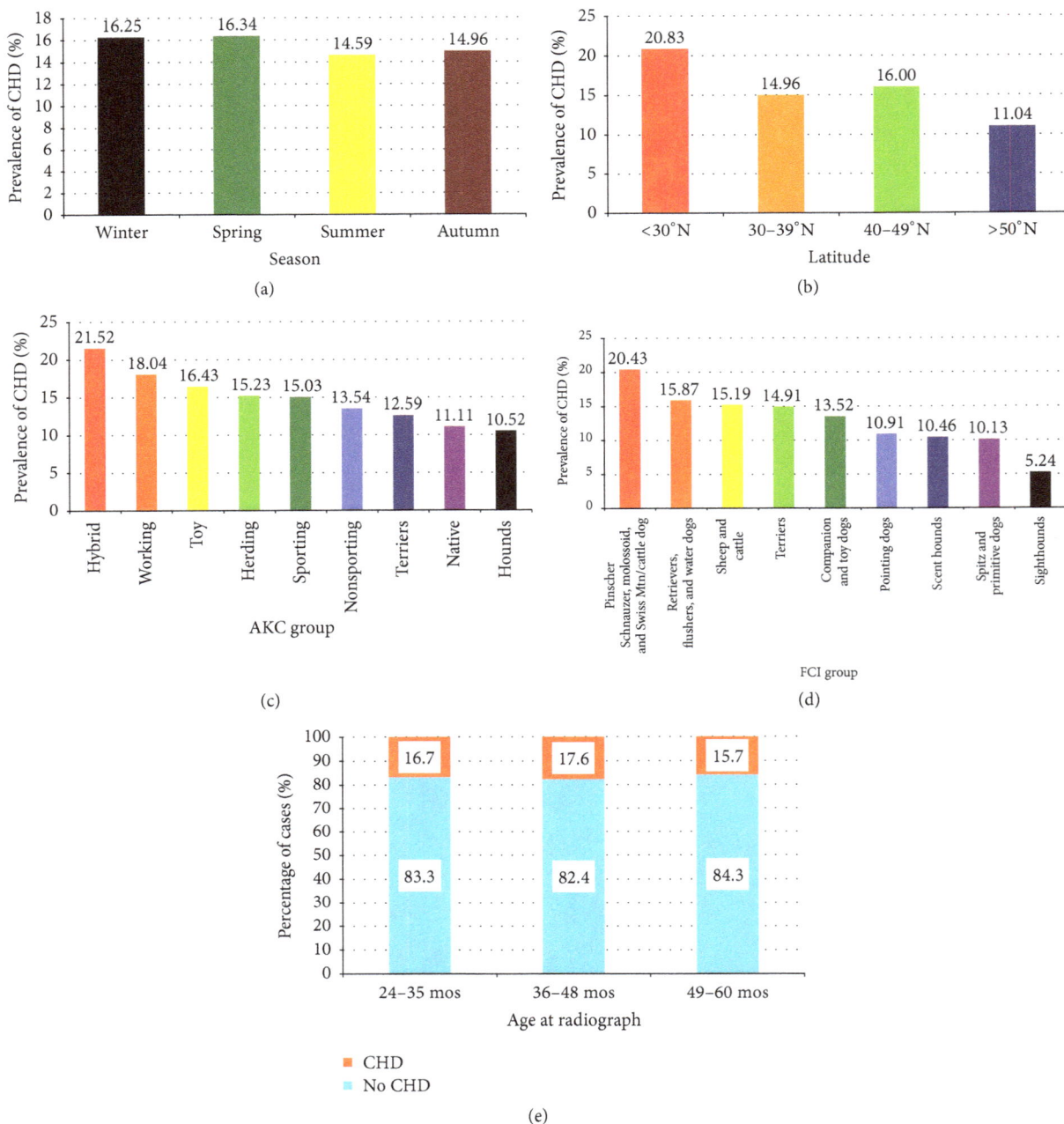

FIGURE 1: Prevalence of CHD by various demographic parameters. (a) By season of birth. (b) By latitude. (c) By AKC groups. (d) By FCI groups. (e) By age at time of radiograph. The numbers in the boxes are the percentage within each column bar.

Those born in spring had the highest risk of CHD (OR 1.14) as well as those living in latitudes < 30°N (OR 2.1), with a minimally higher risk in females (OR 1.05).

3.3. Results by AKC and FCI Groups.
Analyses by each of the AKC and FCI groups were next performed (Table 3). Again, many of the groups showed an increase in CHD in those living in latitudes <30°N, except for toy dogs (where the opposite was noted with a higher risk in the most northern latitudes >50°N); hounds had no variation in CHD by

latitude. When there was an increased OR by season of birth, winter and spring seasons most commonly demonstrated the increased risk with a few demonstrating an autumn increase; no group demonstrated a summer increase. A few groups demonstrated an increased CHD risk in females (AKC herding, working and sporting groups and FCI sheep/cattle and pinscher groups); sighthounds had an increased risk in male dogs.

Analyses within subgroups of AKC and FCI groups (Supplemental Table 2) as well as the most common 25 breeds

TABLE 2: Odds ratios of CHD by AKC/FCI groups, sex, season of birth, and latitude.

(a)

By AKC group	OR	95% CI	p value
Sex			
Female	1.056	(1.069, 1.044)	$<10^{-6}$
Male	1.0 R	—	—
Season of birth			
Autumn	1.025	(1.042, 1.008)	$<10^{-6}$
Winter	1.131	(1.149, 1.112)	0.081
Spring	1.146	(1.165, 1.128)	$<10^{-6}$
Summer	1.0 R	—	—
Latitude			
<30°N	2.116	(2.203, 2.034)	$<10^{-6}$
30–39°N	1.428	(1.477, 1.381)	$<10^{-6}$
40–49°N	1.552	(1.605, 1.501)	$<10^{-6}$
≥50°N	1.0 R	—	—
AKC group			
Herding	1.535	(1.602, 1.470)	$<10^{-6}$
Toy	1.675	(1.788, 1.570)	$<10^{-6}$
Working	1.882	(1.965, 1.804)	$<10^{-6}$
Sporting	1.504	(1.569, 1.442)	$<10^{-6}$
Nonsporting	1.348	(1.415, 1.284)	$<10^{-6}$
Terrier	1.236	(1.311, 1.164)	$<10^{-6}$
Hound	1.0 R	—	—

(b)

By FCI group	OR	95% CI	p value
Sex			
Female	1.053	(1.065, 1.040)	$<10^{-6}$
Male	1.0 R	—	—
Season of birth			
Autumn	1.021	(1.038, 1.004)	0.016
Winter	1.124	(1.142, 1.105)	$<10^{-6}$
Spring	1.143	(1.161, 1.125)	$<10^{-6}$
Summer	1.0 R	—	—
Latitude			
<30°N	2.047	(2.13, 1.967)	$<10^{-6}$
30–39°N	1.410	(1.458, 1.363)	$<10^{-6}$
40–49°N	1.546	(1.599, 1.496)	$<10^{-6}$
≥50°N	1.0 R	—	—
FCI group			
Sheep and cattle	3.229	(3.653, 2.854)	$<10^{-6}$
Pinscher schnauzer, molossoid, and Swiss Mtn/cattle dog	4.618	(5.224, 4.082)	$<10^{-6}$
Terrier	3.163	(3.605, 2.774)	$<10^{-6}$
Spitz and primitive	2.059	(2.334, 1.816)	$<10^{-6}$
Scent hounds	2.096	(2.393, 1.836)	$<10^{-6}$
Pointing dogs	2.184	(2.473, 1.927)	$<10^{-6}$
Retrievers, flushers, and water dogs	3.386	(3.830, 2.994)	$<10^{-6}$
Companion and toy dogs	2.824	(3.204, 2.489)	$<10^{-6}$
Sighthounds	1.0 R	—	—

TABLE 3: Odds ratios of CHD for each AKC/FCI group by sex, season of birth, and latitude*.

| | | Sex | | Latitude | | | | | | Season of birth | | | | | |
	n	Female OR (95% CI)	p value	(<30°N) OR (95% CI)	p value	(30–39°N) OR (95% CI)	p value	(40–49°N) OR (95% CI)	p value	Autumn OR (95% CI)	p value	Winter OR (95% CI)	p value	Spring OR (95% CI)	p value
By AKC group															
Herding	180,911	1.14 (1.171, 1.110)	<10^-6	2.129 (2.323, 1.052)	<10^-6	1.383 (1.489, 1.285)	<10^-6	1.531 (1.648, 1.422)	<10^-6	0.996 (1.035, 0.958)	0.83	1.148 (1.191, 1.107)	<10^-6	1.102 (1.141, 1.063)	<10^-6
Toy	11,011	0.948 (1.052, 0.853)	0.31	0.457 (0.620, 0.339)	<10^-6	0.54 (0.678, 0.430)	<10^-6	0.499 (0.628, 0.397)	<10^-6	0.918 (1.062, 0.794)	0.25	1.073 (1.239, 0.930)	0.34	1.041 (1.200, 0.903)	0.58
Working	216,599	1.069 (1.903, 1.045)	<10^-6	2.345 (2.519, 2.182)	<10^-6	1.489 (1.584, 1.401)	<10^-6	1.558 (1.657, 1.465)	<10^-6	0.979 (1.011, 0.948)	0.19	1.075 (1.109, 1.041)	**0.000008**	1.146 (1.182, 1.111)	<10^-6
Sporting	402,911	1.027 (1.046, 1.009)	**0.0038**	2.179 (2.328, 2.038)	<10^-6	1.523 (1.609, 1.441)	<10^-6	1.7 (1.796, 1.609)	<10^-6	1.082 (1.111, 1.056)	<10^-6	1.189 (1.219, 1.159)	<10^-6	1.195 (1.224, 1.167)	<10^-6
Nonsporting	51,045	0.988 (1.042, 0.938)	0.94	1.588 (1.881, 1.341)	<10^-6	1.258 (1.443, 1.096)	**0.0011**	1.266 (1.454, 1.103)	**0.0008**	0.975 (1.046, 0.938)	0.19	1.004 (1.081, 0.932)	**0.000008**	1.067 (1.146, 0.994)	<10^-6
Terriers	19,156	0.978 (1.071, 0.894)	0.63	2.489 (3.281, 1.887)	<10^-6	1.414 (1.776, 1.126)	**0.0028**	1.492 (1.870, 1.190)	**0.0005**	0.987 (1.118, 0.872)	0.84	1.102 (1.245, 0.975)	0.12	1.082 (1.216, 0.963)	0.19
Hounds	23,974	1.024 (1.114, 0.941)	0.58	1.31 (1.748, 0.980)	0.067	1.044 (1.336, 0.815)	0.74	1.165 (1.493, 0.909)	0.23	0.99 (1.115, 0.879)	0.87	0.933 (1.046, 0.832)	0.23	0.92 (1.031, 0.820)	0.15
By FCI group															
Sheep and cattle	185,366	1.138 (1.169, 1.109)	<10^-6	2.105 (1.295, 1.931)	<10^-6	1.371 (1.475, 1.274)	<10^-6	1.512 (1.623, 1.405)	<10^-6	0.987 (1.026, 0.951)	0.51	1.145 (1.187, 1.105)	<10^-6	1.098 (1.137, 1.060)	<10^-6
Pinscher schnauzer, molossoid, and Swiss Mtn/cattle dog	175,562	1.078 (1.104, 1.053)	<10^-6	2.227 (2.409, 2.059)	<10^-6	1.52 (1.628, 1.419)	<10^-6	1.626 (1.743, 1.518)	<10^-6	1.006 (1.041, 0.972)	0.74	1.076 (1.113, 1.041)	**0.00002**	1.168 (1.207, 1.131)	<10^-6
Terrier	14,507	1.013 (1.115, 0.921)	0.79	2.131 (2.864, 1.585)	**0.000001**	1.287 (1.651, 1.003)	**0.047**	1.412 (1.810, 1.102)	**0.0064**	0.999 (1.142, 0.875)	0.99	1.125 (1.281, 0.988)	0.076	1.089 (1.233, 0.961)	0.18
Spitz and primitive	64,393	1.014 (1.069, 0.961)	0.62	1.709 (2.022, 1.444)	<10^-6	1.121 (1.263, 0.995)	0.06	1.164 (1.31, 1.033)	**0.012**	1.007 (1.081, 0.938)	0.85	1.008 (1.084, 0.937)	0.84	0.92 (0.992, 0.853)	0.031
Scent hounds	16,490	1.095 (1.215, 0.987)	0.085	1.15 (1.573, 0.841)	0.38	0.911 (1.192, 0.700)	0.50	0.922 (1.212, 0.702)	0.56	0.97 (1.121, 0.839)	0.68	1.09 (1.254, 0.947)	0.23	0.939 (1.074, 0.820)	0.36
Pointing dogs	70,962	0.998 (1.048, 0.951)	0.93	1.412 (1.722, 1.164)	**0.0005**	1.179 (1.384, 1.004)	**0.045**	1.288 (1.509, 1.098)	**0.0018**	1.124 (1.207, 1.046)	**0.0014**	1.257 (1.346, 1.173)	<10^-6	1.184 (1.260, 1.112)	<10^-6
Retrievers, flushers, and water dogs	339,651	1.015 (1.035, 0.995)	0.14	2.305 (2.471, 2.149)	<10^-6	1.578 (1.672, 1.488)	<10^-6	1.781 (1.886, 1.681)	<10^-6	1.044 (1.073, 1.016)	**0.0021**	1.15 (1.182, 1.120)	<10^-6	1.188 (1.213, 1.158)	<10^-6
Companion and toy dogs	37,025	0.99 (1.054, 0.930)	0.75	1.02 (1.234, 0.850)	0.83	0.958 (1.102, 0.832)	0.55	0.97 (1.117, 0.842)	0.67	0.938 (1.054, 0.930)	0.14	1.031 (1.123, 0.946)	0.49	1.113 (1.207, 1.026)	**0.001**
Sighthounds	5,111	0.739 (0.945, 0.578)	**0.016**	2.607 (6.622, 1.027)	**0.044**	1.482 (3.421, 0.642)	0.36	2.122 (4.872, 0.924)	0.076	1.45 (2.073, 1.014)	**0.042**	1.24 (1.784, 0.860)	0.25	1.177 (1.661, 0.834)	0.35

*The reference groups were male, latitude ≥50°N, and summer.
The p values for statistically significant variables are in bold type.

(a)

(b)

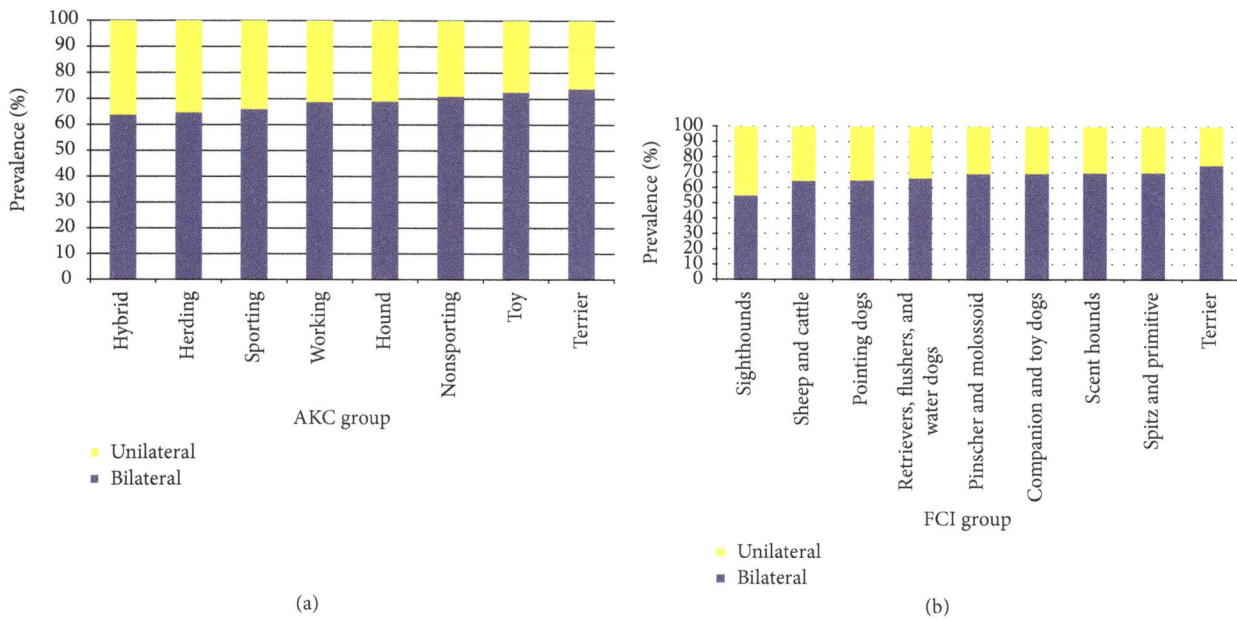

FIGURE 2: Unilateral and bilateral involvement in CHD. (a) By AKC group. (b) By FCI group.

in the data set (Supplemental Table 3) were also performed. Here again, similar findings are as seen for individual AKC and FCI groups. The detailed ORs of CHD for all dogs with $n > 1000$ as well as all dogs with $n > 100$ and a CHD prevalence of >15% (the median value) are given in Supplemental Table 4.

3.4. Severity and Laterality of CHD. For those dogs with CHD, severity of the CHD was analyzed (Table 4). Severe CHD (score of 7) was more common in those with bilateral involvement, AKC groups of herding and working dogs, FCI groups of pinscher and sheep/cattle dogs, those living in the most southern latitudes (<30°N), and those born in spring. Males had a slightly higher proportion of severe CHD. Regarding unilateral or bilateral involvement, bilateral disease was most prevalent in terriers and least prevalent in hybrid dogs within AKC groups (Figure 2(a)); bilateral disease was most prevalent in terriers and least prevalent in sighthounds within FCI groups (Figure 2(b)).

4. Discussion

Limitations of this study need to be acknowledged. Although we used a very large data set, it may not give the true prevalence of CHD, since it only represents the data on those dogs whose radiographs were submitted to the OFA. This predisposes to selection bias as it is not a truly random sample of the canine population [17]. Determination of the "true" prevalence would require a prospective radiographic exam between 2 and 5 years of age of every dog consecutively born, with a population of at least 1 million. Obviously such a study is impossible to perform. The OFA data set is therefore likely the best that can be presently obtained in the North America with the possible exception of the PennHIP™.

With these limitations in mind, there are several important findings. CHD is slightly more common in females, but with a large variation, ranging from 3.36 times more frequent in female Polish Tatra Sheepdogs to 1.63 times more frequent in male Afghan Hounds (Supplemental Table 1). CHD prevalence varies by breed, which was again demonstrated in this study, ranging from 77.7% in the bulldog to 0% in the Italian Greyhound. Many breeds demonstrated a mild increase in risk for CHD when born in winter and spring. CHD was unilateral in 33% of all dogs with CHC. Unilateral involvement was more common in herding/sporting dogs and they had lower hip dysplasia scores. Finally, a new finding is that the prevalence of CHD is more common in dogs living in more southern latitudes.

This study confirms the marked variability in CHD prevalence by breed. In France, the highest prevalence of CHD was in the Cane Corso (59.7%) and the lowest in the Siberian Husky (3.9%) [18]. In a national Veterinary Medical Database from the entire USA [19], the OR of CHD was 10.2 in the Kuvasz with mixed breed dogs being the reference group. In a more recent study using the Veterinary Medical Database [20] the highest prevalence of CHD was 17.16% in the Newfoundland and 0.12% in the Scottish Terrier. In USA veterinary teaching hospitals, the prevalence of CHD was highest in the Rottweiler (35.4%) and lowest in the miniature schnauzer dogs (1.5%) [21]. In a Norwegian study comprised of Newfoundland, Leonberger, Labrador Retriever, and Irish Wolfhounds ($n = 501$), the highest prevalence of CHD was in the Newfoundland and the lowest in the Irish Wolfhound (OR 0.22 that of the Newfoundland) [22]. In Turkey, a study of 484 dogs from 7 different breeds revealed the highest prevalence in Doberman Pinschers (70.6%) and the lowest in Golden Retrievers (50%); the prevalence in Doberman Pinschers in this study in North America was low at 5.1%.

TABLE 4: Severity of CHD by demographic parameters.

Parameter	CHD severity			% severity			p value
	Mild	Moderate	Severe	Mild	Moderate	Severe	
Age (mos ± 1 sd)	31.4 ± 8.4	32.0 ± 8.9	32.5 ± 9.3	—	—	—	$<10^{-6}$
Sex							
Male	55,390	31,452	5,264	60.14	34.15	5.72	$<10^{-6}$
Female	30,931	16,519	2,740	61.63	32.91	5.46	
Laterality							
Bilateral	51,085	36,754	7,537	53.56	38.54	7.90	$<10^{-6}$
Unilateral	35,236	11,217	465	75.10	23.91	0.99	
AKC group							
Herding	17,011	8,906	1,723	61.54	32.22	6.23	
Hound	1,329	427	52	73.51	23.62	2.88	
Working	22,469	14,379	2,371	57.29	36.66	6.05	
Sporting	36,994	20,498	3,232	60.92	33.76	5.32	$<10^{-6}$
Nonsporting	4,452	2,062	413	64.27	29.77	5.96	
Terrier	1,757	605	60	72.54	24.98	2.48	
Toy	1,622	800	105	64.19	31.66	4.16	
FCI group							
Sheep and cattle	17,387	9,106	1,763	61.53	32.23	6.24	
Pinscher schnauzer, molossoid, and Swiss Mtn/cattle dog	20,179	13,430	2,371	56.08	37.33	6.59	
Terrier	1,563	552	53	72.09	25.46	2.44	
Spitz and primitive	4,106	2,120	325	62.68	32.36	4.96	$<10^{-6}$
Scent hounds	1,142	511	74	66.13	29.59	4.28	
Pointing dogs	4,981	2,496	290	64.13	32.14	3.73	
Retrievers, flushers, and water dogs	32,742	18,344	2,976	60.56	33.93	5.50	
Companion and toy dogs	3,710	1,178	126	73.99	23.49	2.51	
Sighthounds	181	85	3	67.29	31.60	1.12	
Geographic group							
<30°N	2,760	1,183	199	66.63	28.56	4.80	
30–39°N	41,628	22,781	3,711	61.11	33.44	5.45	$<10^{-6}$
40–49°N	36,358	20,619	3,498	60.12	34.10	5.78	
≥50°N	5,335	3,235	580	58.31	35.36	6.34	
Season of birth							
Autumn	19,795	10,644	1,722	61.55	33.10	5.35	
Winter	21,512	12,101	1,960	60.47	34.02	5.51	$<10^{-6}$
Spring	24,728	14,456	2,503	59.32	34.68	6.00	
Summer	20,286	10,770	1,819	61.71	32.76	5.53	

It must be remembered that many of these studies used a different grading system than the OFA scores; however, it still confirms marked variability within breeds within each study.

The quoted prevalence of CHD is frequently different between different studies for a particular breed. When comparing the data of Witsberger et al. [20] to ours, the prevalence of CHD for the Newfoundland was 17.2% versus 20.0%, Saint Bernard 14.7% versus 36.8%, Rottweiler 10.3% versus 12.5%, German Shepherd 10.3% versus 16.3%, Golden Retriever 8.5% versus 14.9%, Labrador Retriever 7.4% versus 9.2%, Bulldog 4.4% versus 68.9%, Doberman Pinscher 1.3% versus 5.1%, and Greyhound 0.4% versus 2.1%, respectively. This demonstrates that the sampling technique/composition of the data set markedly impacts the prevalence value as previously mentioned. Prevalence amongst each breed within a country, or region, is likely a result of gene flow, bottle necks, popular sire effects, and the efforts of individuals and breed clubs to impact the prevalence and severity of CHD in a particular breed.

We noted a slight increase in CHD in females with marked differences by breed. Several studies noted no sex difference in the prevalence of CHD. In Norway, Turkey, and the United Kingdom no sex differences were noted for the various breeds studied [22–25]. In Sweden, CHD was 1.14 times more common in female German Shepherds compared to males [26]. In the United States, sex differences were noted in Golden Retrievers [27]; the prevalence of CHD was 5.1% in intact males, 10.3% in males neutered early, 0% in males neutered late, 39% in intact females, 4.5% in females neutered early, and 0% in females neutered late. The status of neutering in the OFA registry is not given, so we cannot compare our findings to those of Torres de la Riva [27].

The prevalence of unilateral CHD was 33% in this study. The prevalence of unilateral CHD was 35% in a New York study of 1022 dogs consisting of Labrador Retrievers, Golden Retrievers, German Shepherds, and crossbreeds [2]. In Pennsylvania, it was 6% in 133 Greyhounds. A recent study of multiple breeds from Italy noted an overall percentage of unilateral CHD of 31.5% [28], strikingly similar to the 33% in this study and the 35% of Lust et al. [2]. This is the first study to investigate the proportion of unilateral CHD by AKC/FCI groups; for AKC groups it was highest in herding dogs (35.4%) and lowest in terriers (27.5%); for FCI groups it was highest in sheep/cattle dogs (35.4%) and lowest in terriers (25.1%) (Table 1).

Few studies discuss season of birth and CHD. In Norway [29], the OR for CHD (Newfoundland, Leonberger, Labrador Retriever, and Irish Wolfhounds) was 3.94 times higher in autumn and 1.85 times higher in winter compared to spring. In another Norwegian study [9], pointers had an increase in CHD in those born in August to February, Labrador Retrievers September to February, with no seasonal effect on CHD in German Shepherds or Golden Retrievers. In Finland [7], German Shepherds born in spring or summer had less CHD. In England [10], Labrador Retrievers and Gordon Setters had less CHD when born in July through October. In New Zealand [8], Labrador Retrievers and Rottweilers had less CHD when born in autumn, but no seasonal variation was observed for German Shepherds or Golden Retrievers. In aggregate, the previous studies in the Northern Hemisphere noted that dogs born in autumn and/or winter months demonstrate a higher prevalence of CHD. In this study we noted an increase of CHD primarily in winter and spring months. When reviewing the data from Supplemental Table 3, 563,403 of the 619,825 dogs (81.4%) showed a seasonal variation. Of these 536,403, 313,202 (55.6%) had the highest percentage in winter, 229,925 (40.8%) in spring, and 20,276 (3.6%) in autumn.

There are several postulated reasons for seasonal differences in CHD. One is the relationship between hip muscle development and season. The most critical time for canine hip joint development is between 3 and 9 months of age [8, 30]; cage confinement during this crucial period has a protective effect on the hip [30]. The proposed explanation is that puppies born in winter spend more time in cages/indoors than in free activities, and indoor confinement may keep the hips in flexion and abduction lessening the development of CHD [29]. The same has been noted in human DDH, where carrying the infant in positions of hip abduction and flexion reduces the incidence of DDH [31–35] while swaddling in extension increases the incidence of DDH [5, 36, 37]. Our

results refute a winter protective effect in CHD. A second explanation is that puppies born in late autumn or early winter, compared to those born in spring or early summer, do not get as much physical exercise. Puppies getting less physical exercise may develop weaker hip musculature than those with a lot of outdoor activity, which when combined with rapid skeletal growth results in weakened constraints on the hip, subsequent subluxation, and CHD [8, 22, 29, 30]. This can explain the increase in CHD in dogs born in late autumn/early winter and corroborates the findings from New Zealand, England, and our study, while conflicting with the data from Norway, Finland, and Sweden.

Another postulated mechanism for CHD seasonal variation is diet and weight gain in puppies. Dogs with limited weight gain in early life have a lower prevalence of CHD [2, 22, 29, 38, 39]. In cold winter months dogs have increased food intake [40, 41], and if not accompanied by an increase in energy consumption (e.g., activity), the dog will gain weight. Increased body weight increases the stress across the developing hip joint leading to subluxation [17, 42, 43]. Vitamin D plays a role in DDH, as humans with homozygosity for the mutant Taq1 vitamin D receptor t allele demonstrate increased acetabular dysplasia [44]. Vitamin D levels may vary by season due to seasonal variation in vitamin D dietary content in both humans and animals [45–52]. Low vitamin D levels and increased body fat in winter may result in more CHD. Finally, various dietary factors differ by season and could result in seasonal differences in hormones in milk (vitamin D, relaxin, and vitamin C) and secondarily influence hip development [52–57].

This is the first description of an increased prevalence of CHD in more southern latitudes. This was true even when multivariate regression logistic analysis was performed adjusting for breed group, gender, and season of birth. One potential explanation is that the generally warmer climate in more southern latitudes may result in a general increase in physical activity at all times, with the hips being less abducted and flexed, resulting in more CHD. Another potential explanation is that the gene pools may be different in different latitudes. Finally, other environmental factors such as diet as discussed above may be involved, resulting in increased CHD. Perhaps the dogs in the more southern latitudes are heavier and place more stress across the hip. It could also be that the dogs in the warmer more southern latitudes grow more rapidly early in life, which is a well-known contributing factor to CHD [38, 39]. This finding and potential explanations will require further study.

There are marked differences and similarities between DDH and CHD (Table 5). The most striking is the difference in incidence/prevalence by race/breed. Prevalence/incidence variation in humans is higher (950-fold difference in Native Americans compared to Africans in Africa) than canines (96-fold difference in the bulldog compared to the whippet) (Supplemental Table 1). DDH occurs predominantly in females (75%) for all races [5], while for CHD the prevalence was only slightly higher in females compared to males (Table 1). However there are large sex variations in CHD which ranged from 3.4 times more frequent in female Polish Tatra Sheepdogs to 1.6 times more frequent

TABLE 5: Comparisons between DDH and CHD.

(a)

Race	Human DDH*					Canine CHD†							
	Incidence per 1000 births	% M	% F	% bilateral	% unilateral	AKC groups	Prevalence	% bilateral	% unilateral	FCI groups	Prevalence	% bilateral	% unilateral
Indigenous peoples						*Sporting dogs*	15.03	66.03	33.87	*Sheep and cattle*	15.19	64.6	35.4
Native American	95.0	30	70	50	50	Retrievers	16.52	65.68	34.32	*Pinscher schnauzer, molossoid, and Swiss mountain/cattle dog*	20.43	69.3	30.7
Sami	40.0					Movers/flushers	12.71	68.7	31.3	*Terrier*	14.91	74.9	25.1
Aboriginal	3.7					Pointers/setters	12.13	65.96	34.04	*Spitz and primitive*	10.00	70.0	30.0
						Versatile sporting	8.42	60.16	39.84	*Scent hounds*	10.13	69.9	30.7
Caucasian						Herding	15.23	64.65	35.35	*Pointing dogs*	10.46	65.0	35.0
Eastern Europe	44.2	21	79	19	81	Working	18.04	68.85	31.15	*Retrievers, flushers, and water dogs*	10.91	66.2	33.8
Mediterranean Islands	14.3					Nonsporting	13.54	71.06	28.94	*Companion and toy dogs*	15.87	69.5	30.5
Australia/New Zealand	12.0	16	84	43	57	*Terrier*	12.59	73.86	26.14	*Sighthounds*	13.52	55.0	45.0
Western Europe	8.1	21	79	19	81	*Toy*	16.43	72.51	27.49				
United Kingdom	8.0					*Hound*	10.52	69.05	30.95				
Scandinavia	7.3	21	79	41	59	Scent hounds	12.97	71.0	29.0				
South America	4.6	24	76	13	87	Sighthounds	4.64	54.2	45.8				
North America	0.8	19	81										
Indo-Mediterranean	5.5	21	79	50	50								
Indo-Malay Africans	0.4												
North America	0.5												
Africa	0.1												

(b)

Seasonal variation[‡]	n	%	Seasonal variation[†]	n	%
Single winter peak	16,425	70.3	Autumn (Sept-Nov)	20,276	2.93
Single summer peak	1,280	5.5	Winter (Dec–Feb)	312,202	45.27
Spring and autumn peaks	3,450	14.8	Spring (March–May)	229,925	33.23
No variation	2,205	9.4	Summer (June–Aug)	0	0
			No variation	128422	18.56

* Data extracted from [5].
‡ Data extracted from [6].
† Present study.

in male Afghan Hounds. DDH is usually unilateral (63.4%) [5] compared to CHD which is usually bilateral (67%). DDH demonstrates a seasonal variation in ~91.0% of cases [6], and 81.4% in CHD, which is remarkably similar. DDH was most prevalent when the baby was born in winter months (70.3%); CHD was most prevalent when the puppy was born in winter and spring. DDH is more common in northern latitudes, while CHD is more common in southern latitudes [5, 6]. This latitudinal difference has also been noted in children with Perthes' disease [58]. Within DDH there are two different types, the typical infantile DDH and the late onset adolescent/adult acetabular dysplasia [59]. The older group, when compared to the infantile group, demonstrated a lower female predominance (88.0 versus 98.0%) with more bilateral involvement (61.2% versus 45.1%). Our findings in CHD more closely mirror the demographics of DDH in the late onset group.

In conclusion, the prevalence of CHD differed markedly by breed, having a slight female predominance but with significant variability by breed, was unilateral in about one-third of cases, and often demonstrated a seasonal variation with a mild increase when the dog was born in spring and winter months. Most interestingly, CHD was more prevalent in the more southern latitudes. This information is important to owners/breeders, suggesting that monitoring of puppies for signs of CHD should be undertaken during the birth months when there is an increased OR of CHD for those affected breeds and/or AKC groups, especially in more southern latitudes. The similarities between CHD and DDH are striking, especially late onset DDH, and suggest that comparative studies of both disorders should lead to a better understanding of a problem that leads to debilitating hip osteoarthritis in both canines and humans.

Conflicts of Interest

The authors declare that they have no conflicts of interest.

Acknowledgments

The authors wish to thank Mr. Eddi Dzuik and Jon Curby, Orthopaedic Foundation for Animals, for granting the authors access to the entire hip dysplasia registry. This research was supported in part by the Garceau Professorship Endowment, Indiana University, School of Medicine, Department of Orthopaedic Surgery, and the Rapp Pediatric Orthopaedic Research Endowment, Riley Children's Foundation, Indianapolis, Indiana.

References

[1] W. H. Riser, "Canine hip dysplasia: cause and control," *Journal of the American Veterinary Medical Association*, vol. 165, no. 4, pp. 360–362, 1974.

[2] G. Lust, J. C. Geary, and B. E. Sheffy, "Development of hip dysplasia in dogs," *American Journal of Veterinary Research*, vol. 34, no. 1, pp. 87–91, 1973.

[3] G. Lust, V. T. Rendano, and B. A. Summers, "Canine hip dysplasia: concepts and diagnosis.," *Journal of the American Veterinary Medical Association*, vol. 187, no. 6, pp. 638–640, 1985.

[4] G. Lust, A. J. Williams, N. Burton-Wurster et al., "Joint laxity and its association with hip dysplasia in Labrador retrievers," *American Journal of Veterinary Research*, vol. 54, no. 12, pp. 1990–1999, 1993.

[5] R. T. Loder and E. N. Skopelja, "The epidemiology and demographics of hip dysplasia," *ISRN Orthopedics*, vol. 2011, Article ID 238607, 46 pages, 2011.

[6] R. T. Loder and C. Shafer, "Seasonal variation in children with developmental dysplasia of the hip," *Journal of Children's Orthopaedics*, vol. 8, no. 1, pp. 11–22, 2014.

[7] M. Leppänen, K. Mäki, J. Juga, and H. Saloniemi, "Factors affecting hip dysplasia in German shepherd dogs in Finland: efficacy of the current improvement programme," *Journal of Small Animal Practice*, vol. 41, no. 1, pp. 19–23, 2000.

[8] A. J. Worth, J. P. Bridges, N. J. Cave, and G. Jones, "Seasonal variation in the hip score of dogs as assessed by the New Zealand Veterinary Association Hip Dysplasia scheme," *New Zealand Veterinary Journal*, vol. 60, no. 2, pp. 110–114, 2012.

[9] I. Hanssen, "Hip dysplasia in dogs in relation to their month of birth," *Veterinary Record*, vol. 128, no. 18, pp. 425–426, 1991.

[10] J. L. N. Wood and K. H. Lakhani, "Effect of month of birth on hip dysplasia in labrador retrievers and Gordon setters," *Veterinary Record*, vol. 152, no. 3, pp. 69–72, 2003.

[11] S. Ohlerth, J. Lang, A. Busato, and C. Gaillard, "Estimation of genetic population variables for six radiographic criteria of hip dysplasia in a colony of Labrador Retrievers," *American Journal of Veterinary Research*, vol. 62, no. 6, pp. 846–852, 2001.

[12] S. Malm, W. F. Fikse, B. Danell, and E. Strandberg, "Genetic variation and genetic trends in hip and elbow dysplasia in Swedish Rottweiler and Bernese Mountain Dog," *Journal of Animal Breeding and Genetics*, vol. 125, no. 6, pp. 403–412, 2008.

[13] D. C. Coile, *Barron's Encyclopedia of Dog Breeds*, Barron's Educational Series, Hauppage, New York, NY, USA, 2nd edition, 2005.

[14] FCI breeds nomenclature, http://www.fci.be/en/Nomenclature/.

[15] H. G. Parker, "Genomic analyses of modern dog breeds," *Mammalian Genome*, vol. 23, no. 1, pp. 19–27, 2012.

[16] M. Rimbault and E. A. Ostrander, "So many doggone traits: mapping genetics of multiple phenotypes in the domestic dog," *Human Molecular Genetics*, vol. 21, no. 1, pp. R52–R57, 2012.

[17] F. H. Comhaire and F. Snaps, "Comparison of two canine registry databases on the prevalence of hip dysplasia by breed and the relationship of dysplasia with body weight and height," *American Journal of Veterinary Research*, vol. 69, no. 3, pp. 330–333, 2008.

[18] J.-P. Genevois, D. Remy, E. Viguier et al., "Prevalence of hip dysplasia according to official radiographic screening, among 31 breeds of dogs in France. A retrospective study," *Veterinary and Comparative Orthopaedics and Traumatology*, vol. 21, no. 1, pp. 21–24, 2008.

[19] E. LaFond, G. J. Breur, and C. C. Austin, "Breed susceptibility for developmental orthopedic diseases in dogs," *Journal of the American Animal Hospital Association*, vol. 38, no. 5, pp. 467–477, 2002.

[20] T. H. Witsberger, J. Armando Villamil, L. G. Schultz, A. W. Hahn, and J. L. Cook, "Prevalence of and risk factors for hip dysplasia and cranial cruciate ligament deficiency in dogs," *Journal of the American Veterinary Medical Association*, vol. 232, no. 12, pp. 1818–1824, 2008.

[21] J. L. Rettenmaier, G. G. Keller, J. C. Lattimer, E. A. Corley, and M. R. Ellersieck, "Prevalence of canine hip dysplasia in a veterinary teaching hospital population," *Veterinary Radiology and Ultrasound*, vol. 43, no. 4, pp. 313–318, 2002.

[22] R. I. Krontveit, A. Nødtvedt, B. K. Sævik, E. Ropstad, H. K. Skogmo, and C. Trangerud, "A prospective study on Canine Hip Dysplasia and growth in a cohort of four large breeds in Norway (1998-2001)," *Preventive Veterinary Medicine*, vol. 97, no. 3-4, pp. 252–263, 2010.

[23] M. Sarierler, "Comparison of femoral inclination angle measurements in dysplastic and nondysplastic dogs of different breeds," *Acta Veterinaria Hungarica*, vol. 52, no. 2, pp. 245–252, 2004.

[24] J. L. N. Wood, K. H. Lakhani, and R. Dennis, "Heritability and epidemiology of canine hip-dysplasia score in flat-coated retrievers and Newfoundlands in the United Kingdom," *Preventive Veterinary Medicine*, vol. 46, no. 2, pp. 75–86, 2000.

[25] B. Freeman, V. B. Evans, and N. R. McEwan, "Canine hip dysplasia in Irish water spaniels: two decades of gradual improvement," *Veterinary Record*, vol. 173, no. 3, pp. 72–73, 2013.

[26] A. Hedhammar, S. E. Olsson, S. A. Andersson et al., "Canine hip dysplasia: study of heritability in 401 litters of German Shepherd dogs," *Journal of the American Veterinary Medical Association*, vol. 174, no. 9, pp. 1012–1016, 1979.

[27] G. Torres de la Riva, B. L. Hart, T. B. Farver et al., "Neutering dogs: effects on joint disorders and cancers in Golden Retrievers," *PLoS ONE*, vol. 8, no. 2, Article ID e55937, 2013.

[28] S. Citi, M. Vignoli, M. Modenato, F. Rossi, and J. P. Morgan, "A radiological study of the incidence of unilateral canine hip dysplasia," *Schweizer Archiv fur Tierheilkunde*, vol. 147, no. 4, pp. 173–178, 2005.

[29] R. I. Krontveit, A. Nødtvedt, B. K. Sævik, E. Ropstad, and C. Trangerud, "Housing- and exercise-related risk factors associated with the development of hip Dysplasia as determined by radiographic evaluation in a prospective cohort of Newfoundlands, Labrador retrievers, Leonbergers, and Irish wolfhounds in Norway," *American Journal of Veterinary Research*, vol. 73, no. 6, pp. 838–846, 2012.

[30] W. H. Riser, "A new look at developmental subluxation and dislocation: hip dysplasia in the dog," *Journal of Small Animal Practice*, vol. 4, no. 6, pp. 421–434, 1963.

[31] M. Janecek, "Congenital hip dislocation in children in Northern Korea," *Acta chirurgiae orthopaedicae et traumatologiae Cechoslovaca*, vol. 23, no. 1, pp. 2–5, 1956.

[32] J. R. Corea, "Is congenital dislocation of the hip rare in Sri Lanka?" *The Ceylon Medical Journal*, vol. 37, no. 3, p. 96, 1992.

[33] J. Edelstein, "Congenital dislocation of the hip in the Bantu," *The Journal of Bone & Joint Surgery—British Volume*, vol. 48, no. 2, p. 397, 1966.

[34] J. C. Griffiths, "Dislocated hip in East African infants and children," *Postgraduate Medical Journal*, vol. 46, no. 532, pp. 86–91, 1970.

[35] A. P. Skirving and W. J. Scadden, "The African neonatal hip and its immunity from congenital dislocation," *Journal of Bone and Joint Surgery - Series B*, vol. 61, no. 3, pp. 339–341, 1979.

[36] S. H. Blatt, "To swaddle, or not to swaddle? Paleoepidemiology of developmental dysplasia of the hip and the swaddling dilemma among the indigenous populations of North America," *American Journal of Human Biology*, vol. 27, no. 1, pp. 116–128, 2015.

[37] R. B. Salter, "Etiology, pathogenesis and possible prevention of congenital dislocation of the hip," *Canadian Medical Association Journal*, vol. 98, no. 20, pp. 933–945, 1968.

[38] R. D. Kealy, S. E. Olsson, K. L. Monti et al., "Effects of limited food consumption on the incidence of hip dysplasia in growing dogs," *Journal of the American Veterinary Medical Association*, vol. 201, no. 6, pp. 857–863, 1992.

[39] R. D. Kealy, D. F. Lawler, J. M. Ballam et al., "Evaluation of the effect of limited food consumption on radiographic evidence of osteoarthritis in dogs," *Journal of the American Veterinary Medical Association*, vol. 217, no. 11, pp. 1678–1680, 2000.

[40] M. D. Finke, "Evaluation of the energy requirements of adult kennel dogs," *Journal of Nutrition*, vol. 121, no. 11, pp. S22–S28, 1991.

[41] J. L. Durrer and J. P. Hannon, "Seasonal variations in caloric intake of dogs living in an arctic environment," *The American Journal of Physiology*, vol. 202, no. 2, pp. 375–378, 1962.

[42] S. L. Sanderson, "The epidemic of canine obesity and its role in osteoarthritis," *Israel Journal of Veterinary Medicine*, vol. 67, no. 4, pp. 195–202, 2012.

[43] A. J. German, "The growing problem of obesity in dogs and cats," *Journal of Nutrition*, vol. 136, no. 7, pp. 1940S–1946S, 2006.

[44] B. Kapoor, C. Dunlop, C. Wynn-Jones, A. A. Fryer, R. C. Strange, and N. Maffulli, "Vitamin D and oestrogen receptor polymorphisms in developmental dysplasia of the hip and primary protrusio acetabuli—a preliminary study," *Journal of Negative Results in BioMedicine*, vol. 6, article 7, 2007.

[45] R. P. Stryd, T. J. Gilbertson, and M. N. Brunden, "A seasonal variation study of 25-hydroxyvitamin D3 serum levels in normal humans," *Journal of Clinical Endocrinology and Metabolism*, vol. 48, no. 5, pp. 771–775, 1979.

[46] M. J. McKenna, "Differences in vitamin D status between countries in young adults and the elderly," *The American Journal of Medicine*, vol. 93, no. 1, pp. 69–77, 1992.

[47] S. S. Harris and B. Dawson-Hughes, "Seasonal changes in plasma 25-hydroxyvitamin D concentrations of young American black and white women," *American Journal of Clinical Nutrition*, vol. 67, no. 6, pp. 1232–1236, 1998.

[48] R. Andersen, C. Mølgaard, L. T. Skovgaard et al., "Teenage girls and elderly women living in northern europe have low winter vitamin D status," *European Journal of Clinical Nutrition*, vol. 59, no. 4, pp. 533–541, 2005.

[49] C. Karohl, S. Su, M. Kumari et al., "Heritability and seasonal variability of vitamin D concentrations in male twins," *American Journal of Clinical Nutrition*, vol. 92, no. 6, pp. 1393–1398, 2010.

[50] G. Snellman, H. Melhus, R. Gedeborg et al., "Seasonal genetic influence on serum 25-hydroxyvitamin D levels: a twin study," *PLoS ONE*, vol. 4, no. 11, 2009.

[51] M. Wacker and M. F. Holiack, "Vitamin D-effects on skeletal and extraskeletal health and the need for supplementation," *Nutrients*, vol. 5, no. 1, pp. 111–148, 2013.

[52] J. E. Parker, K. I. Timm, B. B. Smith et al., "Seasonal interaction of serum vitamin D concentration and bone density in alpacas," *American Journal of Veterinary Research*, vol. 63, no. 7, pp. 948–953, 2002.

[53] C. J. Laing, R. Malik, D. I. Wigney, and D. R. Fraser, "Seasonal vitamin D status of Greyhounds in Sydney," *Australian Veterinary Journal*, vol. 77, no. 1, pp. 35–38, 1999.

[54] P. H. Mäenpää, T. Koskinen, and E. Koskinen, "Serum profiles of vitamins A, E and D in mares and foals during different

seasons," *Journal of animal science*, vol. 66, no. 6, pp. 1418–1423, 1988.

[55] Y. Adkins, A. J. Lepine, and B. Lönnerdal, "Changes in protein and nutrient composition of milk throughout lactation in dogs," *American Journal of Veterinary Research*, vol. 62, no. 8, pp. 1266–1272, 2001.

[56] L. T. Goldsmith, G. Lust, and B. G. Steinetz, "Transmission of relaxin from lactating bitches to their offspring via suckling," *Biology of Reproduction*, vol. 50, no. 2, pp. 258–265, 1994.

[57] C. R. Heinze, L. M. Freeman, C. R. Martin, M. L. Power, and A. J. Fascetti, "Comparison of the nutrient composition of commercial dog milk replacers with that of dog milk," *Journal of the American Veterinary Medical Association*, vol. 244, no. 12, pp. 1413–1422, 2014.

[58] D. C. Perry, D. M. G. MacHin, D. Pope et al., "Racial and geographic factors in the incidence of Legg-Calvé-Perthes' disease: a systematic review," *American Journal of Epidemiology*, vol. 175, no. 3, pp. 159–166, 2012.

[59] C. B. Lee, A. Mata-Fink, M. B. Millis, and Y.-J. Kim, "Demographic differences in adolescent-diagnosed and adult-diagnosed acetabular dysplasia compared with infantile developmental dysplasia of the hip," *Journal of Pediatric Orthopaedics*, vol. 33, no. 2, pp. 107–111, 2013.

25

Body Weight and Scrotal-Testicular Biometry in Three Indigenous Breeds of Bucks in Arid and Semiarid Agroecologies, Ethiopia

Amare Eshetu Gemeda and Kefelegn Workalemahu

College of Veterinary Medicine, Haramaya University, P.O. Box 138, Dire Dawa, Ethiopia

Correspondence should be addressed to Amare Eshetu Gemeda; amare.eshetu@yahoo.com

Academic Editor: Vito Laudadio

The body weight and testicular and epididymal parameters of Afar, Long-eared Somali (LES), and Woyto-Guji (WG) breeds of goat were investigated. A total of 405 randomly selected bucks of Afar ($n = 135$), Long-eared Somali ($n = 135$), and Woyto-Guji ($n = 135$) were included in this study. The overall mean scrotal circumference (SC), testicular volume (TV), testicular length (TL), testicular weight (TW), body weight (BW), epididymal weight (EW), body condition score, and testicular diameter (TD) measurements in all bucks were 20.8 ± 1.94 cm, 68.1 ± 6.18, 4.96 ± 0.79 cm, 70.0 ± 5.66 g, 22.1 ± 2.98 Kg, 9.09 ± 1.88 g, 2.55 ± 0.68, and 4.28 ± 0.45 cm, respectively. Significant ($p < 0.05$) breed differences in SC, TD, TL, TW, BW, EW, and TV were recorded. Long-eared Somali (LES) breed was heaviest and Afar breed was the lightest and Woyto-Guji (WG) had the average BW. In all breeds, the parameters were positively correlated. In Afar breed, the TW had a significant correlation with BW ($r = 0.90$) and SC ($r = 0.65$). In LES BW was highly correlated with TD ($r = 0.96$) and TL ($r = 0.96$). In WG, TW was significantly correlated with TD ($r = 0.94$), EW ($r = 0.90$), TL ($r = 0.89$), and BW ($r = 0.82$). In multiple regression analysis the linear combinations of BCS, SC, and BW significantly predicted TW, TL, TV, TD, and EW in all breeds. In conclusion, Long-eared Somali breed displayed greater BW and scrotal and testicular traits.

1. Introduction

In Ethiopia nearly 22.78 million goats are reared in mixed, pastoral, and agropastoral production systems in extensive farming for different purposes such as sociocultural reasons, milk, meat production, and cash generation [1, 2]. These goats due to their small body size, short reproductive cycle, broad feeding habits, and adaptation strategy to unfavorable environmental conditions such as scarce feed resources are preferred by framers [3–6]. Moreover incorporating goats in grazing systems of a mixed animal species results in efficient use of the natural resources with supple management of livestock environments [5].

Reproductive parameters determine several aspects of goat production including genetic improvement, so adequate data on reproduction in native breeds of goats in Ethiopia is essential for reproductive management and to set up feasible breeding schema [7, 8]. In goat's production, buck fertility influences flock performance and reproductive efficiency compared to the fertility of individual doe [7]; thus, selection of highly fertile bucks is vital for improved goat production [9, 10]. Therefore, to improve goat production in the tropics, the reproductive efficiency and fertility of the bucks require attention [11]. In contrast, fertility studies in livestock have generally tended to focus on the female side with less emphasis on the male [11].

Data on goat reproductive organs morphometric values is useful in breeding soundness evaluation (BSE) to determine fertility potential of breeding males. Such data includes scrotal circumference measurements, an integral part of BSE of animals with a pendulous scrotum [12], particularly, in bulls due to their high correlations with testicular size and sperm production capacity [12, 13]. Parameters such as body size and testicular measurements are also commonly employed in breeding soundness evaluations [14]. Among the selection criteria, testis size is the most suitable parameter to indirectly improve the reproductive performance of females [15, 16]. Furthermore, testicular size is a reliable parameter of the status of reproductive growth, spermatogenesis, and seminal characteristics [17]. However, most works of these natures have been done in bulls but it also relates to other species [18]. Also, information on similar relationship is limited in bucks [13].

The Long-eared Somali, Woyto-Guji, and Afar goats are large-, medium-, and small-sized animals, respectively, that dominate a large part of the arid and semiarid agroecologies of Ethiopia. The Afar breed is distributed in the Rift Valley strip, Danakil depression, Gewane, and northern and western Hararghe, whereas the Long-eared Somali breed is distributed in Ogaden, the lowlands of Bale, Borena, and southern Sidama, and the WG breed is distributed in North and South Omo, southern Sidama, and parts of Wolayta. These goat breeds are adapted to arid and semiarid agroclimates and managed mainly under the pastoral farming systems [19–21]. They represent dominant goat breeds of the slaughter flock in the modern export abattoirs in Ethiopia, which export goat meat to the Middle East [7]. In Ethiopia, prior studies on indigenous goat breeds were focused on the reproductive traits and fertility of female not male goats; as a result, data on fertility and male reproductive traits in indigenous goats in Ethiopia is scant [22, 23]. In view of these, parameters that are relevant to breeding soundness of buck should be assessed. Therefore, the present study was designed and conducted to examine body weight and scrotal and testicular parameters in three indigenous goat breeds in arid and semiarid parts of Ethiopia.

2. Materials and Methods

2.1. Study Area. The study was conducted on apparently health bucks presented for slaughter at Luna Export Abattoir located in Modjo (8°35′N, 39°7′E) town, Lume district, Eastern Shewa Administrative Zone of Oromia Regional State, central Ethiopia. Modjo is located 73 kilometers southeast of Addis Ababa. Luna Export Abattoir exports fresh chilled small ruminant, mainly young male goat meat to the Middle East and African countries [24].

2.2. Study Animals and Data Collection. This study was conducted on apparently healthy bucks which belong to three Ethiopian indigenous goat breeds, namely, Afar locally named Adal or Danakil; Woyto-Guji (WG) locally named Woyto, Guji, and Konso; and Long-eared Somali (LES): its local names Degheir, Galla, Digodi, and Melebo [19, 21]. The breeds of the goat were categorized as per the physical characteristics described by FARM-Africa [19] and ESGPIP [21]. A total of 405 bucks including 135 animals in each breed were randomly selected from a population of bucks presented for slaughter. Accordingly, for respective breed study goats were grouped into three age classes, that is, less than 1 year; 1 to 2 years; and more than 2 years of age. Bucks were grouped according to their age using the dentition method for African

indigenes goat [25]. Each buck considered for this study was assigned an identifier number that was used for both ante- and postmortem examinations. Prior to slaughter of bucks their testes and scrotum were examined for size, symmetry, and consistence as described by [13]. During antemortem examination genital organs of each animal were cautiously examined for the presence of any abnormalities and bucks with signs of clinical problems and gross abnormalities of reproductive organs were omitted from this study [24]. Thus, animals included in this study were confirmed to be free of any gross ante- or postmortem abnormalities and disorders of the genital organs.

At antemortem study prior to the slaughter, live body parameters such as age, body condition score (BCS), body weight (BW, Kg), and scrotal circumference (SC, cm) of each animal were examined and recorded. Body condition score was evaluated as per the method described by Steele [26], Ford et al. [27], and Okere et al. [28]. The scores ranged from 1 = emaciated to 5 = obese. The live body weight (BW; kg) of each animal was recorded before slaughter using a portable balance. Scrotal circumference (SC) was measured according to the method described by Goyal and Memon [13] using nonstretchable measuring tape.

Immediately after bucks were slaughtered, the testes with epididymides of each animal were collected and put into plastic bags labeled with animals particularities and transported in an ice pack to the laboratory where the epididymides were separated from testes and then testicular and epididymal parameters including testicular weights (TW, g), testicular diameter (TD, cm), testicular length (TL, cm), testicular volume (TV), and epididymal weights (EW, g) were measured and recorded for each animal according to methods and procedures adopted from Oyeyemi et al. [29] and Ajao et al. [11]. In brief, testicular weight (TW) and epididymal weight (EW) in gram (g) were measured using a general purpose weighing balance. Testicular diameter (cm) was measured around the widest point at an area that is equidistant to the testicular poles. Testicular length (cm) was also measured along the longitudinal axis of the testis beginning from one pole of the testis to the other pole, while testicular volume (TV, ml) was measured by using a water displacement technique [11, 29, 30].

2.3. Statistical Analysis. The right and left testicular and epididymal measurements were obtained separately; however, the average values of the paired organs were used in the analysis. The data obtained were summarized as mean ± standard deviation and were analyzed using statistical tools of SPSS for Windows version 17.0 (SPSS Inc., Chicago, IL, USA). The effect of breed on body condition (BCS), body weight (BW), and testicular/epididymal measurements was analyzed by one-way analysis of variance (ANOVA). Correlations among the testicular and epididymal parameters with body weight and between the parameters were evaluated. Separate prediction models (multiple regression equations) were developed for each breed to predict testicular and epididymal parameters.

TABLE 1: Mean body weight, body condition, and scrotal and testicular measurements in bucks of three breeds in arid and semiarid agroecologies, Ethiopia (mean ± SD).

Measurements	Breeds			
	Afar (n = 135)	LES (n = 135)	WG (n = 135)	Overall
Scrotal circumference	20.5 ± 2.10[a]	21.4 ± 1.67[b]	20.6 ± 1.93[a]	20.8 ± 1.94
Testicular volume	67.1 ± 6.77[a]	69.8 ± 5.83[b]	67.3 ± 5.92[a]	68.1 ± 6.18
Testicular length	4.47 ± 0.90[a]	5.44 ± 0.55[b]	4.99 ± 0.57[c]	4.97 ± 0.79
Testicular weight	67.6 ± 3.49[a]	74.8 ± 5.81[b]	67.6 ± 3.97[a]	70.0 ± 5.66
Body weight	19.7 ± 2.16[a]	24.5 ± 2.71[b]	21.9 ± 1.84[c]	22.1 ± 2.98
Epididymal weight	10.7 ± 1.20[a]	11.1 ± 1.44[b]	7.92 ± 1.06[c]	9.09 ± 1.88
Testicular diameter	4.06 ± 0.24[a]	4.59 ± 0.49[b]	4.19 ± 0.39[c]	4.28 ± 0.45
Body condition score	2.52 ± 0.71[a]	2.59 ± 0.50[a]	2.54 ± 0.71[a]	2.55 ± 0.68

[a,b,c]Means in the same row and with different superscript have significant difference (p < 0.05). LES: Long-eared Somali; WG: Woyto-Guji.

TABLE 2: Correlations between live weight and testicular/epididymal traits in Afar and Long-eared Somali (LES) breeds.

	BCS	SC	TV	TL	TD	TW	BW	EW
BCS	1	0.13[ns]	0.29[**]	0.18[*]	0.26[**]	0.28[**]	0.17[ns]	0.19[*]
SC	0.42[**]	1	0.44[**]	0.82[**]	0.83[**]	0.65[**]	0.54[**]	0.87[**]
TV	0.27[**]	0.32[**]	1	0.61[**]	0.60[**]	0.64[**]	0.60[**]	0.43[**]
TL	0.48[**]	0.83[**]	0.22[*]	1	0.97[**]	0.86[**]	0.82[**]	0.73[**]
TD	0.38[**]	0.85[**]	0.27[**]	0.92[**]	1	0.80[**]	0.78[*]	0.80[**]
TW	0.49[**]	0.88[**]	0.17[*]	0.90[**]	0.88[**]	1	0.90[**]	0.52[**]
BW	0.41[**]	0.86[**]	0.23[**]	0.96[**]	0.96[**]	0.91[**]	1	0.47[**]
EW	0.36[**]	0.76[**]	0.10[ns]	0.82[**]	0.68[**]	0.80[**]	0.82[**]	1

BSC: body condition score; SC: scrotal circumference; TV: testicular volume; TL: testicular length; TW: testicular weight; BW: body weight; EW: epididymal weight; TD: testicular diameter; [**]p < 0.01; [*]p < 0.05; ns: not significant. Values above the diagonal are for Afar while those below are for Long-eared Somali goats.

The final model fitted was set out using the following equation [31]:

$$Y_i = B_0 + B_1 X_1 + B_2 X_2 + B_3 X_3 + \cdots + B_n X_n, \quad (1)$$

where Y_i is the testicular weights (TW), testicular diameter (TD), testicular length (TL), testicular volume (TV), and epididymal weights (EW); $X_1, \ldots, X_n$ are the body condition, scrotal circumference, and body weight; B_0 is the intercept; $B_1, \ldots, B_n$ are the multiple regression coefficients of the independent variables $X_1, \ldots, X_n$.

3. Results

The mean body weight, scrotal circumference, epididymal weight, and testicular traits with respect to breed are shown in Table 1. The overall scrotal circumference (SC), testicular volume (TV), testicular length (TL), testicular weight (TW), body weight (BW), epididymal weight (EW), body condition score, and testicular diameter (TD) measurements in all bucks were 20.8 ± 1.94 cm, 68.1 ± 6.18, 4.96 ± 0.79 cm, 70.0 ± 5.66 g, 22.1 ± 2.98 Kg, 9.09 ± 1.88 g, 2.55 ± 0.68, and 4.28 ± 0.45 cm, respectively.

Analysis and comparison of measurements in the three indigenous breeds show that Afar, Long-eared Somali (LES), and Woyto-Guji (WG) breeds display significant differences (p < 0.05) in scrotal circumference (SC), testicular volume (TV), testicular length (TL), testicular weight (TW), body

weight (BW), epididymal weight (EW), and testicular diameter (TD). Long-eared Somali (LES) breed scored significantly higher measurement values for most of the traits followed by Woyto-Guji (WG) and Afar breeds.

Results of the correlation analysis between live body and epididymal and testicular measurements as described by Pearson correlation coefficients in Afar, Long-eared Somali, and Woyto-Guji breeds are summarized in Tables 2 and 3. In Afar bucks the testes weight had a highly significant correlation with body weight (r = 0.90, p < 0.01), testicular length (r = 0.86, p < 0.01), testicular diameter (r = 0.80, p < 0.01), testicular volume (r = 0.64, p < 0.01), and scrotal circumference (r = 0.65, p < 0.01). In Long-eared Somali (LES) breed, the highest correlation coefficients were observed for body weight and testicular diameter (r = 0.96, p < 0.01) and body weight and testicular length (r = 0.96, p < 0.01), followed by testicular diameter and testicular length (r = 0.92, p < 0.01) and body weight and testicular weight (r = 0.91, p < 0.01). In Woyto-Guji (WG) breed, testicular weight was highly and significantly correlated with testicular diameter (r = 0.94, p < 0.01), epididymal weight (r = 0.90, p < 0.01), testicular length (r = 0.89, p < 0.01), and body weight (r = 0.82, p < 0.01).

The regression coefficients and R^2 values of testicular variables and epididymal weight from live body parameters estimation with their level of significance using linear regression models for Afar breed are shown in Table 4. The linear

TABLE 3: Correlations between live body measurements and epididymal/testicular traits in Woyto-Guji breed.

	BCS	SC	TV	TL	TD	TW	BW	EW
BCS	1	0.15^{ns}	0.24^{**}	0.36^{**}	0.40^{**}	0.40^{**}	0.37^{**}	0.40^{**}
SC	0.15^{ns}	1	0.67^{**}	0.67^{**}	0.72^{**}	0.77^{**}	0.66^{**}	0.66^{**}
TV	0.24^{**}	0.67^{**}	1	0.38^{**}	0.51^{**}	0.55^{**}	0.41^{**}	0.36^{**}
TL	0.36^{**}	0.67^{**}	0.38^{**}	1	0.96^{**}	0.89^{**}	0.95^{**}	0.98^{**}
TD	0.40^{**}	0.72^{**}	0.51^{**}	0.96^{**}	1	0.94^{**}	0.92^{**}	0.96^{**}
TW	0.40^{**}	0.77^{**}	0.55^{**}	0.89^{**}	0.94^{**}	1	0.82^{**}	0.90^{**}
BW	0.37^{**}	0.66^{**}	0.41^{**}	0.95^{**}	0.92^{**}	0.82^{**}	1	0.94^{**}
EW	0.40^{**}	0.66^{**}	0.36^{**}	0.98^{**}	0.96^{**}	0.90^{**}	0.94^{**}	1

BSC: body condition score; SC: scrotal circumference; TV: testicular volume; TL: testicular length; TW: testicular weight; BW: body weight; EW: epididymal weight; TD: testicular diameter; $^{**}p < 0.01$; ns: not significant.

TABLE 4: Multivariable regression analysis of testicular and epididymal parameters of Afar bucks in Ethiopia.

Parameter	Predictors	B	S. error	Beta	t	Sig.	R	R^2	Adjusted R^2
TW	Constant	33.8	1.27		26.6	***			
	SC	0.38	0.07	0.22	5.79	***	0.93	0.87	0.86
	BW	1.23	0.06	0.77	20.1	***			
	BCS	0.58	0.16	0.12	3.68	***			
TL	Constant	−4.07	0.31		−12.9	***			
	SC	0.24	0.02	0.53	14.7	***	0.94	0.88	0.87
	BW	0.22	0.02	0.53	14.7	***			
	BCS	0.31	0.34	0.02	0.79	ns			
TD	Constant	1.83	0.08		22.1	***			
	SC	0.06	0.004	0.56	14.4	***	0.93	0.86	0.85
	BW	0.05	0.004	0.46	11.6	***			
	BCS	0.03	0.01	0.12	3.43	**			
EW	Constant	−0.5	0.58		−0.86	ns			
	SC	0.52	0.03	0.87	17.2	***	0.87	0.77	0.76
	BW	−0.01	0.03	−0.02	−0.29	ns			
	BCS	0.14	0.07	0.08	1.93	ns			
TV	Constant	22.4	5.18		4.33	***			
	SC	0.54	0.27	0.16	1.99	*	0.65	0.42	0.41
	BW	1.53	0.25	0.49	6.10	***			
	BCS	1.83	0.65	0.19	2.84	**			

BSC: body condition score, SC: scrotal circumference, TV: testicular volume, TL: testicular length, TW: testicular weight, BW: body weight, EW: epididymal weight, and TD: testicular diameter. $^{***}p < 0.001$, $^{**}p < 0.01$, $^{*}p < 0.05$, and ns: not significant.

combinations of body condition, scrotal circumference, and body weight significantly predicted testicular and epididymal traits in Afar bucks ($p < 0.001$). In Afar breed, the standardized beta coefficients suggested that scrotal circumference contributed most to predicting testicular diameter and epididymal weight, whereas body weight stood out as most linear predictor for testicular weight. Testicular length of Afar bucks was best predicted by scrotal circumference and body weight. Testicular volume was best predicted by scrotal circumference, body weight, and body condition. Thus, an Afar bucks, weighing 18 Kg with a BCS of 3 and scrotal circumference of 18 cm, would have testicular weight, testicular length, testicular diameter, epididymal weight, and testicular volume of 64.52 g, 5.14 cm, 3.37 cm, 9.19 g, and 65,15, respectively.

Multivariable regression analysis of testicular and epididymal biometrics on live body parameters in Long-eared Somali bucks was also computed (Table 5). In Long-eared Somali bucks body weight and scrotal circumference were found to be good estimate of testicular weight, length, and diameter and epididymal weight. The predicted testicular weight, testicular length, testicular diameter, epididymal weight, and testicular volume of a Long-eared Somali buck breed weighing 26 kg with a BCS of 4 and scrotal circumference of 24 cm were 80.98 g, 5.71 cm, 4.73 cm, 12.44 g, and 72.94, respectively.

TABLE 5: Multivariable regression analysis of testicular and epididymal parameters of Long-eared Somali bucks in Ethiopia.

Parameter	Predictors	B	S. error	Beta	t	Sig.	R	R^2	Adjusted R^2
TW	Constant	22.4	1.87		11.9	* * *	0.93	0.87	0.87
	SC	1.00	0.17	0.36	5.82	* * *			
	BW	1.19	0.13	0.55	9.02	* * *			
	BCS	0.91	0.28	0.11	3.21	* *			
TL	Constant	0.21	0.14		1.55	ns	0.96	0.92	0.92
	SC	0.01	0.01	0.03	0.06	ns			
	BW	0.19	0.01	0.91	19.2	* * *			
	BCS	0.08	0.02	0.11	4.02	* * *			
TD	Constant	0.17	0.12		1.46	ns	0.96	0.93	0.93
	SC	0.02	0.01	0.90	1.93	ns			
	BW	0.16	0.01	0.89	19.4	* * *			
	BCS	−0.02	0.02	−0.03	−1.09	ns			
EW	Constant	−0.22	0.73		−0.30	ns	0.82	0.68	0.67
	SC	0.15	0.07	0.22	2.21	*			
	BW	0.33	0.05	0.63	6.49	* * *			
	BCS	0.12	0.11	0.01	0.13	ns			
TV	Constant	50.0	4.87		10.3	* * *	0.36	0.13	0.13
	SC	1.14	0.45	0.41	2.54	*			
	BW	−0.41	0.34	−0.19	−1.19	ns			
	BCS	1.56	0.74	1.97	1.97	ns			

BSC: body condition score, SC: scrotal circumference, TV: testicular volume, TL: testicular length, TW: testicular weight, BW: body weight, EW: epididymal weight, and TD: testicular diameter. $^{***}p < 0.001$, $^{**}p < 0.01$, $^{*}p < 0.05$, and ns: not significant.

The R^2 values and regression coefficients of testicular and epididymal traits from body parameters estimation with their level of significance based on linear regression models in Woyto-Guji bucks are shown in Table 6. Body weight contributed most to predicting testicular and epididymal weight, testicular diameter, and length, although scrotal circumference stood out as most linear predictor for testicular volume of Woyto-Guji bucks. Therefore, Woyto-Guji buck with body weight of 20 Kg, scrotal circumference of 20 cm, and a BCS of 3 would have 64.81 g, 3.82 cm, 4.02 cm, 6.96 g, and 66.64 of testicular weight, testicular length, testicular diameter, epididymal weight, and testicular volume, respectively.

4. Discussion

In this study, live body and testicular and epididymal parameters were evaluated in three goat breeds natives to arid and semiarid agroecologies of Ethiopia. The mean (±standard deviation) values of SC (cm), TW (g), TV, TL (cm), TD (cm), and EW (g) were 20.8 ± 1.94, 70.0 ± 5.66, 68.1 ± 6.18, 4.97±0.79, 4.28±0.45, and 9.09±1.88, respectively. The values of the testicular traits obtained in this study are higher than 17.15 ± 1.14 cm, 52.16 ± 10.29 g, and 4.71 ± 0.52 cm reported for scrotal circumference, testicular weight (g), and testicular length, respectively, in Shale bucks in humid zone of Nigeria [29]. But the mean value of testicular diameter in this study is lower than 10.97 ± 0.90 reported in Shale bucks [29]. The discrepancies in values might be due to breed differences, as it has been reported there exist breed differences in the size of the testicular parameters [13].

A measurement of scrotal circumference is an integral part of breeding soundness evaluation of animals with a pendulous scrotum, particularly in bulls [12, 13]. Furthermore, measurements of the SC are viewed as a cheap, repeatable, and objective way to estimate sperm production [32]. In this study the overall mean value of scrotal circumference in bucks was 20.8 ± 1.94 cm and it was observed that the scrotal circumference of Long-eared Somali (21.4 ± 1.67) breed was significantly ($p < 0.05$) higher than that of Afar (20.5 ± 2.10) and Woyto-Guji (20.6 ± 1.93) breeds, but there had been no significant ($p > 0.05$) disparity between Afar and Woyto-Guji breeds. Raji et al. [33] reported SC of 23.99 ± 0.17 and 20.75 ± 0.25 cm in Red Sokoto and Borno White bucks, respectively, in Nigeria which are similar to the results in this study. Furthermore, the mean values of the scrotal circumference in three breeds in the present study are higher than 15.73 cm and 17.15 ± 1.14 cm reported for African Dwarf bucks [34] and Shale bucks [29], respectively, but it was lower than 28 to 39 cm in Nubian buck [13]. These differences might be due to the effect of genotype or breed; similar reports of differences among breeds have been reported in goats [33]. Furthermore, studies suggest that, in addition to breed, season, nutrition, and body weight had an effect on SC of domestic animals [35, 36]. Thus, in this study difference in nutritional managements of bucks could also be responsible for the differences in scrotal circumference among breeds. The larger scrotal circumference value for Long-eared Somali breed, as compared to Afar and Woyto-Guji breeds, might be due to differences in size, as large-sized breeds have greater SC [20, 37]. SC is reliable measurement

TABLE 6: Multivariable regression analysis of testicular and epididymal parameters of Woyito-Guji bucks in Ethiopia.

Parameter	Predictors	B	S. error	Beta	t	Sig.	R	R^2	Adjusted R^2
TW	Constant	22.97	2.05		11.24	* * *			
	SC	0.92	0.11	0.44	8.14	* * *	0.89	0.79	0.78
	BW	1.01	0.13	0.47	8.09	* * *			
	BCS	1.08	0.29	0.16	3.74	* * *			
TL	Constant	−2.21	0.19		−11.4	* * *			
	SC	0.02	0.01	0.07	1.96	ns	0.95	0.91	0.91
	BW	0.28	0.01	0.90	23.9	* * *			
	BCS	0.01	0.03	0.01	0.49	ns			
TD	Constant	0.64	0.12		5.34	* * *			
	SC	0.04	0.01	0.23	5.43	* * *	0.93	0.87	0.87
	BW	0.12	0.01	0.72	16.4	* * *			
	BCS	0.06	0.02	0.12	3.57	* *			
EW	Constant	−4.20	0.39		−10.6	* * *			
	SC	0.05	0.02	0.08	2.08	*	0.94	0.89	0.89
	BW	0.49	0.02	0.86	20.4	* * *			
	BCS	0.12	0.06	0.07	2.18	*			
TV	Constant	24.95	4.80		5.19	* * *			
	SC	2.29	0.27	0.74	8.61	* * *	0.69	0.47	0.46
	BW	−0.48	0.29	−0.15	−1.64	ns			
	BCS	1.83	0.68	0.19	2.72	* *			

BSC: body condition score, SC: scrotal circumference, TV: testicular volume, TL: testicular length, TW: testicular weight, BW: body weight, EW: epididymal weight, and TD: testicular diameter. $^{***}p < 0.001$, $^{**}p < 0.01$, $^{*}p < 0.05$, and ns: not significant.

of reproductive status and seminal characteristics in goats [17]. For instance, a decrease in SC is an indication of an increase in morphologically abnormal sperm in an ejaculate [38]. Hence, Söderquist and Hultén [32] recommended that SC measurements could be applied to estimate testes weight and fertility in rams.

Body weight and condition influence the reproductive potential of domestic animals and body weight itself is affected by breed, age, and nutritional status of bucks [36]. In Ethiopia, Long-eared Somali, Woyto-Guji, and Afar breeds of goats are considered as large-, medium-, and small-sized animals, respectively [19, 21]. In this study the body weight was significantly ($p < 0.05$) varied between breeds. For Long-eared Somali, the mean body weight was 24.5 ± 2.71 kg, Woyto-Guji had intermediate weight of 21.9 ± 1.84 kg, and Afar breed recorded the lightest weight of 19.7 ± 2.16 kg. Breeding soundness examination of male domestic animals should consider body condition because spermatogenesis tends to be limited in poor body condition; thus, sires should be maintained in moderate condition [39]. In this study there were no significant breed ($p > 0.05$) variations in body condition score. However, Long-eared Somali, Woyto-Guji, and Afar breeds had higher body condition score than Arsi-Bale and Central highlands breeds of bucks [20]. The differences might be due to breed difference, nutritional status, and variations in climatic conditions.

Combined with other variables testicular weight can be used to select males for testicular size at puberty since it is a reliable variable for estimating the sperm production capacity [40] but it varies depending on the breed [41]. In

this study the Long-eared Somali breed had a significantly ($p < 0.05$) heavier testes weight than the Woyto-Guji and Afar breeds. The values recorded in the current study are lower than 98.4 ± 1.36 and 92.1 ± 1.88 reported in Red Sokoto and Borno White breeds in a semiarid region of Nigeria [33] but higher than 52.16 ± 10.29 reported for Shale bucks [29]. These differences might be due to differences in breed and nutritional management [41]. It has been reported that animals with heavier testes produce more spermatozoa than those with smaller testes [42]. Furthermore, the mean testes volume of the Long-eared Somali breed was significantly ($p < 0.05$) higher than that of the Woyto-Guji and Afar breeds. These disparities in the mean testes volume for the different breeds recorded in the current study agree with the report of [41] in different breeds of goats in Nigeria. In this study significant ($p < 0.05$) breed difference on epididymal weight, testicular diameter, and testicular length was apparent where Long-eared Somali breed scored significantly higher values for testicular diameter and testicular length followed by Woyto-Guji and the Afar breeds had the least values. On the other hand, epididymal weight was highest in Long-eared Somali breed followed by Afar breed and Woyto-Guji breed scored the least value.

In domestic animals, testes size and sperm production are highly correlated which implies that the larger the testes, the greater the sperm production [18]. Also, SC is good predictor of testicular size along with strong and positive associations between them [18]. In this study, in LES breed, SC had strongest correlations with TW ($r = 0.88$, $p < 0.01$) and body weight ($r = 0.86$, $p < 0.01$), while in Afar breed correlations of SC and TW ($r = 0.65$, $p < 0.01$) and SC and BW ($r = 0.54$, $p < 0.01$) were not that strong compared to that of LES. Furthermore, the correlations of SC with TW ($r = 0.77$, $p < 0.01$) and SC with that of BW ($r = 0.66$, $p < 0.01$) in WG breed were moderate. Raji et al. [33] reported the correlation coefficient of 0.81 between SC and BW in Borno white goats in Nigeria which is similar to that recorded for LES, but higher than values reported for Afar and WG breeds in this study. Furthermore, the correlation coefficients between BW and SC for LES ($r = 0.86$) and WG ($r = 0.66$) are higher than ($r = 0.53$) the correlation reported for Ogaden bucks in Ethiopia [36] which is similar to ($r = 0.54$) correlation recorded for Afar bucks in this study. They were however lower than ($r = 0.94$) correlation reported for Saneen and Jamnapuri crosses [43]. The correlation coefficients of 0.88 and 0.77 between SC and TW for LES and WG breeds, respectively, were comparable to ($r = 0.79$) that reported for red Sokoto bucks [33], which was higher than that ($r = 0.65$) recorded in Afar bucks in this study. But the values obtained in this study were lower than that ($r = 0.96$) reported in Borno white goats [33]. These differences might be due to the effect of genotype or breed [33].

BW had high and significant correlation with TW in LES ($r = 0.91$, $p < 0.001$), Afar ($r = 0.90$, $p < 0.001$), and WG ($r = 0.82$, $p < 0.001$) breeds indicating a good association between BW and TW. Similar reports of BW being significantly correlated with testicular weight were observed in different breeds of goats [11, 44]. These high, positive, and significant correlations between body weight and SC with testicular measurements suggest that either of these variables or their combinations could provide a good estimate for predicting testicular and epididymal traits. Testes weight is known to be very highly correlated with testicular sperm reserves [45]; thus males with larger testes tend to produce more sperm [46]. It has been reported that measurement of scrotal circumference, testes length, weight, and width would be a reliable predictor of the sperm producing capacity of bucks and they can be used to select for improved sperm production and breeding males [47]. In multiple linear regression analysis, simultaneous addition of body condition, scrotal circumference, and body weight were found to increase reliability of predicting testicular parameters in all three breeds. Body weight and SC were found to be a significant and good estimate of testicular measurements and EW with large standardized beta in Afar, Long-eared Somali, and Woyto-Guji breeds.

In conclusion, this study highlighted body weight and reproductive traits in bucks of three breeds native to arid and semiarid agroecologies of Ethiopia. Breed was found to influence body weight, SC, epididymal weight, and testicular biometry in Afar, Long-eared Somali, and Woyto-Guji breeds. Long-eared Somali breed displayed higher body weight, SC, and testicular measurements. The most suitable live body measurements that can be easily measured on live bucks and could be used to predict epididymal and testicular biometry were found to be SC and BW. The findings of this study could be used in breeding soundness assessment to select fertile bucks in their natural environments.

Conflicts of Interest

The authors declared that there are no conflicts of interest concerning this manuscript.

Acknowledgments

The authors would like to acknowledge administration and staffs of the abattoir for their help and support.

References

[1] A. Tesfaye, *Genetic Characterization of Indigenous Goat Populations of Ethiopia Using Microsatellite DNA Markers [Ph.D. thesis]*, NDRI, Karnal, India, 2004.

[2] CSA (Central Statistical Authority), *Agricultural Sample Survey Volume II: Report on Livestock and Livestock Characteristics in Ethiopia*, Addis Ababa, Ethiopia, 2013.

[3] A. K. Misra and K. Singh, "Effect of water deprivation on dry matter intake, nutrient utilization and metabolic water production in goats under semi-arid zone of India," *Small Ruminant Research*, vol. 46, no. 2-3, pp. 159–165, 2002.

[4] IBC (Institute of Biodiversity Conservation), *The State of Ethiopia's Farm Animal Genetic Resources: Country Report. A Contribution to the First Report on the State of the World's Animal Genetic Resources*, IBC, Addis Ababa, Ethiopia, 2004.

[5] A. Hirpa and G. Abebe, "Economic significance of sheep and goat," in *Sheep and Goat Production Handbook for Ethiopia*, A. Yami and and R. C. Merkel, Eds., Ethiopian Sheep And Goat Productivity Improvement Program, pp. 1–4, USAID, 2008.

[6] G. Umeta, M. Duguma, F. Hundesa, and M. Muleta, "Participatory analysis of problems limiting goat production at selected districts of East Showa zone, Ethiopia," *African Journal of Agricultural Research*, vol. 6, no. 26, pp. 5701–5714, 2011.

[7] M. G. Yoseph, *Reproductive Traits in Ethiopian Male Goats with Special Reference to Breed and Nutrition [Ph.D. thesis]*, Swedish University of Agricultural Sciences, Uppsala, Sweden, 2007.

[8] A. T. Alemu, *Phenotypic Characterization of Indigenous Goat Types and Their Production System in Shabelle Zone, South Eastern Ethiopia [M. S. thesis]*, Haramaya University, Dire Dawa, Ethiopia, 2007.

[9] J. Chacón, E. Pérez, E. Müller, L. Söderquist, and H. Rodríguez-Martínez, "Breeding soundness evaluation of extensively managed bulls in Costa Rica," *Theriogenology*, vol. 52, no. 2, pp. 221–231, 1999.

[10] M. A. Memon, W. D. Mickelsen, and H. O. Goyal, "Examination of the reproductive tract and evaluation of potential breeding soundness in bucks," in *Current Therapy in Large Animal Theriogenology 2*, R. S. Youngquist and W. R. Threlfall, Eds., pp. 515–518, Sounder Elsevier, Mo, USA, 2007.

[11] E. O. Ajao, M. O. Akinyemi, E. O. Ewuola, and O. H. Osaiyuwu, "Body measurements of red Sokoto bucks in Nigeria and their relationship with testicular biometrics," *Iranian Journal of Applied Animal Science*, vol. 4, no. 4, pp. 761–767, 2014.

[12] M. R. Jainudeen, H. Wahid, and E. S. E. Hafez, "Sheep and goats," in *Reproduction in Farm Animals*, E. S. E. Hafez and B. Hafez, Eds., pp. 172–181, Blackwell Publishing, Hoboken, NJ, USA, 1993.

[13] H. O. Goyal and M. A. Memon, "Clinical reproductive anatomy and physiology of the buck," in *Current Therapy in Large Animal*

Theriogenology, R. S. Youngquist and W. R. Threlfall, Eds., vol. 2, pp. 511–514, Sounder Elsevier, Mo, USA, 2007.

[14] G. E. Agga, U. Udala, F. Regassa, and A. Wudie, "Body measurements of bucks of three goat breeds in Ethiopia and their correlation to breed, age and testicular measurements," *Small Ruminant Research*, vol. 95, no. 2-3, pp. 133–138, 2011.

[15] J. R. W. Walkley and C. Smith, "The use of physiological traits in genetic selection for litter size in sheep," *Journal of Reproduction and Fertility*, vol. 59, no. 1, pp. 83–88, 1980.

[16] S. J. Schoeman, H. C. Els, and G. C. Combrink, "A preliminary investigation into the use of testis size in cross-bred rams as a selection index for ovulation rate in female relatives," *South African Journal of Animal Sciences*, vol. 17, pp. 144–147, 1987.

[17] C. S. Daudu, "Spermatozoa output, testicular sperm reserve and epididymal storage capacity of the Red Sokoto goats indigenous to northern Nigeria," *Theriogenology*, vol. 21, no. 2, pp. 317–324, 1984.

[18] H. J. Bearden, J. W. Fuquay, and S. T. Willard, *Applied Animal Reproduction*, Pearson Prentice Hall, Upper Saddle River, NJ, USA, 6th edition, 2004.

[19] FARM-Africa, "Goat Types of Ethiopia and Eritrea. Physical Description and Management Systems," Published jointly by FARM-Africa, London, UK, and ILRI (International Livestock Research Institute), Nairobi, Kenya, 1996.

[20] Y. Mekasha, A. Tegegne, A. Abera, and H. Rodriguez-Martinez, "Body size and testicular traits of tropically-adapted bucks raised under extensive husbandry in Ethiopia," *Reproduction in Domestic Animals*, vol. 43, no. 2, pp. 196–206, 2008.

[21] ESGPIP, "Ethiopia Sheep and Goat Productivity Improvement Program, Goat Breeds of Ethiopia: a Guide for Identification And Utilization," Technical Bulletin 27, 2009.

[22] A. Solomon, A. Workalemahu, M. A. Jabbar, M. M. Ahmed, and B. Hurissa, "Livestock marketing in Ethiopia: a review of structure, performance and development initiatives," in *Socioeconomics and Policy Research, Working Paper 52*, pp. 16–20, International Livestock Research Institute, Nairobi, Kenya, 2003.

[23] Y. Lorato, K. M. Ahmed, and B. Belay, "Participatory Ccharacterization of the Woyto-Guji goat and its production environment around Northern Omo, Ethiopia," *Journal of Agriculture and Natural Resources Sciences*, vol. 2, no. 2, pp. 455–465, 2015.

[24] G. Dachasa and A. G. Eshetu, "Gross reproductive organs abnormalities in rams and bucks slaughtered at luna export abattoir, Eastern Shewa Zone, Ethiopia," *Journal of Reproduction and Infertility*, vol. 6, no. 2, pp. 41–47, 2015.

[25] R. T. Wilson and J. W. Durkin, "Age at permanent incisor eruption in indigenous goats and sheep in semi-arid Africa," *Livestock Production Science*, vol. 11, no. 4, pp. 451–455, 1984.

[26] M. Steele, *The Tropical Agriculturalist (Goats)*, Macmillan, London, UK, 2nd edition, 1996.

[27] J. D. Ford, C. Okere, and O. Bolden-Tiller, "Libido test scores, body conformation and traits in Boer and Kiko goat bucks," *ARPN Journal of Agricultural and Biological Sciences*, vol. 4, pp. 54–61, 2009.

[28] C. Okere, P. Bradley, E. R. Bridges, O. Bolden-Tiller, D. Ford, and A. Paden, "Relationships among body conformation, testicular traits and semen output in electro-ejaculate pubertal Kiko goat bucks," *ARPN Journal of Agricultural and Biological Sciences*, vol. 6, pp. 43–48, 2011.

[29] M. O. Oyeyemi, A. P. Fayomi, D. A. Adeniji, and K. M. Ojo, "Testicular and epididymal parameters of Sahel buck in the humid zone of Nigeria," *International Journal of Morphology*, vol. 30, no. 2, pp. 489–492, 2012.

[30] F. Toe, J. E. O. Rege, E. Mukasa-Mugerwa et al., "Reproductive characteristics of Ethiopian highland sheep I. Genetic parameters of testicular measurements in ram lambs and relationship with age at puberty in ewe lambs," *Small Ruminant Research*, vol. 36, no. 3, pp. 227–240, 2000.

[31] N. L. Leech, K. C. Barrett, and G. A. Morgan, *SPSS for Intermediate Statistics: Use and Interpretation*, Lawrence Erlbaum Associates Publishers, London, UK, 2nd edition, 2005.

[32] L. Söderquist and F. Hultén, "Normal values for the scrotal circumference in rams of Gotlandic breed," *Reproduction in Domestic Animals*, vol. 41, no. 1, pp. 61–62, 2006.

[33] A. O. Raji, J. U. Igwebuike, and J. Aliyu, "Testicular biometry and its relationship with body weight of indigenous goats in a semi-Arid region of Nigeria," *ARPN Journal of Agricultural and Biological Science*, vol. 3, no. 4, pp. 6–9, 2008.

[34] A. H. Abu, I. A. Okwori, T. Ahemen, and L. D. Ojabo, "Evaluation of scrotal and testicular characteristics of west african dwarf bucks fed guava leaf meal," *Journal of Animal Science Advances*, vol. 6, no. 4, pp. 1636–1641, 2016.

[35] W. D. Mickelsen, L. G. Paisley, and J. J. Dahmen, "The effect of season on the scrotal circumference and sperm motility and morphology in rams," *Theriogenology*, vol. 16, no. 1, pp. 45–51, 1981.

[36] Y. Mekasha, A. Tegegne, and H. Rodriguez-Martinez, "Sperm morphological attributes in indigenous male goats raised under extensive husbandry in Ethiopia," *Animal Reproduction*, vol. 4, no. 1-2, pp. 15–22, 2007.

[37] A. M. Al-Ghalban, M. J. Tabbaa, and R. T. Kridli, "Factors affecting semen characteristics and scrotal circumference in Damascus bucks," *Small Ruminant Research*, vol. 53, no. 1-2, pp. 141–149, 2004.

[38] W. D. Mickelsen, L. G. Paisley, and J. J. Dahmen, "Seasonal variations in scrotal circumference, sperm quality, and sexual ability in rams," *Journal of the American Veterinary Medical Association*, vol. 181, no. 4, pp. 376–380, 1982.

[39] T. Parkinson, "Fertility, subfertility and infertility in male animals," in *Veterinary Reproduction and Obstetrics*, D. E. Noakes, T. J. Parkinson, and G. C. W. England, Eds., pp. 705–730, Sounders Elsevier, Philadelphia, Pa, USA, 9th edition, 2009.

[40] G. H. Coulter, L. L. Larson, and R. H. Foote, "Effect of age on testicular growth and consistency of Holstein and Angus bulls," *Journal of Animal Science*, vol. 41, no. 5, pp. 1383–1389, 1975.

[41] A. A. Ibrahim, J. Aliyu, R. M. Ashiru, and M. Jamilu, "Biometric study of the reproductive organs of three breeds of sheep in Nigeria," *International Journal of Morphology*, vol. 30, no. 4, pp. 1597–1603, 2012.

[42] L. F. C. Brito, A. E. D. F. Silva, M. M. Unanian, M. A. N. Dode, R. T. Barbosa, and J. P. Kastelic, "Sexual development in early- and late-maturing Bos indicus and Bos indicus x Bos taurus crossbred bulls in Brazil," *Theriogenology*, vol. 62, no. 7, pp. 1198–1217, 2004.

[43] T. A. Bongso, M. R. Jainudeen, and A. S. Zahrah, "Relationship of scrotal circumference to age, body weight and onset of spermatogenesis in goats," *Theriogenology*, vol. 18, no. 5, pp. 513–524, 1982.

[44] Y. Abba and I. O. Igbokwe, "Testicular and related size evaluations in nigerian sahel goats with optimal cauda epididymal sperm reserve," *Veterinary Medicine International*, vol. 2015, Article ID 357519, 5 pages, 2015.

[45] S. O. Ogwuegbu, B. O. Oko, M. O. Akusu, and T. A. Arie, "Gonadal and extra gonadal sperm reserves of the Maradi (Red Sokoto) goats," *Bulletin of Animal Health and Production in African*, vol. 33, pp. 139–141, 1985.

[46] O. E. Okwun, G. Igboeli, J. J. Ford, D. D. Lunstra, and L. Johnson, "Number and function of Sertoli cells, number and yield of spermatogonia, and daily sperm production in three breeds of boar," *Journal of Reproduction and Fertility*, vol. 107, no. 1, pp. 137–149, 1996.

[47] L. Keith, C. Okere, S. Solaimam, and O. Tiller, "Accuracy of predicting body weights from body conformation and testicular morphometry in pubertal Boer goats," *Research Journal of Animal Sciences*, vol. 3, no. 2, pp. 26–31, 2009.

26

Acute Phase Response and Neutrophils: Lymphocyte Ratio in Response to Astaxanthin in Staphylococcal Mice Mastitis Model

Tshering Dolma, Reena Mukherjee, B. K. Pati, and U. K. De

Division of Medicine, Indian Veterinary Research Institute, Izatnagar, Uttar Pradesh 243122, India

Correspondence should be addressed to Reena Mukherjee; drbapai1959@gmail.com

Academic Editor: Fulvio Riondato

The purpose of the study was to determine the immunotherapeutic effect of astaxanthin (AX) on total clinical score (TCS), C-reactive protein (CRP), and neutrophil:lymphocyte ratio in mice mastitis model challenged with pathogenic *Staphylococcus aureus*. Twenty-four lactating mice were divided in 4 equal groups: group I mice served as normal healthy control, group II, positive control, were challenged with pathogenic *S. aureus*, group III mice were challenged and treated with AX, and group IV were treated with amoxicillin plus sulbactum. The TCS was higher in postchallenged mice; however it was significantly higher in group II untreated mice as compared to group III and group IV mice. The neutrophil was higher and lymphocyte count was lower in group II mice at 120 hrs post challenge (PC). The CRP was positive in all the challenged group at 24 hrs PC, but it remained positive till 120 hrs PC in group II. The parameters are related to enhancement of the mammary defense and reduction of inflammation. Hence AX may be used alone or as an adjunct therapy with antibiotic for amelioration of mastitis. Development of such therapy may be useful to reduce the antibiotic burden in management of intramammary infection.

1. Introduction

Bovine mastitis is the inflammation of the mammary gland frequently resulting from *Staphylococcus aureus* colonization in the mammary parenchyma causing high economic losses despite intensive research and preventive measures [1]. *In vitro* antibacterial sensitivity of commonly used antibiotic-swas demonstrated by several researchers for *S. aureus* isolates [2]; however the pathogen remains difficult to eradicate with the available antibiotics. Failure in treatment could be due to nonavailability or weak penetration of the antibiotics as the organism survives intracellularly. The greatest demerits of antibiotic treatment are the development of multiple drug resistant bacterial strains and residues in the milk which possess human health hazard. World Health Organization [3] emphasizes need of judicial use of antimicrobials to combat antimicrobial resistance and also to encourage the development of novel preventive and therapeutic aids. Hence search is going on globally for an alternative to antibiotic, or to reduce its dose and duration for therapy. Astaxanthin (AX) is a xanthophyll carotenoid, predominantly of marine origin and naturally obtained from the chlorophyte algae *Haematococcus pluvialis* [4]. Astaxanthin is a highly potent antioxidant apart from it, it anti-inflammatory, immunomodulatory and antibacterial activities [5–8]. Therefore, the present study was undertaken to determine the effect of AX on acute phase protein, neutrophils:lymphocyte ratio, histopathological changes, and clinical recovery in murine staphylococcal mastitis model.

2. Materials and Methods

2.1. Antibiotic Sensitivity Test (ABST) and Minimum Inhibitory Concentration (MIC) of AX. Astaxanthin was procured from a reputed pharmaceutical company (Zenith Pharmaceuticals, Bangalore, India). Ten mg powder was reconstituted in 10 mL sterile saline solution (NSS), filtered through membrane filter (0.22 μm pore size), and stored in sterile vials. ABST of astaxanthin was done by the disc diffusion method as described by NCCLS [9] against pathogenic *Staphylococcus aureus* isolated from mastitis milk samples and the standard

TABLE 1: Therapeutic plan of astaxanthin (AX) in lactating mice challenged with pathogenic *Staphylococcus aureus*.

Groups	Number of mice	Treatment	Dose	Frequency	Route	Interval
Group I	6	Normal healthy mice	—	—	—	—
Group II	6	Positive control	—	—	—	—
Group III	6	AX*	16 mg/kg body weight	Twice daily	Orally	Oral drenching of AX for 5 days PC twice a day
Group IV	6	Antibiotic**	12.5 mg/kg body weight	Twice daily	Intramuscular	5 days post challenge/twice a day

AX* was drenched orally after reconstitution in sterile normal saline solution, at the rate of 16 mg/kg body weight 10 days prior to challenge and continued 5 days post challenge.
**Amoxicillin + sulbactam—via intramuscular route, at 12.5 mg/kg body weight.

reference *S. aureus* strain (MTCC number 96, Microbial Type Culture Collection, Chandigarh, India). The dose of astaxanthin was calculated by conducting the MIC against *Staphylococcus aureus* by tube dilution method as described in previous papers [10, 11]. For oral drenching in mice, the dosage (in mg/kg) was calculated as per the formulae given below:

$$\text{Dosage (mg/kg) of Astaxanthin} = \text{MIC} \times 20. \quad (1)$$

2.2. Isolation and Characterization of Staphylococcus aureus.
The dairy cows were screened for mastitis by California Mastitis Test [12]. Isolation and identification of pathogenicorganism from the mastitic milk samples was done as per the standard procedure [13]. The *S. aureus* organism was initially identified on the basis of colony morphology on 5% blood agar as [14] and later by Gram staining and growth on selective media like mannitol salt agar (MSA) and Baird Parker agar plates and further subjected to coagulase test; in brief, 2 test tubes were filled up with 0.5 mL of diluted rabbit plasma; to the first tube 0.1 mL of overnight broth culture of test organism was added and to the second tube 0.1 mL of sterile broth was added and incubated at 37°C for 4 hrs and observed for the coagulation of plasma if positive [14]. Biochemical tests were performed with standard kits (HiStaph Identification Kit, HiMedia, India). However, molecular characterization was not performed. The dose of organism for intramammary challenge was calculated by surface viable count as per the method described elsewhere [15]. Eighteen-hour grown broth culture of *S. aureus* at the rate of 5×10^5 bacteria was taken for challenge in mice in each mammary gland.

2.3. Experimental Design and Procurement of Mice.
Healthy adult lactating Swiss albino mice weighing around 30–40 grams were procured from the institute's vivarium, after weaning their pups, maintained in the divisional animal shed, and housed in animal cages, providing ad libitum water and feed, under standard temperature, ventilation, and humidity. The experimental trial was conducted in lactating mice using the left fourth (L4) and right fourth (R4) inguinal mammary gland. The mice were grouped into four groups with 6 mice in each group. Group I mice served as healthy negative control. Group II were challenged with *S. aureus* and served

as positive control. In group III, astaxanthin was drenched after reconstitution in sterile normal saline solution at the rate of 16 mg/kg body weight from 8 days prior to challenge and continued for 5 days PC orally; group IV was treated with amoxicillin plus sulbactam at the dose rate of 12.5 mg/kg body weight twice daily for 3 days by intramuscular route as depicted in Table 1.

2.4. Challenge of Mice with Pathogenic Staphylococcus aureus.
All the mice of group II, group III, and group IV were inoculated with 18 hrs old culture of *S. aureus* via intramammary route at the rate of 5×10^6 bacteria per teat, under general anesthesia with ketamine at 65 mg/kg and xylazine at 4 mg/kg.

2.5. Total Clinical Scores (TCS).
Mammary glands of mice were screened for mastitis by visual examination [16] followed by total clinical score card.

2.6. Collection of Blood for Serum Collection and Hematological Parameters.
Around 1 mL of blood was collected from the mice using micro capillary tubes on day 0, 24, 72 and 120 hrs post challenge from retrobulbar venous plexus behind the eyeball taking special care not to damage the ocular membrane structure [17]. Serum separation was done for CRP. Simultaneously thin blood smear was made stained with Giemsa stain for differential leukocyte count (DLC) to determine neutrophil : lymphocyte ratio [18].

2.7. C-Reactive Protein (CRP).
C-reactive protein was done in serum using a standard kit (CRP kit, Latex Agglutination Method, Span Diagnostics LTD., Mumbai, India) by the manufacturer's instruction.

2.8. Histopathological Examination.
The mice from each of the four groups were sacrificed after 120 hours PC using xylazine-ketamine combination as injectable anesthesia. Mammary glands L4 and R4 were carefully removed from the skin flaps using blunt scissors and were spread onto a prelabeled glass slide without any air bubbles or hair and stored in 10% (v/v) formalin and further processed for Hematoxylin and Eosin (H&E) staining to visualize the histopathological changes in the tissue section. Mice of all 4 groups were

TABLE 2: Clinical score card of mice at 0 hr, 24 hrs, 48 hrs, 72 hrs, and 120 hrs post challenge in posttreated mice (mean ± SE).

Groups	0 hr	24 hrs	48 hrs	72 hrs	120 hrs
Group I	$0 \pm .00^{a,x}$	$0 \pm .00^{a,x}$	$0 \pm .00^{a,x}$	$0 \pm .00^{a,x}$	$0 \pm .00^{a,x}$
Group II	$0 \pm .00^{a,x}$	$2 \pm .00^{b,z}$	$2.5 \pm .25^{b,y}$	$3.25 \pm .25^{c,z}$	$3 \pm .00^{c,z}$
Group III	$0 \pm .00^{a,x}$	$1.25 \pm .25^{b,y}$	$1.25 \pm .25^{b,y}$	$1 \pm .25^{b,y}$	$.9 \pm .00^{a,y}$
Group IV	$0 \pm .00^{a,x}$	$1.25 \pm .00^{b,y}$	$1 \pm .00^{a,y}$	$1 \pm .00^{a,y}$	$.9 \pm .00^{a,y}$

*Mean values with dissimilar superscripts in the row (a, b, and c) and column (x, y, and z) vary significantly at $P < 0.05$.

sacrificed at 120 hrs post challenge. Tissue sections of mammary gland of group I lactating mice revealed normal healthy lactating alveoli with no signs of inflammation. In group II mice multiple focal micro abscess predominated by neutrophil and fibrinous exudates in the mammary parenchyma was observed with complete disruption of mammary cellular details. In mice of group III that received astaxanthin, mammary gland was normal with no inflammatory reaction except at the hypodermic adipose tissue and muscularis junction. In group IV mice, the mammary gland tissue section showed relatively less pathological changes as compared to group II. Cellular inflammatory infiltration was mild.

2.9. Statistical Analysis. The data collected on each parameter was analyzed by standard statistical methods. Level of significance was set ($P < 0.05$) by applying Friedman test for total clinical scores. Level of significance was set ($P < 0.05$) by applying two-way ANOVA for DLC, using statistical software SPSS (Version 17).

3. Results

3.1. ABST and MIC of Astaxanthin. The zone of inhibition against isolated *S. aureus* was 26 mm for astaxanthin, whereas it was 32 mm for amoxicillin. The MIC of astaxanthin was 750 μg against isolated *S. aureus*.

3.1.1. Isolation and Biochemical Characterization of S. aureus. The Gram staining revealed characteristic Gram positive cocci arranged in small bunches (Staphylo). Confirmation was carried out by performing biochemical test for *Staphylococcus aureus*. Organisms showing positive for catalase, maltose fermentation, coagulase positive, haemolysis of blood agar, oxidation fermentation, methyl red and Voges-Proskauer test were confirmed as *S. aureus*.

3.2. Total Clinical Scores (TCS). There was no variation in TCS at 0 hr, 24 hrs, 48 hrs, 72 hrs, and 120 hrs of observational period in group I mice, whereas in group II, mild inflammation of the mammary glands was observed at 24 hrs PC. At 48 hrs PC in group II mice showed profound depression with appreciable swelling, enlargement, and reddish discoloration with extravasations of blood stained exudates; at 72 and 120 hrs mortality was 60%. On the contrary in group III treated mice there were little inflammatory changes at 48 and 72 hrs PC, with signs of recovery at 120 hrs PC; similarly mild inflammatory changes in mammary gland could be observed

at 48 and 72 hrs PC in group IV mice with recovery at 120 hrs PC (Table 2).

3.3. DLC in Blood. DLC was done in all groups at 0 hr, 24 hrs, 48 h, 72 hrs, and 120 hrs post challenge, respectively. At 0 hr lymphocyte count was more and neutrophils count was lesser in all the 4 groups, whereas neutrophil count increased and lymphocyte count decreased significantly in all the infected groups (group II, group III, and group IV) as compared to healthy group (group I) at 24 hrs PC. In group II animals the mean neutrophil count increased to an extent of 66.07% at 120 hrs PC as compared to 0 hr count. Similarly in group III and group IV significantly higher count to an extent of 48.6% and 40.6% could be observed at 24 hrs, respectively; however the neutrophil count at 48 h, 72 hrs, and 120 hrs PC did not differ significantly, whereas the lymphocyte counts in group II animals decreased to an extent of 63% at 120 hrs PC as compared to 0 hr count. Similarly in group III and group IV significantly lower count to an extent of 18.9% and 31.6% could be observed at 24 hrs, respectively; however the lymphocyte count at 48 hrs, 72 hrs, and 120 hrs PC did not differ significantly (Figure 1).

3.4. CRP in Serum. The CRP was estimated in serum. On day 0 and 120 hrs post challenge the CRP was negative in all groups. Positive CRP was observed in group II at 24, 48, and 76 hrs PC, whereas in group III the CRP positive reaction was recorded at 24 hrs PC only, whilst the CRP reaction was negative in group IV at 24 hrs PC.

3.5. Histopathological Examination. Mice were sacrificed at 120 hrs PC forhistopathological examination of mammary tissue. Tissue sections of mammary gland of group I mice revealed normal healthy lactating alveoli with no signs of inflammation. In group II mice multiple focal micro abscess predominated by neutrophil and fibrinous exudates in the mammary parenchyma was seen with complete disruption of mammary cellular details. In group III receiving astaxanthin, there were few inflammatory cells with no exudation and the tissue structure was normal. Similarly in group IV cellular inflammatory infiltration was mild and mammary parenchyma appeared normal.

4. Discussion

So far antibiotics are the only proven method for the treatment of mastitis; however, antibiotic therapy has got several

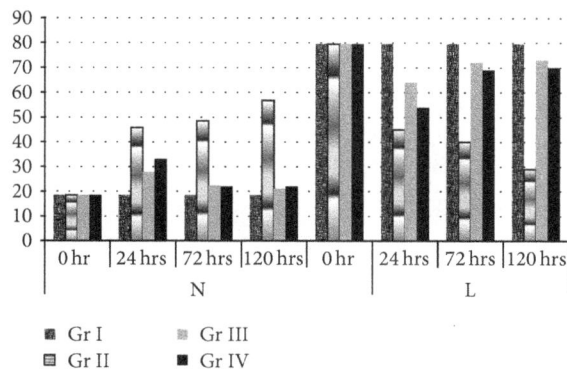

FIGURE 1: Percent neutrophil and lymphocyte in blood in response to the treatment with astaxanthin (group III) and amoxicillin plus sulbactam (group IV) and in positive control (group II) and in normal healthy mice (group I) (mean ± SE).

demerits including the harmful drug residue in food chain. The clinical efficacy of the nonantibiotic agents is recently being researched extensively with promising results; these include bacterial enzymes, antimicrobial peptides, bioresponse modifiers, cytokines, micronutrients, vitamins, and medicinal herbs [18, 19].

Astaxanthin is a xanthophyll carotenoid, naturally obtained from the chlorophyte algae *Haematococcus pluvialis* [4]. In the present trial the immunotherapeutic effect of astaxanthin (AX) was studied in mice staphylococcal mastitis. In the astaxanthin treated mice, the clinical score was almost normal; in the tissue sections of mammary gland the cellular details were almost normal with negligible infiltration of inflammatory cell and little exudation in H&E stained section. AX treatment also resisted the intramammary challenge of pathogenic *S. aureus*; hence no pathological changes could be observed and clinical recovery was 100%. In our experiment AX revealed 26 mm zone of inhibition against isolated *S. aureus*. Kumari and Ramanujan [8] also demonstrated the antibacterial activity of AX against *S. aureus*. The CRP is an acute phase protein and is expressed in early stages of infection, acute phase response was higher in post challenge nontreated mice till 72 hrs PC, whereas the CRP was lower in AX treated mice at 48 and 72 hrs PC; it could be due to the anti-inflammatory potential of AX. Astaxanthin is a potent antioxidant and powerful scavenger of free radicals like superoxide and signet oxygen [20]. It suppresses varied inflammatory mediators like TNF-α, IL-1β, cyclooxygenase-2, and nitric oxide synthase [21, 22]. In the present study the neutrophil count in post challenge nontreated mice was significantly higher, whereas it significantly decreased after 48 hrs PC in AX treated mice. The AX treatment also increased the lymphocyte count; it indicates the immunomodulatory potential of AX. Kurihara et al. [7] demonstrated the immunomodulatory property of astaxanthin; the authors suggested that astaxanthin treatment in diseased mice inhibited the suppressor of NK cell activity and lipid peroxidation.

5. Conclusion

In conclusion, this study represents an initial investigation on the therapeutic use of astaxanthin in mice mastitis model challenged with highly pathogenic *S. aureus*. The results of the present study indicate the antibacterial, anti-inflammatory, and immunomodulatory activity of AX treatment against intramammary challenge with pathogenic bacteria. AX treatment significantly reduced the neutrophil count and acute phase protein and enhanced the lymphocyte count and improved early clinical recovery with no pathological changes in the mammary parenchyma. The present drug trial determines the potential benefits of the AX therapy in intramammary infection in mice model as well as standardization of nonantibiotic agent to reduce antibiotic residue from food chain.

Conflict of Interests

The authors declare that there is no conflict of interests regarding the publication of this paper.

Acknowledgments

Tshering Dolma is thankful to Indian Council of Agriculture Research, New Delhi, for providing the financial assistance in form of Junior Research Fellowship. Authors are also thankful to the director of the institute for providing the facilities.

References

[1] S. Taponen and S. Pyörälä, "Coagulase-negative staphylococci as cause of bovine mastitis-Not so different from *Staphylococcus aureus*?" *Veterinary Microbiology*, vol. 134, no. 1-2, pp. 29–36, 2009.

[2] D. C. Oliveira, S. W. Wu, and H. De Lencastre, "Genetic organization of the downstream region of the *mecA* element in methicillin-resistant *Staphylococcus aureus* isolates carrying different polymorphisms of this region," *Antimicrobial Agents and Chemotherapy*, vol. 44, no. 7, pp. 1906–1910, 2000.

[3] WHO, Antimicrobial resistance: global report on surveillance, 2014, http://www.who.int/drugresistance/en/.

[4] M. Olaizola and M. E. Huntley, "Recent advances in commercial production of astaxanthin from microalgae," in *Biomaterials and Bioprocessing*, M. Fingerman and R. Nagabhushanam, Eds., Science Publishers, 2003.

[5] Y. Ikeda, S. Tsuji, A. Satoh, M. Ishikura, T. Shirasawa, and T. Shimizu, "Protective effects of astaxanthin on 6-hydroxydopamine-induced apoptosis in human neuroblastoma SH-SY5Y cells," *Journal of Neurochemistry*, vol. 107, no. 6, pp. 1730–1740, 2008.

[6] M. Bennedsen, X. Wang, R. Willén, T. Wadström, and L. P. Andersen, "Treatment of *H. pylori* infected mice with antioxidant astaxanthin reduces gastric inflammation, bacterial load and modulates cytokine release by splenocytes," *Immunology Letters*, vol. 70, no. 3, pp. 185–189, 2000.

[7] H. Kurihara, H. Koda, S. Asami, Y. Kiso, and T. Tanaka, "Contribution of the antioxidative property of astaxanthin to its protective effect on the promotion of cancer metastasis in

mice treated with restraint stress," *Life Sciences*, vol. 70, no. 21, pp. 2509–2520, 2002.

[8] U. Kumari and R. Ramanujan, "Isolation of astaxanthin from shrimp metapenaeus dobsoni and study of its pharmacological activity," *Journal of Current Chemical and Pharmaceutical Science*, vol. 3, no. 1, pp. 60–63, 2013.

[9] NCCLS, "Performance standards for antimicrobial susceptibility testing, 9th informational supplements," Document M100-S9, NCCLS, Wayne, Pa, USA, 1999, (vol. 19, no. 1, Table 21).

[10] L. A. Chitwood, "Tube dilution antimicrobial susceptibility testing: efficacy of a microtechnique applicable to diagnostic laboratories," *Applied Microbiology*, vol. 17, no. 5, pp. 707–709, 1969.

[11] J. H. Jorgensen, "Selection criteria for an antimicrobial susceptibility testing system," *Journal of Clinical Microbiology*, vol. 31, no. 11, pp. 2841–2844, 1993.

[12] O. W. Schalm and D. O. Noorlander, "Experiments and observations leading to development of the California mastitis test," *Journal of the American Veterinary Medical Association*, vol. 130, no. 5, pp. 199–204, 1957.

[13] T. K. Griffin, F. H. Dodd, F. K. Neave, D. R. Westgarth, R. G. Kingwil, and C. D. Wilson, "A method of diagnosing intramammary infection in dairy cows for large experiments," *Journal of Dairy Research*, vol. 44, no. 1, pp. 25–45, 1977.

[14] R. Cruickshank, *Mackie and Mc Cartney's Handbook of Bacteriology*, E & S.Livingstone limited, Edinburgh, UK, 10th edition, 1962.

[15] A. A. Miles, S. S. Misra, and J. O. Irwin, "The estimation of the bactericidal power of the blood," *The Journal of Hygiene*, vol. 38, no. 6, pp. 732–749, 1938.

[16] Sridevi, *Studies on isolation, characterization and therapeutic use of bacteriophages against Streptococcus agalactiae associated with ruminant mastitis [M.V.Sc. thesis]*, Indian Veterinary Research Institute, Izatnagar, India, 2005.

[17] N. C. Jain, *Schalm's Veterinary Hematology*, Lea and Febrriger, Philadelphia, Pa, USA, 4th edition, 1986.

[18] R. Mukherjee, G. C. Ram, P. K. Dash, and T. Goswami, "The activity of milk leukocytes in response to a water-soluble fraction of Mycobacterium phlei in bovine subclinical mastitis," *Veterinary Research Communications*, vol. 28, no. 1, pp. 47–54, 2004.

[19] R. Mukherjee, P. K. Dash, and G. C. Ram, "Immunotherapeutic potential of *Ocimum sanctum* (L) in bovine subclinical mastitis," *Research in Veterinary Science*, vol. 79, no. 1, pp. 37–43, 2005.

[20] S. Goto, K. Kogure, K. Abe et al., "Efficient radical trapping at the surface and inside the phospholipid membrane is responsible for highly potent antiperoxidative activity of the carotenoid astaxanthin," *Biochimica et Biophysica Acta*, vol. 1512, no. 2, pp. 251–258, 2001.

[21] K.-E. Eilertsen, H. K. Mæhre, I. J. Jensen et al., "A wax ester and astaxanthin-rich extract from the marine copepod *Calanus finmarchicus* attenuates atherogenesis in female apolipoprotein E-deficient mice," *The Journal of Nutrition*, vol. 142, no. 3, pp. 508–512, 2012.

[22] S.-J. Lee, S.-K. Bai, K.-S. Lee et al., "Astaxanthin inhibits nitric oxide production and inflammatory gene expression by suppressing IκB kinase-dependent NF-κB activation," *Molecules and Cells*, vol. 16, no. 1, pp. 97–105, 2003.

27

Prevalence of *Calodium hepaticum* and *Cysticercus fasciolaris* in Urban Rats and Their Histopathological Reaction in the Livers

Bharathalingam Sinniah, Muniandy Narasiman, Saequa Habib, and Ong Gaik Bei

Laboratory Based Medicine, Faculty of Medicine, Universiti Kuala Lumpur Royal College of Medicine Perak, No. 3 Jalan Greentown, 30450 Ipoh, Perak, Malaysia

Correspondence should be addressed to Bharathalingam Sinniah; bsinniah@unikl.edu.my

Academic Editor: Carlos González-Rey

Humans can get infected with several zoonotic diseases from being in close contact with rats. This study was aimed at determining the prevalence and histopathological changes caused by *Calodium hepaticum* and *Cysticercus fasciolaris* in infected livers of wild caught urban rats. Of the 98 urban rats (*Rattus rattus diardii* and *Rattus norvegicus*) autopsied, 64.3% were infected; 44.9% were infected with *Caladium hepatica*, 39.3% were infected with *Cysticercus fasciolaris*, and 20.4% were infected with both parasites. High infection rates suggest that urban rats are common reservoir for both parasites, which are potentially a threat to man. *Calodium hepaticum* infections were identified by the presence of ova or adults in the liver parenchyma. They appear as yellowish white nodules, measuring 1–7 mm in diameter or in streaks scattered widely over the serosal surface of the liver. *Cysticercus fasciolaris* infections are recognized morphologically by their shape (round or oval) and are creamy white in colour. Histological studies of *Calodium hepaticum* showed areas of granulomatous lesions with necrotic areas around the dead ova and adults. In almost all cases, the rats appeared robust, looked healthy, and showed no visible signs of hepatic failure despite the fact that more than 64.0% of their livers were infected by either one or both parasites.

1. Introduction

Rats are the most common and widespread of all mammals in the world, making it difficult to estimate their numbers, which probably run into the billions. They are responsible for the transmission of several zoonotic diseases to man, which include parasites and microbes. Man gets infected with many rodent pathogens primarily through bites, scratches, and the consumption of food or drinks contaminated with rodent droppings or urine. Besides transmitting diseases, they eat almost anything and destroy properties. Currently, most large cities and towns in developing and developed countries face a growing menace from the rat population. Rats are definitive host for *Calodium hepaticum* and intermediate host for *Cysticercus fasciolaris*. The nematode parasite *Calodium hepaticum* (syn. *Capillaria hepatica*, Bancroft, 1983) has a global distribution and is commonly reported in rodents [1, 2] and to a lesser extent in dogs [3, 4], cats [5], primates

[6], and humans [5, 7–9]. *Calodium hepaticum* is a common parasite which infects rodents worldwide but rarely in humans. Currently 163 human cases of *Calodium hepaticum* (72 reports of hepatic capillariasis, 13 serologically confirmed infections, and 78 observations of spurious infections) have been reported from different parts of the world [9, 10]. *Calodium hepaticum* ova are deposited by female worms in clusters in the parenchyma tissue of the liver and are only released into the environment following the death of its host due to natural causes, predation cannibalism, or decay. Consumption of infected livers is the main cause of spurious infection, where the eggs are released in the faeces without causing disease. Human infection with *Taenia taeniaeformis* is rare and only few cases have been reported [11]. Hepatic calodiasis is mainly diagnosed by liver biopsy or necropsy. *Cysticercus fasciolaris* is the larval stage of the cestode, *Taenia taeniaeformis* (Batsch, 1786) (syn. *Hydatigera taeniaeformis*) also known as cat tapeworm. The pathogenesis of these two

parasites is distinct. *Calodium hepaticum* infection causes multifocal granulomatous inflammation and is directly associated with the presence of live, dying, or dead worms or their eggs. Septal fibrosis is commonly seen in animals infected with *C. hepaticum* [12–14]. *Cysticercus fasciolaris* infections induce vigorous fibroplasia and progressive inflammation within the liver parenchyma [12, 13]. The aim of this study was to determine the prevalence of *Cysticercus fasciolaris* and *Calodium hepaticum* coinfection and their pathology in rodent livers to help better understand the infection in humans.

2. Materials and Methods

A total of 104 rodents, comprising 52 *Rattus norvegicus*, 46 *Rattus rattus diardii*, and 6 *Mus musculus,* were trapped from the urban areas of Ipoh, Malaysia. Ipoh was chosen as the area of study as there was a campaign by the local municipal council to control the rat population because rats were becoming a big public health problem. The rodents were trapped in the vicinity of wet markets and drains behind restaurants and food courts. Rats were captured using wire traps that measured 29 × 22 × 50 cm. For bait, we used either dried salted fish, or slices of bread spread with peanut butter or cheese. Data of each rodent necropsied were recorded, including locality, date of capture, and gender. Fifty-one female and forty-seven males were trapped at night and transported to the laboratory in the morning. The rats were necropsied and examined within 24 hours of capture. Animal procedures were conducted in adherence to the Ethical Committee of the University. Each trap with the live rat inside was individually placed into a big bucket with a lid. The animals were anaesthetized by placing cotton wool soaked with chloroform into the bucket and covered for 2-3 minutes. The anaesthetized rat was removed from the cage and sacrificed by severing the aorta. Gross examination of the liver was initially conducted to screen for *Calodium hepaticum* and *Cysticercus fasciolaris* infections. A small portion of the infected liver was removed from each rat, fixed in 10.0% neutral-buffered formal-saline (pH 6.9), and processed for paraffin embedding. The tissues were sectioned at 5 μm in thickness. In addition, all macroscopic abnormalities were also examined. The cut sections were stained with haematoxylin and eosin (H&E) and examined under light microscopy for histopathological reactions. Infections were confirmed by demonstrating the presence of ova or adults of *C. hepaticum* in the liver and *Cysticercus fasciolaris* was confirmed by breaking the cyst and exposing the larva.

3. Results

Of the 98 rats examined, 64.0% were infected, of which 44.9% were positive with *Calodium hepaticum*, 39.3% were positive with *Cysticercus fasciolaris*, and 20.4% were positive with both as shown in Table 1. None of the six shrews examined were infected with these two parasites. Gross examination of the infected livers showed firm whitish yellow nodules (1–7 mm) or appeared in patches or as irregular streaks, randomly

TABLE 1: Prevalence of *Calodium hepaticum* and *Cysticercus fasciolaris* in liver of 98 urban rats.

Liver parasite	Number of positive	% positive
Single infection		
Calodium hepaticum	24/98	24.5
Cysticercus fasciolaris	19/98	19.4
Double infection		
C. hepaticum + *C. fasciolaris*	20/98	20.4
Total *C. hepaticum* infection	44/98	44.9
Total *C. fasciolaris* infection	39/98	39.3
Total liver infected	63/98	64.3

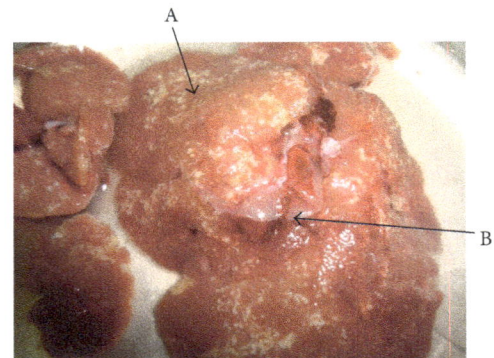

FIGURE 1: Liver of urban wild rodent showing coinfection with *Calodium hepaticum* and *Cysticercus fasciolaris*. *Calodium hepaticum* (A) appears as yellowish white patches/tracts or streaks on the liver surface. The cysts of *Cysticercus fasciolaris* (B) are embedded in the liver (arrow) containing the larva.

scattered in the serosal surface. *Cysticercus fasciolaris* cysts measured, on an average, 9–14 mm in diameter. Each cyst contained a single larva measuring 14–31 cm in length, with a scolex containing two rows of hooks, 4 suckers followed by a very long neck. The infected rats mostly had multiple cysts, which appeared creamy white in colour, oval or round in shape, embedded within the liver as shown in Figure 1. Prior to necropsy, none of the rats exhibited any adverse clinical signs. Histopathological studies showed that encapsulation by *Cysticercus fasciolaris* caused very little fibrotic changes in the rats. In some signs of inflammation with periportal eosinophil infiltrates, microabscesses and prominent Kupffer cells were seen. In some livers, the larvae were seen encapsulated by connective tissue surrounded by mild to moderate inflammatory infiltrates predominantly composing lymphocytes, macrophages, moderate eosinophils, and few large scattered fibroblasts. In few livers, mild fibrotic lesions were seen around the cyst, as shown in Figure 2. *Calodium hepaticum* ova are barrel-shaped and unembryonated and have typical bipolar plugs on either end with prominent radial striations on the outer layer of the egg shell. The eggs measured, on an average, 22 μm in width and 51 μm in length as shown in Figure 3. Histopathological section of infected livers showed areas of granulomatous reaction. These responses were more profound around the ova of *Calodium hepaticum* infection with fibrous inflammatory reaction, as

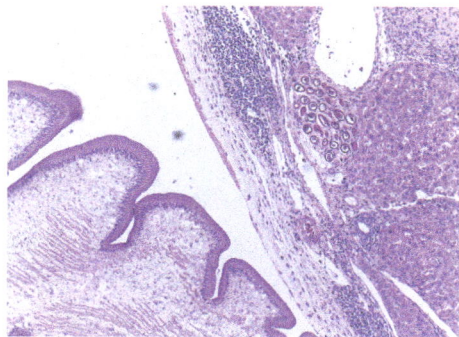

FIGURE 2: *Cysticercus fasciolaris* is within a cyst which is surrounded by connective tissues and inflammatory cells. Eggs of *Calodium hepaticum* are shown in a cluster within the parenchyma tissues (haematoxylin and eosin stain: ×10).

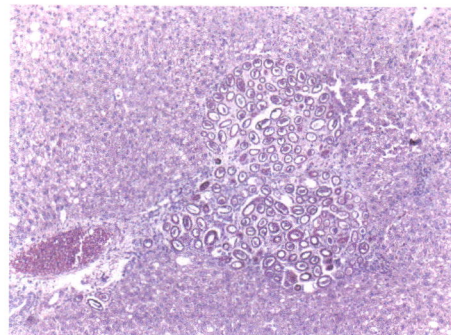

FIGURE 4: Clusters of *C. hepaticum* eggs surrounded by granulomatous lesions (H&E stain ×10).

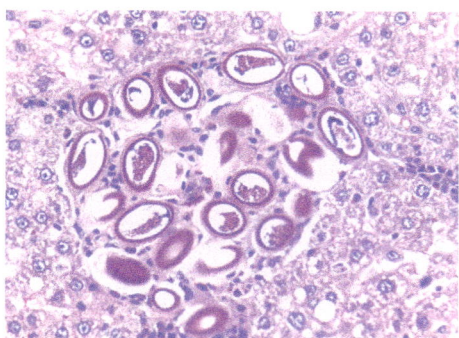

FIGURE 3: Cluster of *Calodium hepaticum* eggs surrounded by granulomatous lesion. Bioperculated ova with polar prominence at each end that are characteristic of *C. hepaticum* are seen (haematoxylin and eosin stain: ×40).

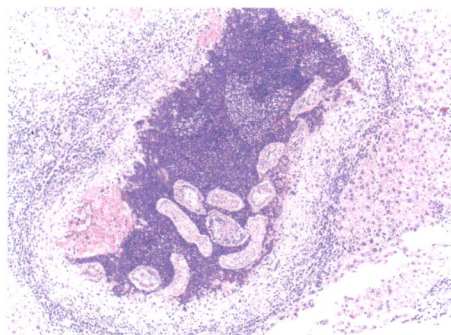

FIGURE 5: Dead worms and eggs are surrounded by an acute inflammatory reaction containing a central area of necrosis, calcification, and fibrosis (H&E stain: ×10).

4. Discussion

shown in Figure 4. Tissue reaction around dead *Calodium hepaticum* worms or ova consisted of a large numbers of inflammatory cells, mainly mononuclear leukocytes, few polymorphs, and eosinophils, as shown in Figure 5. Microscopic studies showed multiple nodular microgranulomas and coalescing macrogranulomas with intralesional parasitic eggs. Occasionally adult worms were seen scattered in the liver. Small granulomas (microgranulomas) in the liver of some rats are comprised of solid aggregates of epithelioid macrophages surrounded by lymphocytes and eosinophils. In few cases, the granulomas contained no fragments of worms, eggs, or any trace of worm derived material. Thin and thick peripheral lesions are most commonly characterized by fibrous capsules, containing lymphocytes, small to moderate amounts of neutrophils, and plasma cells. The core of the nodules contained mainly neutrophils with necrotic debris, epithelioid cells, few multinucleated cells, eosinophils, and occasionally calcified materials. In addition the central hepatic vein was moderately dilated while the surrounding sinusoids in the livers contained erythrocytes and a few inflammatory cells. Fibrocellular septae, separated the hepatic parenchyma into irregular portions, were noted in the vicinity of granulomatous reaction. Periportal inflammatory infiltration and hepatocyte regeneration were also observed.

Calodium hepaticum infection in rodents has been reported worldwide with prevalence rates ranging from 7.9% to more than 88.0% [1, 8, 10, 15]. In this study, 44.9% of rats were infected with *Calodium hepaticum* and 39.3% with *Cysticercus fasciolaris*. The adult female *Calodium hepaticum* deposits ova in clusters in the liver parenchyma and these eggs become encapsulated as a result of chronic inflammatory response of the host. The ova are lemon-shaped with thick egg shells and are striated with polar plugs at each end, measuring on average 22 μm in width and 51 μm in length. Macroscopically, infected livers showed diffuse, irregular yellowish white patches that appeared in streaks or small nodules on the external surface and within the liver, and in some cases adult worms and egg masses were found, in line with earlier reports [16–18]. Adult male worms die approximately forty days after infection, whereas females die within 60 days. Dead worms disintegrate and become "walled off" due to host response and gradually destroyed.

The clusters of ova which are trapped within the liver undergo fibrotic tissue responses [17, 19]. The worm material inside the fibrotic reaction may be viewed as a protective response. In the present study, we observed heavy lymphocytic infiltrates at the periphery of the egg containing granulomas. Our observations are consistent with studies conducted in other countries that showed similar granulomatous inflammation in the livers of naturally infected rats [8, 20]. This response is precipitated by dying and disintegrating adult worms and ova. The granuloma (macrogranuloma) formation is said to have an immunological basis and occurs as a consequence of an immune response mounted by the host, against egg-derived antigens [15, 21]. In support of such an idea, Solomon and Soulsby [22] reported finding circulating antibodies to egg antigens in infected mouse. Focal lesions with septal fibrosis are very often seen associated with *C. hepaticum* infections [17]. Septal fibrosis is commonly seen in more than 90.0% of infected livers and is represented by thin, straight fibrocellular/fibrous tissue septa that divide the liver parenchyma into hepatic nodules. Septal fibrosis extends from portal spaces and spreads toward neighbouring portal spaces and central veins, finally involving the entire organ, thus creating a septate mosaic pattern in the infected liver [17, 19, 23].

In rats, *Cysticercus fasciolaris* cysts can occur singly or in numerous numbers. The cyst wall is rough, and in chronic infections, it can cause irritation to the hepatic tissues, inducing slight local inflammatory reaction due to immune-related activities [24]. Microscopic observations showed mild inflammatory reactions around the cysts, infiltrated by lymphocytes, macrophages, eosinophils, and few scattered large fibroblasts. Rats infected with *Cysticercus fasciolaris* and other cestode larvae have the capacity to stimulate immune responses, which allow the larval stage to become invasive [25]. This irritation may stimulate and promote the hepatic cells around the cyst to develop and exhibit carcinogenic behaviour. The chemical reactions caused between the larvae and hepatic tissues may induce cellular changes which may develop into fibrosarcomas [26].

Histopathological observations in chronic infections showed plenty of fibroblasts with neoplastic characteristics similar to fibrosarcomas. [27, 28]. In chronic infection where the hepatic cysts are more than three months old, the larvae may induce fibrosarcomas in the liver tissue [24, 27, 28]. In man, *Calodium hepaticum* may cause the loss of liver cells, thereby resulting in the loss of liver function. Dead adult parasites can stimulate a rapid immune response in the host, leading to inflammation and encapsulation in collagen fibres leading to septal fibrosis and cirrhosis [15].

5. Conclusion

As of today there are no good policies on the control of rats for health and economic benefits. The laws for proper sanitation are not effectively implemented. As a result the prevalence of *Calodium hepaticum* and *Cysticercus fasciolaris* in rodents is high in many tropical countries and poses a health threat as large populations of humans live in close proximity to the rodent population. These rodents act as reservoir hosts for these parasites and are a potential risk for human infections in Malaysia as well as in other countries in the region. Cases of human infections reported from this region are from Thailand [29], India [30], Korea [31], and China [32–35]. In view of this and with the high prevalence of rats in this country, steps should be taken to prevent human infections. The effective solution lies in the hands of the communities. To achieve this there is a need to mobilize the communities to promote better health through self-help and group activities.

Conflict of Interests

The authors declare that there is no conflict of interests regarding the publication of this paper.

Acknowledgments

The authors thank Universiti Kuala Lumpur Royal College of Medicine Perak for STRG Grant no. 12016 to conduct this research. They thank Mr. Joechim Francis Antony for his assistance in trapping the rats.

References

[1] B. Sinniah, M. Singh, and K. Anuar, "Preliminary survey of *Capillaria hepatica* (Bancroft, 1893) in Malaysia," *Journal of Helminthology*, vol. 53, no. 2, pp. 147–152, 1979.

[2] D. M. Spratt and G. R. singleton, "Studies on the life-cycle, infectivity and clinical effects of *Capillaria hepatica* (Bancroft) (Nematoda) in mice (*Mus musculus*)," *Australian Journal of Zoology*, vol. 34, no. 5, pp. 663–675, 1986.

[3] R. Stokes, "*Capillaria hepatica* in a dog," *Australian Veterinary Journal*, vol. 49, no. 2, p. 109, 1973.

[4] S. Lloyd, C. M. Elwood, and K. C. Smith, "*Capillaria hepatica* (*Calodium hepaticum*) infection in a British dog," *Veterinary Record*, vol. 151, no. 14, pp. 419–420, 2002.

[5] A. R. Resendes, A. F. S. Amaral, A. Rodrigues, and S. Almeria, "Prevalence of *Calodium hepaticum* (Syn. *Capillaria hepatica*) in house mice (*Mus musculus*) in the Azores archipelago," *Veterinary Parasitology*, vol. 160, no. 3-4, pp. 340–343, 2009.

[6] T. K. Graczyk, L. J. Lowenstine, and M. R. Cranfield, "*Capillaria hepatica* (Nematoda) infections in human-habituated mountain gorillas (*Gorilla gorilla beringei*) of the Parc National de Volcans, Rwanda," *Journal of Parasitology*, vol. 85, no. 6, pp. 1168–1170, 1999.

[7] R. Piazza, M. O. Correa, and R. N. Fleury, "On a case of human infestation with *Capillaria hepatica*," *Revista do Instituto de Medicina Tropical de São Paulo*, vol. 5, pp. 37–41, 1963.

[8] R. Ceruti, O. Sonzogni, F. Origgi et al., "*Capillaria hepatica* infection in wild brown rats (*Rattus norvegicus*) from the urban area of Milan, Italy," *Journal of Veterinary Medicine*, vol. 48, no. 3, pp. 235–240, 2001.

[9] H.-P. Fuehrer, P. Igel, and H. Auer, "*Capillaria hepatica* in man—an overview of hepatic capillariosis and spurious infections," *Parasitology Research*, vol. 109, no. 4, pp. 969–979, 2011.

[10] H.-P. Fuehrer, "An overview of the host spectrum and distribution of *Calodium hepaticum* (syn. *Capillaria hepatica*): part 1—Muroidea," *Parasitology Research*, vol. 113, no. 2, pp. 619–640, 2014.

[11] E. P. Hoberg, "*Taenia* tapeworms: their biology, evolution and socioeconomic significance," *Microbes and Infection*, vol. 4, no. 8, pp. 859–866, 2002.

Prevalence of Calodium hepaticum and Cysticercus fasciolaris in Urban Rats...

199

[12] J. R. Georgi and M. E. Georgi, "Histopathological diagnosis," in *Parasitology for Veterinarians*, pp. 359–395, WB Saunders, Philadelphia, Pa, USA, 5th edition, 1990.

[13] H. Mehlhorn and V. Walldorf, "Liver cycles," in *Parasitology in Focus: Facts and Trends*, H. Mehlhorn, Ed., pp. 192–199, Springer, Berlin, Germany, 1998.

[14] S. B. de Andrade and Z. A. Andrade, "Experimental hepatic fibrosis due to *Capillaria hepatica* infection (differential features presented by rats and mice)," *Memorias do Instituto Oswaldo Cruz*, vol. 99, no. 4, pp. 399–406, 2004.

[15] A. T. Gomes, L. M. Cunha, C. G. Bastos, B. F. Medrado, B. C. A. Assis, and Z. A. Andrade, "Capillaria hepatica in rats: focal parasitic hepatic lesions and septal fibrosis run independent courses," *Memorias do Instituto Oswaldo Cruz*, vol. 101, no. 8, pp. 895–898, 2006.

[16] G. W. Luttermoser, "An experimental study of *Capillaria hepatica* in the rat and the mouse," *American Journal of Epidemiology*, vol. 27, no. 2, pp. 321–340, 1938.

[17] L. A. Ferreira and Z. A. Andrade, "Capillaria hepatica: a cause of septal fibrosis of the liver," *Memorias do Instituto Oswaldo Cruz*, vol. 88, no. 3, pp. 441–447, 1993.

[18] B. M. Gotardo, R. G. Andrade, and Z. A. Andrade, "Hepatic pathology in *Capillaria hepatica* infected mice," *Revista da Sociedade Brasileira de Medicina Tropical*, vol. 33, no. 4, pp. 341–346, 2000.

[19] M. M. de Souza, M. Tolentino Jr., B. C. A. Assis, A. C. de Oliveira Gonzalez, T. M. C. Silva, and Z. A. Andrade, "Significance and fate of septal fibrosis of the liver," *Hepatology Research*, vol. 35, no. 1, pp. 31–36, 2006.

[20] B. Davoust, M. Boni, D. Branquet, J. D. de Lahitte, and G. Martet, "Research on three parasitic infestations in rats captured in Marseille: evaluation of the zoonotic risk," *Bulletin de l'Academie Nationale de Medecine*, vol. 181, no. 5, pp. 187–195, 1997.

[21] S. F. el-Nassery, W. M. el-Gebali, and N. Y. Oweiss, "Capillaria hepatica: an experimental study of infection in white mice," *Journal of the Egyptian Society of Parasitology*, vol. 21, no. 2, pp. 467–478, 1991.

[22] G. B. Solomon and E. J. L. Soulsby, "Granuloma formation to *Capillaria hepatica* eggs. I. Descriptive definition," *Experimental Parasitology*, vol. 33, no. 3, pp. 458–467, 1973.

[23] R. F. Oliveira and Z. A. Andrade, "Worm load and septal fibrosis of the liver in *Capillaria hepatica*-infected rats," *Memórias do Instituto Oswaldo Cruz*, vol. 96, no. 7, pp. 1001–1003, 2001.

[24] K. P. Jithendran and R. Somvanshi, "Experimental infection of mice with *Taenia taeniaeformis* eggs from cats, course of infection and pathological studie," *Parasitology Research*, vol. 81, no. 2, pp. 103–108, 1995.

[25] H. O. Bogh, M. W. Lightowlers, N. D. Sullivan, G. F. Mitchell, and M. D. Rickard, "Stage-specific immunity to *Taenia taeniaeformis* infection in mice. A histological study of the course of infection in mice vaccinated with either oncosphere or metacestode antigens," *Parasite Immunology*, vol. 12, no. 2, pp. 153–162, 1990.

[26] K. Al- Jashamy, K. El-Salihi, A. Sheikh, and H. Saied, "Cysticercosis in rat infected with *C. fasciolaris*," in *Proceedings of the 9th National Conference on Medical Sciences*, p. 185, University Sciences Malaysia, Kubang Kerian, Malaysia, May 2004.

[27] A. R. Irizarry-Rovira, A. Wolf, and M. Bolek, "Taenia taeniaeformis-induced metastatic hepatic sarcoma in a pet rat (*Rattus norvegicus*)," *Journal of Exotic Pet Medicine*, vol. 16, no. 1, pp. 45–48, 2007.

[28] M. A. Hanes and L. J. Stribling, "Fibrosarcomas in two rats arising from hepatic cysts of *Cysticercus fasciolaris*," *Veterinary Pathology*, vol. 32, no. 4, pp. 441–444, 1995.

[29] S. Tesana, A. Puapairoj, and O.-T. Saeseow, "Granulomatous, hepatolithiasis and hepatomegaly caused by *Capillaria hepatica* infection: first case report of Thailand," *Southeast Asian Journal of Tropical Medicine and Public Health*, vol. 38, no. 4, pp. 636–640, 2007.

[30] H. Govil and M. Desai, "Capillaria hepatica parasitism," *Indian Journal of Pediatrics*, vol. 63, no. 5, pp. 698–700, 1996.

[31] G. Choe, J.-Y. Chai, S.-H. Lee, and J. G. Chi, "Hepatic capillariasis: first case report in the Republic of Korea," *American Journal of Tropical Medicine and Hygiene*, vol. 48, no. 5, pp. 610–625, 1993.

[32] P. C. Fan, W. C. Chung, and E. R. Chen, "Capillaria hepatica: a spurious case with a brief review," *The Kaohsiung Journal of Medical Sciences*, vol. 16, no. 7, pp. 360–367, 2000.

[33] B. K. Xu and D. N. Lin, "General condition of a rare human parasite in China," *Zhonghua Yixue Zachi*, vol. 59, pp. 286–296, 1979.

[34] X. M. Lim, H. Li, X. D. Zhoa, and Y. Deng, "1 Case of *Capillaria hepatica* infection," *Zhongguo Jisheng Chongbing Fangzhi Zahi*, vol. 17, article 230, 2004.

[35] J. N. Huang and J. X. Lin, "The pathological diagnosis of first case of *Capillaria hepatica* in Fujian Province," *Zhongguo Renshou Gonghuanbing*, vol. 20, article 556, 2004.

28

Phenotypical and Genotypical Properties of an *Arcanobacterium pluranimalium* Strain Isolated from a Juvenile Giraffe (*Giraffa camelopardalis reticulata*)

Karin Risse,[1] **Karen Schlez,**[1] **Tobias Eisenberg,**[1] **Christina Geiger,**[2] **Anna Balbutskaya,**[3] **Osama Sammra,**[3] **Christoph Lämmler,**[3] **and Amir Abdulmawjood**[4]

[1] *Landesbetrieb Hessisches Landeslabor, Schubertstraße 60, 35392 Gießen, Germany*
[2] *Frankfurt Zoo, Bernhard-Grzimek-Allee 1, 60316 Frankfurt, Germany*
[3] *Institut für Pharmakologie und Toxikologie, Justus-Liebig-Universität Gießen, Schubertstraße 81, 35392 Gießen, Germany*
[4] *Institut für Lebensmittelqualität und-sicherheit, Stiftung Tierärztliche Hochschule Hannover, Bischofsholer Damm 15, 30173 Hannover, Germany*

Correspondence should be addressed to Christoph Lämmler; christoph.laemmler@vetmed.uni-giessen.de

Academic Editor: Daniel A. Feeney

The present study was designed to characterize phenotypically and genotypically an *Arcanobacterium pluranimalium* strain (*A. pluranimalium* 4868) following necropsy from a juvenile giraffe. The species identity could be confirmed by phenotypical investigations and by MALDI-TOF MS analysis, by sequencing the 16S rDNA, pluranimaliumlysin encoding gene *pla*, and glyceraldehyde-3-phosphate dehydrogenase encoding gene *gap* with sequence similarities to *A. pluranimalium* reference strain DSM 13483[T] of 99.2%, 89.9%, and 99.1%, respectively. To our knowledge, the present study is the first phenotypic and genotypic characterization of an *A. pluranimalium* strain isolated from a giraffe.

1. Introduction

Genus *Arcanobacterium* was described by Collins et al. 1982 [1] as a group of facultative anaerobic, asporogenous, and Gram-stain positive rods. According to Yassin et al. (2011) [2], this genus consists of four species, namely, *Arcanobacterium haemolyticum*, *Arcanobacterium hippocoleae*, *Arcanobacterium phocae*, and *Arcanobacterium pluranimalium*. More recently, *Arcanobacterium canis* and *Arcanobacterium phocisimile*, two species which were most closely related to *A. haemolyticum*, were described as novel species of this genus [3, 4].

The original species characterization of *A. pluranimalium* was performed with two strains isolated from a dead harbour porpoise and a dead fallow deer [5]. In the following years *A. pluranimalium* could also be isolated from a dog with pyoderma [6], from ovine specimens on 33 occasions, and

from a milk sample of a single cow with mastitis [7]. More recently several *A. pluranimalium* strains recovered from various specimens were identified phenotypically and by using various molecular targets [8].

2. Material and Methods

The present study was focused on the characterization of an *A. pluranimalium* strain following necropsy from a juvenile giraffe by various phenotypic properties, by MALDI-TOF MS analysis, and genotypically by sequencing 16S rDNA and the *A. pluranimalium*-specific target genes *pla* and *gap*.

The 80.5 kg female giraffe (*Giraffa camelopardalis reticulata*) of the present study was born in 2013. The giraffe was not accepted by its mother or wet nurse and did not accept hand rearing attempts and, because of general weakness, was euthanized three days after birth. The subsequent postmortem analysis revealed an acute hyperemia of lung and liver and a focal emphysema of the lung. The acute pneumonia was caused by a bacterial infection associated with aspirated foreign bodies.

Bacteriological investigations yielded the isolation of A. pluranimalium and Escherichia coli, partly together with coagulase negative staphylococci, α-haemolytic streptococci, and Pseudomonas fluorescens from liver, spleen, kidney, and lung. A moderate to high growth of E. coli was generally noted (++, +++); A. pluranimalium grew only in low numbers (+). The A. pluranimalium strain 4868, originally obtained from the spleen, was used for further studies. The bacterial strain was investigated phenotypically and by MALDI-TOF analysis [6, 9] and genotypically by amplification and sequencing of 16S rDNA using universal oligonucleotide primer 16 UNI-L (5′-AGA-GTT-TGA-TCA-TGG-CTC-AG-3) and 16 UNI-R (5′-GTG-TGA-CGG-GCG-GTG-TGT-AC-3) for amplification, under the following PCR conditions: (×1 (95°C, 600 sec), ×30 (95°C, 30 sec, 58°C, 60 sec, 72°C, 60 sec), and using oligonucleotide primer 533-F (5′-GTG-CCA-GCM-GCC-GCG-GTA-A′-3) and 907R (5′-CCG-TCA-ATT-CMT-TTG-AGT-TT-3′) for sequencing. The strain was also characterized by amplification of the target gene pla with the oligonucleotide primer pla-F: 5′-GTT GAT CTA CCA GGA TTG ACG C-3′ and pla-R: 5′-TTG TCG GGG TGT CCA TTG CC-3′ and gene gap with the oligonucleotide primer gap-F 5′-TTG ACC GAC AAC AAG ACC CT-3′ and gap-R 5′-CCA TTC GTT GTC GTA CCA AG-3′as described [8, 10]. Alignment studies were performed using DNASTAR Lasergene Version 8.0.2 (DNASTAR Inc., Madison, WI, USA), Clustal W method. For MALDI-TOF MS the isolates were prepared using the direct smear method as well as an extraction protocol provided by the manufacturer. Briefly, freshly grown bacteria were harvested and diluted in ethanol, centrifuged (2000 ×g), air-dried, and resuspended in aqueous volumes of 70% formic acid and acetonitril followed by a vortex step. Five microliters was directly transferred to the steel target. Analysis was performed on a MALDI-TOF MS Biotyper Version V3.3.1.0. The database used (DB 4613, Bruker Daltonics) comprised 45 spectra from A. pluranimalium DSM 13483[T].

3. Results and Discussions

A. pluranimalium 4868 investigated in the present study was identified by determination of hemolysis and CAMP-like hemolytic reactions, by using a commercial identification system as well as various other phenotypical tests. The CAMP-like hemolytic reactions with Staphylococcus aureus β-hemolysin, Rhodococcus equi, and Arcanobacterium haemolyticum as indicator strains are known as typicalcharacteristics of this species [6, 8, 11]. Comparable to

previously investigated A. pluranimalium [6, 8] the phenotypical tests also revealed the typical biochemical properties of this species (Table 1). It was of interest that A. pluranimalium 4868 of the present study was catalase negative. This was observed previously for A. pluranimalium of bovine origin [8].

As shown by numerous authors MALDI-TOF MS is a powerful tool for species identification of a broad spectrum of bacteria including Gram-positive and Gram-negative bacteria [12–14]. Comparable to the previously conducted MALDI-TOF MS analysis of bacteria of genera Arcanobacterium and Trueperella (formerly belonging to genus Arcanobacterium [9, 15]), MALDI-TOF MS allowed the identification of A. pluranimalium 4868 of the present study to the species level matching to A. pluranimalium reference strain DSM 13483[T] with a log score value of 2.28.

Sequencing 16S rDNA, the potentially cytolytic toxin pluranimaliumlysin encoding target gene pla and the glyceraldehyde-3-phosphate dehydrogenase encoding target gene gap revealed a sequence similarity of 99.2%, 89.9%, and 99.1% to the respective sequences of A. pluranimalium DSM 13483[T]. All three sequences of A. pluranimalium 4868 were deposited in GenBank (HG794511, HG423389, and HG423390). A typical dendrogram of the sequencing results of the genes pla and gap is shown in Figures 1 and 2. Comparable to gene plo of T. pyogenes, which appeared to be a constant characteristic of all investigated T. pyogenes [16–19], pla of A. pluranimalium seems to be also constantly present in all strains of this species and could be used, as described previously [8], and in the present study for molecular identification of A. pluranimalium. More recently, Moser et al. 2013 [20] also described pla as novel target for molecular identification of this species.

Sequencing of gene gap had already been described for molecular identification of staphylococcal species [21] and more recently for identification of an A. haemolyticum strain isolated from a donkey [10]. In the present study gene gap could also be used as novel target for identification of A. pluranimalium. Further studies will give information about the constant presence and sequence similarities of both target genes pla and gap, respectively.

4. Conclusion

The clinical importance of A. pluranimalium of the present study, which was isolated from various organs of the giraffe together with in high number appearing E. coli, remains unclear. Since, beside aspiration pneumonia, no other pathological findings could be detected, this might represent the route of infection. However, the isolation of this bacterial species from giraffe and the hitherto described origin harbor porpoise, fallow deer, dog, sheep, and cow emphasizes the species name A. pluranimalium.

TABLE 1: Biochemical properties of *A. pluranimalium* 4868 investigated in the present study and *A. pluranimalium* DSM 13483[T].

Biochemical properties	*A. pluranimalium* 4868	*A. pluranimalium* DSM 13483[T**]
Hemolysis on sheep blood agar	+	+
CAMP-like reaction with:[*]		
Staphylococcus aureus β-hemolysin	+	+
Streptococcus agalactiae	−	−
Rhodococcus equi	+	+
Arcanobacterium haemolyticum	+	+
Reverse CAMP reaction	−	−
Nitrate reduction	−[1]	−[1]
Pyrazinamidase	+[1]	+[1]
Pyrrolidonyl arylamidase	+[1]	+[1,2]
Alkaline phosphatase	−[1]	−[1,2]
β-Glucuronidase (β-GUR)	+[1,2,3]	+[1,2,3]
β-Galactosidase (β-GAL)	−[1], (+)[3]	−[1], (+)[3]
α-Glucosidase (α-GLU)	−[1,2,3]	−[1,2,3]
β-Glucosidase (β-GLU)	+[2]	+[2]
N-Acetyl-β-glucosaminidase (β-NAG)	−[1,3]	−[1,3]
Esculin (β-glucosidase)	(+)[1]	+[1]
Urease	−[1]	−[1]
Gelatine	+[1]	+[1]
Fermentation of:		
Glucose	+[1]	+[1]
Ribose	+[1]	+[1]
Xylose	(+)[1]	−[1]
Mannitol	−[1]	−[1]
Maltose	−[1]	(+)[1]
Lactose	−[1]	−[1]
Saccharose	−[1]	−[1]
Glycogen	−[1]	−[1]
α-Mannosidase	−[2]	+[2]
Catalase	−	+

The reactions are shown as follows: [*]synergistic CAMP-like reaction with indicator strains; [**]results mostly obtained from Ülbegi-Mohyla et al., 2010 [6]; +: positive reaction; (+): weak positive reaction; −: negative reaction. [1]Api-Coryne test system (Biomerieux, Nürtingen, Germany); [2]tablets containing substrates (Rosco Diagnostica A/S, Taastrup, Denmark); [3]4-methylumbelliferyl conjugated substrates (Sigma, Steinheim, Germany).

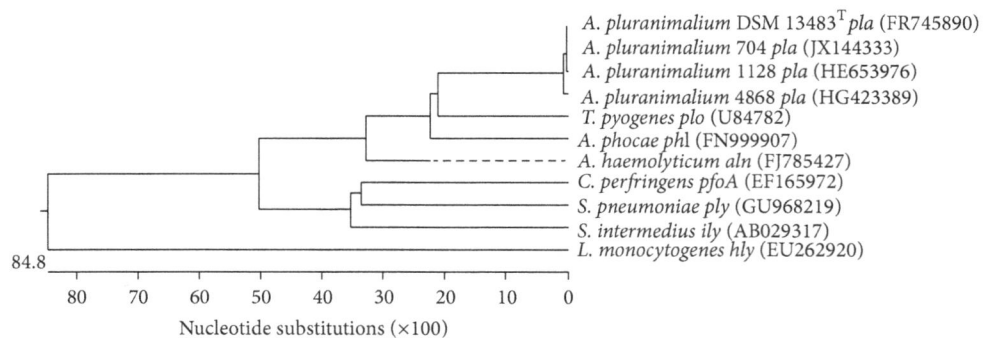

FIGURE 1: Dendrogram of sequences of gene *pla* of *A. pluranimalium* 4868 of the present study, three additional *A. pluranimalium*, and various other cytolytic toxin encoding genes obtained from GenBank.

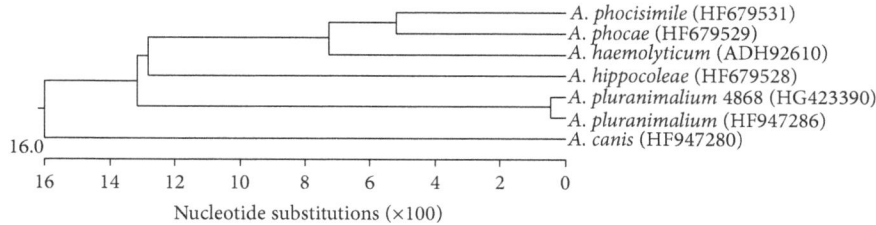

FIGURE 2: Dendrogram of gene *gap* of *A. pluranimalium* 4868, reference strain *A. pluranimalium* DSM 13483^{T}, and various other species of genus *Arcanobacterium* obtained from GenBank.

Conflict of Interests

The authors declare that they have no competing interests. The authors certify that they have no affiliation with or financial involvement in any organization or entity with a direct financial interest in the subject matter or materials discussed in this paper.

References

[1] M. D. Collins, D. Jones, and G. M. Schofield, "Reclassification of "Corynebacterium haemolyticum" (MacLean, Liebow & Rosenberg) in the genus Arcanobacterium gen.nov. as Arcanobacterium haemolyticum nom.rev., comb.nov.," *Journal of General Microbiology*, vol. 128, no. 6, pp. 1279–1281, 1982.

[2] A. F. Yassin, H. Hupfer, C. Siering, and P. Schumann, "Comparative chemotaxonomic and phylogenetic studies on the genus Arcanobacterium Collins et al. 1982 emend. Lehnen et al. 2006: proposal for Trueperella gen. nov. and emended description of the genus Arcanobacterium," *International Journal of Systematic and Evolutionary Microbiology*, vol. 61, no. 6, pp. 1265–1274, 2011.

[3] M. Hijazin, E. Prenger-Berninghoff, O. Sammra et al., "Arcanobacterium canis sp. nov., isolated from otitis externa of a dog, and emended description of the genus Arcanobacterium Collins et al. 1983 emend. Yassin et al. 2011," *International Journal of Systematic and Evolutionary Microbiology*, vol. 62, pp. 2201–2205, 2012.

[4] M. Hijazin, O. Sammra, H. Ülbegi-Mohyla et al., "Arcanobacterium phocisimile sp. nov., isolated from harbour seals," *International Journal of Systematic and Evolutionary Microbiology*, vol. 63, pp. 2019–2024, 2013.

[5] P. A. Lawson, E. Falsen, G. Foster, E. Eriksson, N. Weiss, and M. D. Collins, "Arcanobacterium pluranimalium sp. nov., isolated from porpoise and deer," *International Journal of Systematic and Evolutionary Microbiology*, vol. 51, no. 1, pp. 55–59, 2001.

[6] H. Ülbegi-Mohyla, A. A. Hassan, J. Alber et al., "Identification of Arcanobacterium pluranimalium isolated from a dog by phenotypic properties and by PCR mediated characterization of various molecular targets," *Veterinary Microbiology*, vol. 142, no. 3-4, pp. 458–460, 2010.

[7] G. Foster and B. Hunt, "Distribution of Arcanobacterium pluranimalium in animals examined in veterinary laboratories in the United Kingdom," *Journal of Veterinary Diagnostic Investigation*, vol. 23, no. 5, pp. 962–964, 2011.

[8] A. Balbutskaya, O. Sammra, S. Nagib et al., "Identification of Arcanobacterium pluranimalium by matrix-assisted laser desorption ionization-time of flight mass spectrometry and, as

novel target, by sequencing pluranimaliumlysin encoding gene pla," *Veterinary Microbiology*, vol. 168, no. 2–4, pp. 428–431, 2014.

[9] M. Hijazin, A. A. Hassan, J. Alber et al., "Evaluation of matrix-assisted laser desorption ionization-time of flight mass spectrometry (MALDI-TOF MS) for species identification of bacteria of genera Arcanobacterium and Trueperella," *Veterinary Microbiology*, vol. 157, no. 1-2, pp. 243–245, 2012.

[10] O. Sammra, A. Balbutskaya, S. Nagib et al., "Properties of an Arcanobacterium haemolyticum strain isolated from a donkey," *Berliner und Münchener Tierärztliche Wochenschrift*, vol. 127, no. 1-2, pp. 10–14, 2014.

[11] H. Ülbegi-Mohyla, A. A. Hassan, T. Kanbar et al., "Synergistic and antagonistic hemolytic activities of bacteria of genus Arcanobacterium and CAMP-like hemolysis of Arcanobacterium phocae and Arcanobacterium haemolyticum with Psychrobacter phenylpyruvicus," *Research in Veterinary Science*, vol. 87, no. 2, pp. 186–188, 2009.

[12] P. Seng, M. Drancourt, F. Gouriet et al., "Ongoing revolution in bacteriology: routine identification of bacteria by matrix-assisted laser desorption ionization time-of-flight mass spectrometry," *Clinical Infectious Diseases*, vol. 49, no. 4, pp. 543–551, 2009.

[13] P. R. Murray, "Matrix-assisted laser desorption ionization time-of-flight mass spectrometry: usefulness for taxonomy and epidemiology," *Clinical Microbiology and Infection*, vol. 16, no. 11, pp. 1626–1630, 2010.

[14] A. Bizzini, K. Jaton, D. Romo, J. Bille, G. Prod'hom, and G. Greub, "Matrix-assisted laser desorption ionization—time of flight mass spectrometry as an alternative to 16S rRNA gene sequencing for identification of difficult-to-identify bacterial strains," *Journal of Clinical Microbiology*, vol. 49, no. 2, pp. 693–696, 2011.

[15] M. Hijazin, H. Ülbegi-Mohyla, J. Alber et al., "Identification of Arcanobacterium (Trueperella) abortisuis, a novel species of veterinary importance, by matrix-assisted laser desorption ionization-time of flight mass spectrometry (MALDI-TOF MS)," *Berliner und Münchener tierärztliche Wochenschrift*, vol. 125, no. 1-2, pp. 32–37, 2012.

[16] S. J. Billington, B. H. Jost, W. A. Cuevas, K. R. Bright, and J. G. Songer, "The Arcanobacterium (Actinomyces) pyogenes hemolysin, pyolysin, is a novel member of the thiol-activated cytolysin family," *Journal of Bacteriology*, vol. 179, no. 19, pp. 6100–6106, 1997.

[17] H. B. Ertaş, A. Kiliç, G. Özbey, and A. Muz, "Isolation of Arcanobacterium (Actinomyces) pyogenes from abscessed cattle kidney and identification by PCR," *Turkish Journal of Veterinary & Animal Sciences*, vol. 29, no. 2, pp. 455–459, 2005.

[18] H. Ülbegi-Mohyla, M. Hijazin, J. Alber et al., "Identification of *Arcanobacterium pyogenes* isolated by post mortem examinations of a bearded dragon and a gecko by phenotypic and genotypic properties," *Journal of Veterinary Science*, vol. 11, no. 3, pp. 265–267, 2010.

[19] M. Hijazin, H. Ülbegi-Mohyla, J. Alber et al., "Molecular identification and further characterization of *Arcanobacterium pyogenes* isolated from bovine mastitis and from various other origins," *Journal of Dairy Science*, vol. 94, no. 4, pp. 1813–1819, 2011.

[20] A. Moser, R. Stephan, J. Sager, S. Corti, and A. Lehner, "*Arcanobacterium pluranimalium* leading to a bovine mastitis: species identification by a newly developed *pla* gene based PCR," *Schweizer Archiv für Tierheilkunde*, vol. 155, no. 6, pp. 373–375, 2013.

[21] J. Yugueros, A. Temprano, B. Berzal et al., "Glyceraldehyde-3-phosphate dehydrogenase-encoding gene as a useful taxonomic tool for *Staphylococcus* spp," *Journal of Clinical Microbiology*, vol. 38, no. 12, pp. 4351–4355, 2000.

Permissions

List of Contributors

Daniel Oladimeji Oluwayelu, Adebowale Idris Adebiyi, Ibukunoluwa Olaniyan and Phyllis Ezewele
Department of Veterinary Microbiology and Parasitology, University of Ibadan, Ibadan 20005, Nigeria

Oluwasanmi Aina
Department of Veterinary Anatomy, University of Ibadan, Ibadan 20005, Nigeria

Sara Sechi, Nicoletta Spissu, Filippo Fiore and Raffaella Cocco
Department of Veterinary Medicine, Pathology and Veterinary Clinic Section, Via Vienna 2, 07100 Sassari, Italy

Francesca Chiavolelli, Sergio Canello and Gianandrea Guidetti
SANYpet S.p.a., Research and Development Department, Via Austria 3, Bagnoli di Sopra, 35023 Padua, Italy

Alessandro Di Cerbo
School of Specialization in Clinical Biochemistry, "G. d'Annunzio" University, Via dei Vestini 31, 66100 Chieti, Italy

OluremiMartha Daudu, Rahamatu Usman Sani, Iyetunde Ifeyori Adedibu, Gideon Shaibu Bawa and Taiye Sunday Olugbemi
Department of Animal Science, Faculty of Agriculture, Ahmadu Bello University, Zaria 810107, Nigeria

Lawrence Anebi Ademu
Department of Animal Production and Health, Federal University Wukari, 641111, Nigeria

Patrick D.Mathews
Department of Parasitology, Institute of Animal Biology, University of Campinas, 13083-862 Campinas, Brazil

Antonio F.Malheiros
Department of Biological Science, University of State of Mato Grosso, 78200-000 Cáceres, Brazil

Narda D. Vasquez
Department of Tropical Aquaculture, Institute of Biology, National University of the Peruvian Amazon, 765 Iquitos, Peru

Milton D. Chavez
Department of Health, Safety and Environment, Enersul Limited Partnership, Calgary, Canada T2H 1M5

A. Deubelbeiss, M.-L. Zahno, M. Zanoni, D. Bruegger and R. Zanoni
Institute of Virology and Immunology, 3012 Berne, Switzerland

Masato Fujimura and Hironobu Ishimaru
Fujimura Animal Allergy Hospital, Aomatanihigashi 5-10-26, Minou-shi, Osaka 562-0022, Japan

L. DeTolla
Departments of Pathology, Medicine, Epidemiology and Public Health and the Program of Comparative Medicine, School of Medicine, University of Maryland, Baltimore, MD, USA

R. Sanchez and E. Khan
Program of Comparative Medicine, School of Medicine, University of Maryland, Baltimore, MD, USA

B. Tyler and M. Guarnieri
Johns Hopkins School of Medicine Department of Neurological Surgery, 1550 Orleans Street CRB-264, Baltimore, MD 21231, USA

H. A. Umar, I. A. Lawal and O. O. Okubanjo
Department of Veterinary Parasitology and Entomology, Faculty of Veterinary Medicine, Ahmadu Bello University, Zaria 2222, Nigeria

A.M.Wakawa
Department of Avian Medicine, Faculty of Veterinary Medicine, Ahmadu Bello University, Zaria 2222, Nigeria

Meucci Valentina, Guidi Grazia, Melanie Pierre, Breghi Gloria and Lippi Ilaria
Department of Veterinary Clinics, University of Pisa, San Piero a Grado, Via Livornese Lato Monte, 56122 Pisa, Italy

Kreangsak Prihirunkit
Department of Pathology, Faculty of Veterinary Medicine, Kasetsart University, Bangkok 10900,Thailand

Amornrate Sastravaha and Chalermpol Lekcharoensuk
Department of Small Animal Sciences, Faculty of Veterinary Medicine, Kasetsart University, Bangkok 10900, Thailand

Phongsak Chanloinapha
Veterinary Teaching Hospital, Kasetsart University, Bangkok 10900, Thailand

Dharma Purushothaman, Shu-Biao Wu and Wendy Yvonne Brown
School of Environmental and Rural Science, Department of Animal Science, University of New England, Armidale, NSW 2351, Australia

Barbara A. Vanselow
NSW Department of Primary Industries, Beef Industry Centre, University of New England, Armidale, NSW 2351, Australia

Sarah Butler
North Hill Vet Clinic, Armidale, NSW 2350, Australia

Jeremiah Easley, Desiree Shasa and Eileen Hackett
Department of Clinical Sciences, Colorado State University Veterinary Teaching Hospital, 300West Drake Road, Colorado State University, Fort Collins, CO 80523, USA

María-Guadalupe Gordillo-Pérez
Unidad de Investigacion Medica en Enfermedades Infecciosas y Parasitarias, Hospital de Pediatria, Centro Medico Nacional Siglo XXI, Instituto Mexicano del Seguro Social, 07300 Mexico City, Mexico

Carolina Guadalupe Sosa-Gutierrez
Unidad de Investigacion Medica en Enfermedades Infecciosas y Parasitarias, Hospital de Pediatria, Centro Medico Nacional Siglo XXI, Instituto Mexicano del Seguro Social, 07300 Mexico City, Mexico
Departamento de Parasitologia, Facultad de Medicina Veterinaria y Zootecnia, Universidad Nacional Autonoma de México, Mexico City, Mexico

Maria Teresa Quintero Martinez
Departamento de Parasitologia, Facultad de Medicina Veterinaria y Zootecnia, Universidad Nacional Autonoma de México, Mexico City, Mexico

SoilaMaribel Gaxiola Camacho and Silvia Cota Guajardo
Departamento de Parasitologia, Facultad de Medicina Veterinaria y Zootecnia, Universidad Autonoma de Sinaloa, SIN, Mexico

Maria D. Esteve-Gassent
Department of Veterinary Pathobiology, College of Veterinary Medicine and Biomedical Sciences, Texas A&M University, TX, USA

Ngonda Saasa and Ethel M'kandawire
Department of Disease Control, University of Zambia, School of Veterinary Medicine, Lusaka, Zambia

King Shimumbo Nalubamba and Joyce Siwila
Department of Clinical Studies, University of Zambia, School of Veterinary Medicine, 10101 Lusaka, Zambia

Sylvester Ochwo, Mathias Afayoa, Frank Norbert Mwiine, Ikwap Kokas, Julius Boniface Okuni, Ann Nanteza and Lonzy Ojok
College of Veterinary Medicine, Animal Resources and Biosecurity, Makerere University, Kampala, Uganda

David Kalenzi Atuhaire
College of Veterinary Medicine, Animal Resources and Biosecurity, Makerere University, Kampala, Uganda
National Agricultural Research Organization, National Livestock Resources Research Institute, Tororo, Uganda

Loyce Okedi
National Agricultural Research Organization, National Livestock Resources Research Institute, Tororo, Uganda

Eugene Arinaitwe, Rose Anna Ademun-Okurut and Christosom Ayebazibwe
Ministry of Agriculture, Animal Industry and Fisheries, National Animal Disease Diagnostics and Epidemiology Centre, Entebbe, Uganda

William Olaho-Mukani
African Union-Inter African Bureau for Animal Resources, Nairobi, Kenya

N. R. Senthil, K. M. Palanivel and R. Rishikesavan
Department of Veterinary Epidemiology and Preventive Medicine, Veterinary College and Research Institute and Tamilnadu Veterinary and Animal Sciences University, Tamilnadu, Namakkal 637002, India

Kamilius A. Mamiro, Henry B.Magwisha and Elpidius J. Rukambile
Central Veterinary Laboratory, TVLA, Dar Es Salaam, Tanzania

Martin R. Ruheta
Directorate of Veterinary Services, Dar Es Salaam, Tanzania

Expery J. Kimboka
District Veterinary Office, Utete, Rufiji, Tanzania

Deusdedit J.Malulu and Imna I.Malele
Vector & Vector Borne Diseases Institute (VVBD), Tanga, Tanzania

Kristin A. Clothier
California Animal Health & Food Safety Lab System, School of Veterinary Medicine, University of California, Davis, Davis, CA 95616, USA
Departments of Pathology, Microbiology, and Immunology, School of Veterinary Medicine, University of California, Davis, Davis, CA 95616, USA

Barbara A. Byrne
Departments of Pathology, Microbiology, and Immunology, School of Veterinary Medicine, University of California, Davis, Davis, CA 95616, USA
Veterinary Medical Teaching Hospital, School of Veterinary Medicine, University of California, Davis, Davis, CA 95616, USA

Carlos Hermosilla, Liliana M. R. Silva and Anja Taubert
Institute of Parasitology, Justus Liebig University Giessen, 35392 Giessen, Germany

Mauricio Navarro
Institute of Pathology, University Austral of Chile, Valdivia, Chile
University of California Davis School of Veterinary Medicine, Sacramento, CA 95616, USA

M. Guarnieri, R. Sarabia-Estrada and B. Tyler
Johns Hopkins School of Medicine, Department of Neurological Surgery, Baltimore, MD, USA

C. Brayton
Johns Hopkins School of Medicine, Department of Molecular and Comparative Pathobiology, Baltimore, MD, USA

P. McKnight
George Mason University, Fairfax, VA, USA

L. DeTolla
University of Maryland School of Medicine, Departments of Pathology, Medicine, Epidemiology and Public Health and the Program of Comparative Medicine, Baltimore, MD, USA

Braniff de la Torre Valdovinos and Nancy Elizabeth Franco Rodriguez
Department of Computer Science, CUCEI, Universidad de Guadalajara, Avenida Revolucion No. 1500 Building M, Laboratory 212, 44430 Guadalajara, JAL, Mexico

Judith Marcela Duenas Jimenez
Department of Physiology, CUCS Universidad de Guadalajara, Sierra Mojada 950, Building PThird Floor, 44290 Guadalajara, JAL, Mexico

Ismael Jimenez Estrada
Department of Physiology Biophysics and Neurosciences, Centro de Investigacion y Estudios Avanzados IPN, Avenida Instituto Politecnico Nacional 2508, 07360 Mexico City, DF, Mexico

Jacinto Banuelos Pineda
Department of Veterinary and Medicine, CUCBA Universidad de Guadalajara, Camino Ing. Ramon Padilla Sanchez 2100, 45110 Zapopan, JAL, Mexico

Jose Roberto Lopez Ruiz, Laura Paulina Osuna Carrasco, Ahiezer Candanedo Arellano and Sergio Horacio Duenas Jimenez
Department of Neuroscience, CUCS Universidad de Guadalajara, Sierra Mojada 950, Building P Third Floor, 44290 Guadalajara, JAL, Mexico

B. Shumbusho
Department of Veterinary Medicine, University of Rwanda, Musanze, Rwanda

J. P. Mpatswenumugabo
Department of Veterinary Medicine, University of Rwanda, Musanze, Rwanda Department of Veterinary Pathology, Microbiology and Parasitology, University of Nairobi, Kangemi, Kenya

L. C. Bebora and G. C. Gitao
Department of Veterinary Pathology, Microbiology and Parasitology, University of Nairobi, Kangemi, Kenya

V. A. Mobegi
Department of Biochemistry, University of Nairobi, Nairobi, Kenya

B. Iraguha
Rwanda Dairy Competitiveness Program II, Kigali, Rwanda

O. Kamana
Department of Food Safety and Food Quality Management, University of Rwanda, Musanze, Rwanda

Mude Shecho and Naod Thomas
School of Veterinary Medicine, Wolaita Sodo University, Wolaita Sodo, Ethiopia

Jelalu Kemal and Yimer Muktar
College of Veterinary Medicine, Haramaya University, Dire Dawa, Ethiopia

Randall T. Loder
Department of Orthopaedic Surgery, Indiana University School of Medicine and James Whitcomb Riley Children's Hospital, Indianapolis, IN 46202, USA

Rory J. Todhunter
Department of Clinical Sciences, College of Veterinary Medicine, Cornell University, Ithaca, NY 14853-6401, USA

Amare Eshetu Gemeda and Kefelegn Workalemahu
College of Veterinary Medicine, Haramaya University, Dire Dawa, Ethiopia

Tshering Dolma, Reena Mukherjee, B. K. Pati and U. K. De
Division of Medicine, Indian Veterinary Research Institute, Izatnagar, Uttar Pradesh 243122, India

Bharathalingam Sinniah, Muniandy Narasiman, Saequa Habib and Ong Gaik Bei
Laboratory Based Medicine, Faculty of Medicine, Universiti Kuala Lumpur Royal College of Medicine Perak, No. 3 Jalan Greentown, 30450 Ipoh, Perak, Malaysia

Karin Risse, Karen Schlez and Tobias Eisenberg
Landesbetrieb Hessisches Landeslabor, Schubertstraße 60, 35392 Gießen, Germany

Christina Geiger
Frankfurt Zoo, Bernhard-Grzimek-Allee 1, 60316 Frankfurt, Germany

Anna Balbutskaya, Osama Sammra and Christoph Lämmler
Institut für Pharmakologie und Toxikologie, Justus-Liebig-Universität Gießen, Schubertstraße 81, 35392 Gießen, Germany

Amir Abdulmawjood
Institut für Lebensmittelqualität und-sicherheit, Stiftung Tierärztliche Hochschule Hannover, Bischofsholer Damm 15, 30173 Hannover, Germany

Index